Monte Carlo Simulation for the Pharmaceutical Industry

Concepts, Algorithms, and Case Studies

Chapman & Hall/CRC Biostatistics Series

Editor-in-Chief

Shein-Chung Chow, Ph.D.
Professor
Department of Biostatistics and Bioinformatics
Duke University School of Medicine
Durham, North Carolina

Series Editors

Byron Jones
Senior Director
Statistical Research and Consulting Centre
(IPC 193)
Pfizer Global Research and Development
Sandwich, Kent, U.K.

Jen-pei Liu
Professor
Division of Biometry
Department of Agronomy
National Taiwan University
Taipei, Taiwan

Karl E. Peace
Georgia Cancer Coalition
Distinguished Cancer Scholar
Senior Research Scientist and
Professor of Biostatistics
Jiann-Ping Hsu College of Public Health
Georgia Southern University
Statesboro, Georgia

Bruce W. Turnbull
Professor
School of Operations Research
and Industrial Engineering
Cornell University
Ithaca, New York

Chapman & Hall/CRC Biostatistics Series

Published Titles

Chapman & Hall/CRC Biostatistics Series

Monte Carlo Simulation for the Pharmaceutical Industry

Concepts, Algorithms, and Case Studies

Mark Chang

Amag Pharmaceuticals
Lexington, Massachusetts, U.S.A.

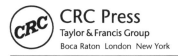

CRC Press
Taylor & Francis Group
Boca Raton London New York

CRC Press is an imprint of the
Taylor & Francis Group, an **informa** business

A CHAPMAN & HALL BOOK

CRC Press
Taylor & Francis Group
6000 Broken Sound Parkway NW, Suite 300
Boca Raton, FL 33487-2742

First issued in paperback 2018

ISBN-13: 978-1-4398-3592-0 (hbk)
ISBN-13: 978-1-138-37438-6 (pbk)

Library of Congress Cataloging-in-Publication Data

Chang, Mark.
  Monte Carlo simulation for the pharmaceutical industry : concepts, algorithms, and case studies / Mark Chang.
    p. ; cm. -- (Chapman & Hall/CRC biostatistics series ; 36)
  Includes bibliographical references and index.
  ISBN 978-1-4398-3592-0 (hardcover : alk. paper)
    1. Drug development--Computer simulation. 2. Monte Carlo method. I. Title. II. Series: Chapman & Hall/CRC biostatistics series ; 36.
    [DNLM: 1. Drug Industry--methods. 2. Computer Simulation. 3. Drug Design. 4. Monte Carlo Method. 5. Technology, Pharmaceutical--methods. QV 736 C4555m 2011]

RM301.25.C46 2011
615'.19--dc22   2010019530

Visit the Taylor & Francis Web site at
http://www.taylorandfrancis.com

and the CRC Press Web site at
http://www.crcpress.com

To my teachers and my family.

Contents

Preface

Drug development, aimed at improving people's health, becomes more costly every year. The pharmaceutical industry must join its efforts with government and the health professions to seek new, innovative, and cost-effective approaches in the development process. During this evolutionary process over the next decades, computer simulations will no doubt play a critical role. Computer simulation or Monte Carlo simulation is the technique of simulating a dynamic system or process using a computer program. Computer simulations, as an efficient and effective research tool, have been used in virtually every area of engineering, science, mathematics, etc.

In this book, I present *concepts*, *theories*, *algorithms*, and *cases studies* of Monte Carlo simulation in the pharmaceutical and health industries. The concepts refer not only to simulation in general, but also to various types of simulations in drug development. The theory will include virtual data sampling, game theory, deterministic and stochastic decision theories, adaptive design methods, Petri net, genetic programming, resampling methods, and other strategies. These theories and methods are necessary either to carry out the simulations or to make the simulations more efficient, even though there are many practical problems that can be simulated directly in an ad hoc fashion without any theory about their efficiency or convergence considerations. The algorithms, which can be descriptive, computer pseudocode, or a combination of both, provide the basis for implementation of simulation methods. The case studies or applications are simplified versions of real-world problems. These simplifications are necessary because a single case could otherwise occupy the whole book, preventing readers from exploring broad issues. There are also examples of how simulation can be formulated to address interesting questions that have not been studied before. In my view, building simulation models is, to a large extent, a creative process; it is an innovation in application, which can impact our lives more positively than other innovations or creations. Simulation often requires knowledge in several disciplines, including mathematics/statistics, programming, and the subject field.

The overarching goals of this book are not limited just to the scope of simulation methodologies and computer algorithms, but also include sharing personal thoughts, experiences, and views about how to become a visionary, to be creative, a logical thinker and, a skillful "simulator." Being visionary can be helpful in formulating the questions and building simulation models; on the other hand, using simulations we can answer visionary questions. Being visionary requires having a big-picture view and understanding the issues profoundly. Being visionary is helpful in facilitating communications and getting one's ideas across to key stockholders in a company. This belief is reflected in the chapters on meta-simulation and macro-simulation, and throughout the book. Being creative requires wide knowledge in the field and cross-disciplines and skill in identifying the similarities among different things and making analogies. For this reason, I decided to cover a broad range of problems in drug development and to provide introductory examples from many different fields. Being logical implies being capable of abstract thought. Simulation processes often appear to be intuitive and concrete. However, to build the model or convert a practical problem into a simulation problem and develop an algorithm require a high degree of abstract thinking and the ability to visualize all the steps in the simulation process. After the algorithm is developed, implementation using any computer language or software is a relatively straightforward task if one knows the programming language well.

Many academic and industry professionals, myself included, share the view that, despite our great efforts, there is still a gap between what students learn in school and what they actually need in their work. To narrow this gap, teaching materials or books that can bridge the gap between academia and industry are necessary. This book is an attempt in this direction. The style of the book is unique in the sense that it is a mix of textbook and monograph. Having said that, industry statisticians, scientists, and software engineers/programmers are intended to be its primary readers.

The second unique characteristic of this book is the broad coverage of subject fields from drug discovery (molecular design, disease modeling, and biological pathway simulation), preclinical aspects (pharmacokinetics, pharmacodynamics), clinical development (adaptive clinical trials, trial management, and execution), and prescription drug commercialization. In contrast, most monographs deal with only a very specific field.

Before discussing specific Monte Carlo techniques, background information, and the issues and/or trends in the field are covered. This is particularly important for Monte Carlo model building and for communicating simulation results back to the team or any concerned parties. You will be amazed when you find out, in a successful Monte Carlo project, how much more time and effort are expended on team communication than on actual simulations. Most simulation books are either completely mathematical/statistical oriented or resemble a software user manual, and neglect the background topics altogether.

The third unique feature is in the exercises. Typically, exercises in a textbook are provided with all the information for students to answer the questions. However, in the real world, especially in drug development, virtually every challenging problem requires that we make judgments on what information is needed and where to get it in order to solve the problem at hand, and most times appropriate assumptions are also required. Because of the assumptions and uncertainties of source information, how to interpret the results also becomes an essential part of the task, which, from my experience, is often overlooked in the classroom and by students. In light of this, for many exercises in this book, readers are expected to make a judgment as to whether the information provided is sufficient or not; if not, they must identify and use other sources or make appropriate assumptions, and then finally use the methods/tools discussed to solve the problem.

Road Map

The book studies a broad category of computer simulations, virtually covering the whole spectrum of drug development in the thirteen chapters.

Chapter 1, Simulation, Simulation Everywhere, covers the general concepts of simulations, emphasizing the importance of analogy and simulation using various examples from daily life, art, music, bilingualism, strategies for commuting, economics, math, science, finance, optimization, and others.

Chapter 2, Virtual Sampling Techniques, discusses general methods for the generation of random numbers, methods for variance reduction, and methods for generating random numbers from specific distributions. The discussions are brief, especially on methods for specific distributions.

Chapter 3, Overview of Drug Development, provides basic knowledge about different stages of drug development, from discovery through preclinical and clinical development. This knowledge is important to readers who have little knowledge about drug development and want to develop the ability to confidently model a practical problem as a Monte Carlo problem.

Simulations are divided into meta, macro, and micro simulations. Chapter 4, Meta-Simulation for the Pharmaceutical Industry, investigates the characteristics of competition and collaboration between independent business entities or pharmaceutical companies using simulations, including pharmaceutical gaming and prescription drug global pricing. Those simulation methods are constructed on the basis of game theory; therefore, the chapter also serves as an introduction to game theory.

Chapter 5, Meta-Simulation for Pharmaceutical Research and Development, studies meta-simulation, in which different stages of drug development and different drug candidates are considered simultaneously in simulation models. The simulation approaches are constructed based on the Markov decision process. The chapter provides materials to smoothly transfer from a deterministic sequential decision process, to a Markov decision process, to a pharmaceutical decision process, and to extensions of Markov decision processes.

Chapter 6, Clinical Trial Simulations (CTS), deals with simulations in classical and adaptive trials, which is of the most interest to the pharmaceutical industry and where simulation finds most of its applications in drug development. Unified adaptive design methods are also introduced.

Chapter 7, Clinical Trial Management and Execution, focuses on the various challenges in clinical trial management and execution (e.g., trial management, patient recruitment, adaptive randomization, dynamic drug supply, and adaptive trial monitoring) and the reformulation of the problems into Monte Carlo simulation in conjunction with other theoretical methods such as critical path analysis.

Chapter 8, Prescription Drug Commercialization, covers the dynamics of prescription drug marketing, the stock-flow dynamic model for brand planning, and a competitive drug marketing strategy. Different models such as a stochastic market game are discussed in the simulations.

Chapter 9, Molecular Design and Simulation, comprises various topics including why molecular design and simulation, molecular similarity search, overview of molecular docking, small molecule conformation analysis, ligand–receptor interaction, docking algorithms, and scoring functions.

Chapter 10, Disease Modeling and Biological Pathway Simulation, discusses computational system biology, petri nets, and biological pathway simulation with PN.

Chapter 11, Pharmacokinetic Simulation, gives an overview of abortion, distribution, metabolism, and excretion (ADEM) and their modeling, especially physiologically based pharmacokinetic modeling.

Chapter 12, Pharmacodynamic Simulation, provides an overview of pharmacodynamics, enzyme kinetics, pharmacodynamic models, drug–drug interactions, and case studies.

Chapter 13, Monte Carlo for Inference and Beyond, includes several important topics, including sorting algorithms, resampling methods, and genetic programming.

In the appendices, implementations of three algorithms, representing easy, moderate, and difficult levels of coding, are presented as examples, in Javascript language. The code is embedded in an html file; thus only Internet Explorer is needed to run the programs. More algorithms are implemented and made available at www.statisticians.org.

The book deals with multiple disciplines employing different syntax conventions. There is a balance between being syntax consistent throughout the book and respecting syntax/conventions in the individual subject fields. Since the levels of Monte Carlo development in different areas of the pharmaceutical industry are very different, I try to not overstress consistency in the complexity level of the mathematical models or in the simulation technologies actually used. For example, clinical trial simulations are more developed, but simulation in prescription drug commercialization is relatively naive from a mathematical perspective. As a second example, the subject of molecular design and simulation is usually accomplished using commercial software, not because of the mathematical complexity but because of the necessarily lengthy coding for ligand-protein 3D geometry, molecular or quantum mechanics, and the software user interface. Thus, I spend less time in discussing the algorithms, but focus instead on the issues concerned when conducting these kinds of simulations.

I candidly admit that my goals are ambitiously high, and my approach in this book needs to be tested. Therefore, any comments or criticisms are encouraged. I can be reached at www.statisticians.org.

Finally, thanks to Dr. Robert Pierce; his valuable comments have greatly improved the manuscript. Thanks also to Acquisitions Editor David Grubbs from Taylor & Francis for providing me the opportunity to work on this project.

Mark Chang

Lexington, MA, USA
www.statisticians.org

Chapter 1

Simulation, Simulation Everywhere

This chapter will cover the following topics:

- Modeling and Simulation
- Introductory Monte Carlo Examples
- Simulations in Drug Development

1.1 Modeling and Simulation

1.1.1 *The Art of Simulations*

Simulation is the imitation of a physical or conceptual system (process) in order to gain insight into its functioning and to optimize its performance. The act of simulating generally entails representing certain key characteristics or behaviors of a selected physical or abstract system. Key issues in simulation include acquisition of valid source of information about the referent, selection of key characteristics and behaviors, the use of simplifying approximations and assumptions within the simulation, and fidelity and validity of the simulation outcomes.

A Monte Carlo method, also called Monte Carlo, Monte Carlo simulation, or computer simulation, is a technique that usually involves using computer-generated random numbers and theory of probability to solve problems. The term Monte Carlo method was coined by S. Ulam and Nicholas Metropolis in reference to games of chance, a popular attraction in Monte Carlo, Monaco (Hoffman, 1998; Metropolis and Ulam, 1949).

The term simulation is often associated with the term modeling. Modeling can be mechanical modeling, mathematical or statistical modeling, or analogy. Mathematical or statistical modeling of phenomena can have analytical closed form solutions or more often numerical solutions. For many complicated situations the solutions have to be obtained with the assistance

1

of computer simulation.

The terms modeling and simulation are often used interchangeably because they both use analogy. However, there are some fine differences — simulations often involve repetitions of virtual random data sets, whereas modeling often applies to an observed data set. In practice, modeling and simulation are often combined to effectively solve problems. In engineering, modeling can mimic behavior using a different scale from the original object being modeled. As an example, before constructing a large dam for a reservoir, engineers usually use a physical model (prototype) in 1:100 to 1:1000 scale in the laboratory and evaluate the safety of the dam as it undergoes various forces. They use the results to infer the performance of the actual dam to be built. This is reasonable because there are underlying relationships between the model and the original object. The theory of the study of the relationships is called dimensional analysis in mechanics (Szirtes, 2007). Spaceship launching is another example: before the launch, numerous tests or simulations have to be carried out.

Like many other fields, computer simulation can also be an art — there are many ways to achieve the goal, and some are better than others. In addition to the necessary mathematical/statistical and computer knowledge, the keys to a successful simulation are the ability to make analogies and a reasonably good knowledge of the subject field. If you can use logic and analogy to transfer the problem into a sensible Monte Carlo simulation, you are halfway to solving the problem. Given the importance of basic subject knowledge, I have included as a chapter in this book background materials for drug development, so that the reader can fully understand the Monte Carlo methods without frequently referring to other texts. Simulation in drug development often requires strong interaction among people from different disciplines, and this subject knowledge will help facilitate your communications. You will be amazed how much time and effort you need to put into collaboration — getting input for your model and convincing others of your proposal.

Before we discuss simulation techniques in the pharmaceutical and health industries, it is helpful to take a glance at some entertaining examples. These examples are selected because they are simple, but also because they demonstrate the amazing power of simulations.

1.1.2   *Genetic Programming in Art Simulation*

Simulation can be used in many fields (with or without mathematical modeling): science, engineering, finance, art, and music (Romero & Machdo, 2008; Cope, 2001). The portrait of Lisa Gherardini (the Mona Lisa) in the

Louvre in Paris, painted by Leonardo da Vinci during the Italian Renaissance, is perhaps the most famous and iconic painting in the world. Roger Alsing used a special Monte Carlo method called genetic programming (GP) to successfully reproduce the portrait with only 50 semi-transparent polygons (see Figure 1.1). The result is astonishing! One implication of this successful simulation using GP is that GP can be used to compress/zip the picture with truly tiny computer storage — only information containing 50 semi-transparent polygons in this case! We will return to GP later in this section.

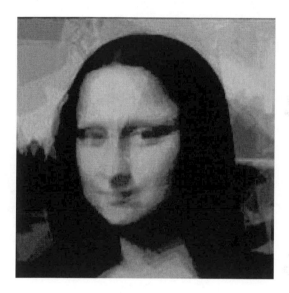

Figure 1.1:   The Mona Lisa Generated Using GP

1.1.3   *Artificial Neural Network in Music Machinery*

Virtual music represents a broad category of machine-created composition which attempts to replicate the style but not the actual notes of existing music (Cope, 1993). One of the first formal types of algorithms in music theory, and another good example of virtual music, is the eighteenth century Musikalisches Wurfelspiel, or musical dice game. The idea behind this musically sophisticated game involved composing a series of measures of music that could be recombined in many different ways and still be stylistically viable — virtual music. Following this process, even a very simple piece becomes a source of innumerable new works (Cope, 2001).

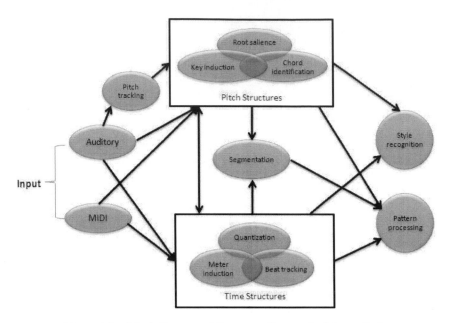

Figure 1.2:   Music Scores and Structure Process for Monte Carlo
(Source: Adapted from Rowe, 2001)

Rowe (2001) used an artificial neural network to simulate the subsymbolic process (Figure 1.2). Neural networks are a class of algorithms that learn relations between inputs and outputs. Their structure is derived from a schematic model of the neurons of the brain. A typical artificial neural network (ANN) consists of layers of connected nodes. A weight is placed on each connection in a neural network. Activation travels from one node to another across a connection. The weighted sum of activations from nodes at a previous layer is compared to a threshold to determine the activation of the current node.

The initial connection weights can be set arbitrarily. One of the great attractions of ANNs is that they are able to learn: the weights can be adjusted automatically from data. To accomplish this, a training set of input data with known answers attached is presented to the network. Over the course of a training session, the connection weights are gradually adjusted by the neural network itself until they reach convergence. If the training set captures the regularities of a wider class of inputs, the trained network will then be able to correctly classify inputs not found in the training set as well. Such a process is an example of supervised learning, in which a teacher (the training set) is used to guide the network in acquiring the necessary knowledge (connection weights).

After the ANN is well trained, it can be used as a music teacher to classify musical works in teaching and can even become a virtual musician, producing music pieces of various kinds. As far as the applications of ANN in drug development, we will discuss the topic in detail in later chapters of this book.

1.1.4 Bilingual Bootstrapping in Word Translation

Li and Li (2004) developed an effective machine learning technique (bilingual bootstrapping) for word translation disambiguation. It makes use of a small amount of classified data and a large amount of unclassified data in both the source and the target languages. It repeatedly constructs classifiers in the two languages in parallel and boosts the performance of the classifiers by classifying unclassified data in the two languages and by exchanging information regarding classified data between the two languages (Figure 1.3).

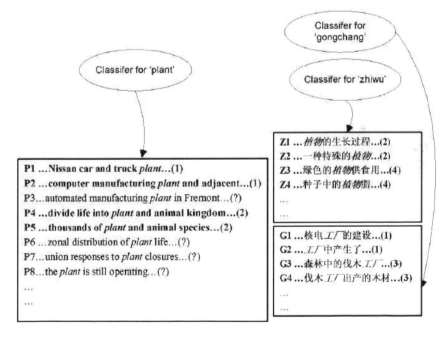

Figure 1.3: Bilingual Bootstrapping
(Source: Li and Li, 2004)

Bootstrapping is a statistical method for estimating the sampling distribution of an estimator by sampling with replacement from the original sample, most often with the purpose of deriving robust estimates of standard errors and confidence intervals of a population parameter such as a mean, median, proportion, odds ratio, correlation coefficient, or regression coefficient. It can also be used for constructing hypothesis tests. It is often used as a robust alternative to an inference based on parametric assumptions when those assumptions are in doubt, or where parametric inference is impossible or requires very complicated formulas for the calculation of standard errors. When large data sets are available, we can use random sampling with or without replacement to validate the neural network method. We will discuss more about bootstrapping methods in Chapter 13.

1.2 Introductory Monte Carlo Examples

The best way to describe Monte Carlo simulation may be through examples. In the next section, we give some simple examples, walking through the steps taken to solve the problems using Monte Carlo simulation. Keep in mind that to solve problems effectively, Monte Carlo simulations are often combined with other modeling methods or theories, such as game and decision theories. In addition, basic knowledge of the subject field of the underlying problem is critical to the success of the simulation.

1.2.1 *USA Territory*

Suppose we are asked to find the size of the USA's territory. The only thing we have is a map (Figure 1.4), in 1:20000 scale, on a rectangular piece of paper of 24 in × 36 in. Can we accomplish the mission?

Let's analyze the situation: The map has an irregular shape and there seems no simple and direct way to calculate the size (area). However, if we can find the ratio of map size to rectangle size, the size of the USA's territory can be calculated using the following equation:

$$A_{usa} = R A_{reg} S_{map} = 20000 R A_{reg} \qquad (1.1)$$

where R is the ratio of the areas (USA over the rectangle) $\frac{A_{usa}}{A_{reg}}$; S_{map} is the scale of the map; A_{reg} is the area of the rectangle, which is easy to measure.

It is clear that the key to the problem is to find the ratio

$$R = \frac{A_{usa}}{A_{reg}}. \qquad (1.2)$$

Among other alternatives, we can use mechanical simulation to estimate the ratio through the following steps: (1) Cut the map into many small

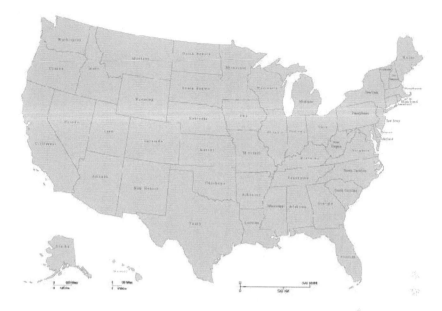

Figure 1.4:   Map of the US

pieces randomly. Based on the dominant color on the piece, some of the pieces will be considered white and some gray (the map part). (2) Fully mix all the pieces. (3) Randomly draw a piece N times with replacement and record the number of gray pieces (N_{usa}). A simple probabilistic fact tells us that when $n \to \infty$, the following equation holds with a probability of 1:

$$R = \frac{A_{usa}}{A_{reg}} = \frac{N_{usa}}{N}. \tag{1.3}$$

But what if we don't want to destroy the map? Well, that is easy too. Get a small object, e.g., a needle; throw it randomly toward the map many times; record the number of times (N_{usa}) the needle tip falls on the USA map and the number of times (N) the needle tip falls on the entire rectangle; (1.3) and (1.1) are still valid. Note that the paper used to draw the map does not have to be a rectangle, but can be any shape. For convenience, we call the paper or area that covers the map the "majorization space."

1.2.2 π *Simulation*

We now consider how we can use computer simulation to perform this type of simulation more efficiently. To make it more interesting, let's estimate the constant π. To this end, we change the USA map to a disk with a known radius (for simplicity let the radius $r = 1$ and the majorization space be a square with side length of $2r = 2$). See Figure 1.5. From (1.2), the ratio of the areas can be expressed as

$$R = \frac{\pi r^2}{(2r)^2} = \frac{\pi}{4}. \tag{1.4}$$

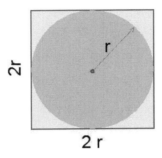

Figure 1.5:   Pi by Simulation

From (1.4), we have the equality $\pi = 4R$ for the π simulation specified below:

(1) Generate two random numbers independently from $U(0, 1)$, the uniform distribution over range $[0, 1]$, representing a point (x, y) in an XY plane.
(2) Check if the point falls in the circle (i.e., if $(x-0.5)^2 + (y-0.5)^2 < 0.25$).
(3) If the point falls in the circle, increase the count n by 1.
(4) Repeat steps (1)–(3) m times.
(5) Calculate the final ratio $R = \frac{n}{m}$ and the estimate $\pi = 4R$.

Let's write the steps using computer pseudocode or an algorithm:

Algorithm 1.1: Pi Simulation
Objective: return an estimate for the constant π
input number of simulation nRuns
$m := 0$
For $iRun := 1$ **To** nRuns
    Generate x from $U(0, 1)$
    Generate y from $U(0, 1)$
    $d := (x - 0.5)^2 + (y - 0.5)^2$

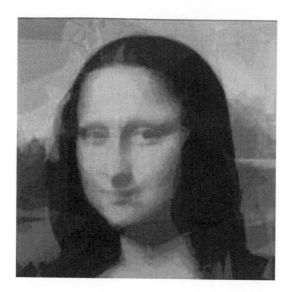

Figure 1.1:   Mona Lisa Generated Using GP

If $d < 0.25$ **Then** $m := m + 1$
Endfor
$Pi := 4 \frac{m}{\text{nRuns}}$
Return Pi
§

There are other simulation algorithms for calculating π up to 2398 digits (e.g., Press, et al. 2007, p. 1194). The most famous example of π simulation is the Buffon Needle experiment.

1.2.3 Definite Integrals

Suppose we want to calculate the integral

$$I = \int_a^b f(x)dx, (c \geq f(x) \geq 0, b > a). \tag{1.5}$$

The interpretation of the integral is the area under curve $f(x)$ (Figure 1.6), which naturally links to the previous simulations. Indeed, we can develop a simulation algorithm similar to Algorithm 1.1 to calculate the integral. Note that the area of the majorization space is $c \times (b - a)$ in the current case.

Algorithm 1.2 Monte Carlo for a Definite Integral
Objective: return the numerical value of integral I defined by (1.5)
Input number of simulation nRuns
$m := 0$
For $iRun := 1$ **To** nRuns
    generate x from $U(a, b)$
    generate y from $U(0, c)$
    If $y < f(x)$ **Then** $m := m + 1$
Endfor
$I := c(b - a) \frac{m}{\text{nRuns}}$
Return I
§

A better simulation approach is to calculate the mean value $\bar{f}$ of $f(x)$ over (a, b) and then obtain $I = (b - a) \bar{f}$. The mean $\bar{f}$ can be estimated using simulation as $\bar{f} \approx \frac{1}{m_{\max}} \sum_{i=1}^{m_{\max}} f(x_i)$, where x_i is a random number from the uniform distribution $U(a, b)$. We formalize this approach in Algorithm 1.3.

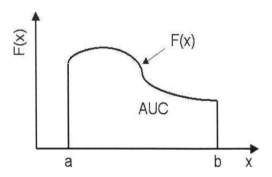

Figure 1.6:   Area Under Curve (AUC)

Algorithm 1.3 Improved Monte Carlo for a Definite Integral
Objective: return the numerical value of integral I defined by (1.5)
input number of simulation nRuns
$sum := 0$
For $iRun := 1$ **To** nRuns
     generate x from $U(a, b)$
     $sum := sum + f(x)$
Endfor
$I := (b - a)\frac{sum}{\text{nRuns}}$
Return I
§

We can see that only one random number is needed for each simulation run using Algorithm 1.3, whereas two random numbers are required for each simulation run in Algorithm 1.2.

The validity of the algorithm is based on the law of large numbers in statistics, which ensures:

$$\frac{1}{b-a} \int_a^b f(x)\, dx \approx \bar{f}. \tag{1.6}$$

Theorem 1.1   *Weak Law of Large Numbers:* *Suppose that the expectation $E(X)$ of X is finite. Then the sample mean $\bar{X}_m$ converges in probability to $E(X)$; thus $\lim_{m \to \infty} P\left(\left|\bar{X}_m - E(X)\right| > \varepsilon\right) = 0$ for every $\varepsilon > 0$, where $\bar{X}_m = \frac{1}{m} \sum_{i=1}^m X_i$.*

Theorem 1.2   *Strong Law of Large Numbers:* *Suppose that the expectation $E(X)$ of X is finite and then converges almost surely to $E(X)$. Thus $\lim_{m \to \infty} P\left(\bar{X}_m = E(X)\right) = 1$.*

Theorem 1.3 *Central Limit Theory: For any* $\lambda_\alpha > 0$,

$$P\left(\left|\bar{X}_m - I\right| < \frac{\lambda_\alpha \sigma}{\sqrt{m}}\right) \approx \frac{2}{\sqrt{2\pi}} \int_0^{\lambda_\alpha} \exp\left(-\frac{t^2}{2}\right) dt = 1 - \alpha. \qquad (1.7)$$

In other words,

$$\sqrt{m}\left(\hat{I}_m - I\right) \to N\left(0, \sigma^2\right), \text{ in distribution,}$$

where $\sigma^2 = var\left\{g\left(x\right)\right\}$, $g\left(\cdot\right) = $ real *function.*

Therefore the error of this Monte Carlo approximation for an integral is $O\left(\sqrt{m}\right)$ regardless of the dimension of the integral. This a major advantage of using simulation for a high-dimensional definite integral in comparison to numerical integration.

An interesting question is: how does the size of the majorization space affect the efficiency of the program? Will the simulation reach its maximum efficiency when the ratio of areas is close to 0.5? We leave the reader to find the answer (Exercise 1.2). In Chapter 2, we will discuss how to improve the efficiency of the sampling procedure.

1.2.4 *Fastest Route*

Industry and technology revolution do not always make life easier. Traffic jams often make one think: I am better off riding a bicycle. Using backward induction (see Chapter 5 for details) in decision theory, we can easily find the shortest route back home from the office. However, finding the fastest route is a quite different story, and much more challenging because there is random traffic involved. You may use Yahoo or Google Map to search for the shortcut, but whether this "shortcut" is real or not is dependent on how many other drivers utilize the same information. If every driver uses the same information and takes the same "shortcut," it will not be the fastest path at all. In real life, people often try different roads and record (by heart) the driving time taken each time. If they find a trip is faster than a previous trip on a different path, they may increase the probability of taking this road. By doing this, they hope to find the best path or strategy in the long run or on average. Can we prove this strategy works (and how well it works) using Monte Carlo? Many practical problems involve this type of competition and are well studied in game theory (see Chapter 4). In fact, this commuting problem is similar to the random-play-the-winner strategy in Casino and the response-adaptive randomization in clinical trial design (Chang, 2007b, 2008 and Chapter 9 of this book). But for now, let's develop an algorithm (Algorithm 1.4) to find the fastest path before we leave home today.

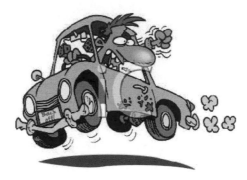

Figure 1.7:   Finding the Fastest Route

To fit the scope of this introductory chapter, we need to make some necessary assumptions to simplify the problem so that we have a concise algorithm. The assumptions in Algorithm 1.4 are: all paths have the same distance, driver k may (but not necessarily) switch his/her path with the probability of switching $= \frac{n_{ij}}{n_{i-1,j}+n_{ij}}$, where n_{ij} = number of cars on the jth road on the ith day. $U(M)$ is the probability mass function or random number generator that generates integers 1 to M with equal probability. For a typical day i, on a typical path j, we need to determine whether a typical car k will switch paths based on the probability of switching $\frac{n_{ij}}{n_{i-1,j}+n_{ij}}$. If yes, the path he/she is switching to is based on the probability $U(M)$. Note that even if a driver intends to switch, there is still a $1/M$ probability that he will turn out to be a nonswitcher. Therefore the actual switching probability is $\frac{M-1}{M}\frac{n_{ij}}{n_{i-1,j}+n_{ij}}$. When a switch does occur, the number of cars on the two paths involved in the switching need to be updated (reduced or increased by 1) for the next day. Here is the algorithm in computer pseudocode.

Algorithm 1.4: The Fastest Route
Objective: return $\{n_{ij}\}$ the number of cars on the jth path on day i.
Input nRuns (days of drive), M (number of paths available).
Assign any initial n_{1j} cars on each path j on day 1
For $i := 1$ **To** nRuns
    For $j := 1$ **To** M
        For $k := 1$ **To** n_{ij}
            Generate x from $U(0,1)$

If $x \leq \frac{n_{ij}}{n_{i-1,j}+n_{ij}}$ **Then**

generate m from $U(M)$

$n_{i+1,m} := n_{im} + 1$

$n_{i+1,k} := n_{ik} - 1$

Endif

Endfor

Endfor

Endfor

Return $\{n_{ij}\}$

§

We always make decisions based on previous experiences when we are facing a set of options; therefore this kind of Monte Carlo can be used in many situations within and outside drug development (see Chapters 4 and 5). One can build very interesting scenarios to study how the drug industry and even the global economy works.

1.2.5 *Economic Globalization*

Globalization in its literal sense is the transformation of local or regional phenomena into global ones. It can be described as a process by which the people of the world are unified into a single society and function together. This process is a combination of economic, technological, sociocultural, and political forces. Globalization is often used to refer to economic globalization, that is, integration of national economies into the international economy through trade, foreign direct investment, capital flows, migration, and the spread of technology (Wikipedia, 2009). Advances in communication and transportation technology, combined with free-market ideology, have given goods, services, and capital unprecedented mobility.

Despite the complicated reasons behind individual cases, there is a very general statistical or mathematical model for such globalization processes, i.e., random (Brownian) motion at the microscopic level or the diffusion equation at the macroscopic level.

At the macroscopic level, diffusion can be modeled by the differential equation:

$$\frac{du}{dt} = -ku, \tag{1.8}$$

where u is the quantity of interest, e.g., electrical voltage or the level of technology or knowledge in different regions. The solution for (1.8) is the exponential function

$$u = u_0 e^{-kt},$$

where u_0 is determined by the initial condition.

Equation (1.8) states that when there is no external force, there is a general tendency that quantity u moves from an area with a higher value to another with a lower value. The speed of this homogenization process (diffusion) is characterized by a constant, k. In the globalization process, government policies of a country play a critical role in determining the value of k.

Diffusions are everywhere — we can say that if there is a difference, there will be a diffusion: water flow from higher to lower, technology diffusion from first world countries to third world countries, diffusion due to the difference in labor costs between the US and China. The difference in the percentage of English speakers in the US and China will also create diffusion; even overall cultural differences in two countries can lead to diffusion. These multi-channel diffusion processes from one region to another are not isolated or statistically dependent, but are governed by the following multi-dimension diffusion equation:

$$\frac{du_i}{dt} = -k_{ij}u_j, \tag{1.9}$$

where the diffusion coefficients k_{ij} are usually a function of u_{ij}, which means (1.9) is a nonlinear differential equation system. Such a system is virtually impossible to solve analytically, but can be easily solved using Monte Carlo simulation. Many commercial and noncommercial software tools (e.g., ExtendSim) are available for Monte Carlo simulations. Algorithm 1.7 later in this chapter can be used to find the steady state solution for this problem.

In Chapter 11 (Pharmacokinetic Simulation), we will discuss how microscopic Brownian motion turns out mathematically to be a diffusion equation at the macroscopic level and we present Monte Carlo algorithms for multi-channel diffusion of drug substances.

The diffusion model is a deterministic approach, which models the mean or overall behavior without variability considerations. In contrast, Monte Carlo simulations at the microscopic level provide both mean and variability evaluations for random phenomena.

1.2.6　*Percolation and Chaos*

In physics, chemistry, materials science, and geography, percolation concerns the movement of fluids through porous materials or random media.

Examples include the movement of solvents through filter paper and the seepage or movement of liquids (e.g., water or petroleum) through soil. Electrical analogs include the flow of electricity through random networks. Another interesting application is coffee percolation, where the solvent is water, the permeable substance is the coffee grounds, and the soluble constituents are the chemical compounds that give coffee its color, taste, and aroma.

Percolation is recognized as important in studying random media because when it happens the system will degenerate into chaos. A simple question to ask is: what is the average proportion of void-ratio (void volume to solid volume) that will cause percolation? Let's develop a Monte Carlo algorithm to answer the question.

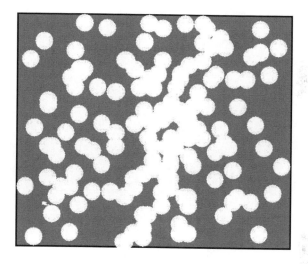

Figure 1.8: Simulation of Percolation

The basic idea of percolation simulation is, in a bounded space (e.g., a square, representing a piece of solid material), continually generate small disks (holes) at random locations in each other until the piece of material is percolated (Figure 1.8). The void ratio at percolation is then calculated. The occurrence of percolation can be either visually identified or computed in the simulation. To compute the percolation condition, a simple way is to use a "laser-beam" to scan the area, e.g., from left (top) to right (bottom), whenever a new disk is generated. Every time the laser beam moves right a very small unit it checks if it hits or intersects any disk; if no intersection, no percolation; if the laser beam always intersects some disk(s) during the scanning, it is percolated. Algorithm 1.5 is developed from this idea.

Algorithm 1.5: Simulation of Percolation

Objective: return average number of random holes at percolation.

Input: nRuns, small disk radius r

$nAve := 0$

For $iRun := 1$ **To** nRuns

    $i := 0$

    percolation := False

    While Not percolation:

        Generate x from $U(0, 1)$

        Generate y from $U(0, 1)$

        Draw a circle centered at (x, y) with radius r

        $i := i + 1$

        Check percolation

        If percolation **Then** $nAve := nAve + i/\text{nRuns}$

    Endwhile

Endfor

Return $nAve$

§

Note that we have ignored the disk overlapping in Algorithm 1.5 for simplicity. The line Check percolation is brief. The analytic solution is found to be 1/3 when the defects are completely random or uniformly distributed over the 3D space.

1.2.7 *Fish Pond*

If you want to measure the volume of water (V_w) in a pond, an easy way is to pour a cup (volume v) of a (colored) testing liquid into a pond and let it sufficiently mix (diffuse). Then take a cup of water from the pond and measure the concentration (c) of the test liquid. We now can calculate the volume of water in the pond: $V = \frac{v}{c} - v$ because the concentration is $c = v/(v + V)$.

Suppose we want to estimate the number of fish in a pond without pumping out the water (Figure 1.9). We can use a similar approach. Get a certain number (n_1) of fish (not from the pond), mark them, and put them into the pond. On the next day, we catch some (n_2) of the fish, and find r out of n_2 have been marked (r/n_2 equivalent to c). We now can estimate the total number of fish in the pond: $n = \frac{n_1 n_2}{r} - n_1$.

However, a commonly used method for solving this kind of problem is the so-called mark-recapture method (MRM). The simplest version of this method is the two-sample method: Capture some fish (n_1), mark them, and put them back into the pond. On the next day you capture some fish (n_2). Of these, r were marked the day before. Then the estimated population size (N) is given by

$$N = \frac{n_1 n_2}{r}.$$ (1.10)

An approximately unbiased variance of N, or $var(N)$, can be estimated as:

$$var(N) = \frac{(n_1 + 1)(n_2 + 1)\,(n_1 - r)\,(n_2 - r)}{(r + 1)^2\,(r + 2)}.$$ (1.11)

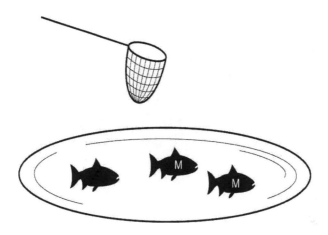

Figure 1.9:   Capture-Recapture Method
(Source: www.figurethis.org)

This method is called the Lincoln–Petersen method. It can be used to estimate population size if (1) only two independent samples are taken, (2) each individual has an equal probability of being selected (or captured), and (3) the study population is closed, meaning no deaths or births and no migration between visits.

MRM is a method commonly used in ecology to estimate population size, population vital rates (i.e., survival, movement, and growth), and the number of people needing particular services (e.g., people infected with HIV). MRM can also be used to study the error rate in software source code, in clinical trials, databases, etc. This approach is useful when the total population size is unknown.

1.2.8   Competing Risks

Medical science and health technology have been improved dramatically in the past decades. The resulting health status and life-expectancy changes are particularly interesting to us. According to National Vital Statistics Reports (Vol. 56, No. 10, April 24, 2008), the five leading causes of death in the USA for 2005 were heart disease (652,091), cancer (559,312), stroke (143,579), chronic lower respiratory diseases (130,933), and accidents (unintentional injuries, 117,809). Among the fifteen leading causes of death, age-adjusted death rates decreased significantly from 2004 to 2005 for the top three leading causes, heart disease, cancer, and stroke, as long-term decreasing trends for these causes continued. Significant increases occurred for chronic lower respiratory diseases, unintentional injuries, Alzheimer's disease, influenza and pneumonia, hypertension, Parkinson's disease, and homicide. Despite the disease spectrum shifts, the life expectancy of the US population was 77.8 years, the same as that in 2004. What does it mean that life expectancies remained unchanged for the total population? Are our great efforts in medicine and health being balanced out by increasing negative causes (war, pollution, epidemiological disease)? Is it a phenomenon of simultaneous age-adjusted life expectancy? Is it because we allocate our health resources inefficiently? In what follows we will study how to allocate health resources appropriately and see the impact of inappropriate allocations.

We all face potential multiple causes of death. A cancer patient's response to cancer treatment effectively may fail due to other diseases such as stroke. To study the mechanism of life expectancy in disease complication is an interesting topic to governments for resource allocation. Algorithm 1.6 can be used to study the effect of single-cause life expectancy change on overall life expectancy ($aveLife$). This algorithm can be easily used for resource allocation purposes as described in the following: Suppose we just consider two causes of death, cancer and heart disease. Assume life expectancy will be T_1 without heart disease and T_2 without cancer. The cost for an increase of 1% in T_1 is C_1 (cancer treatment cost) and the cost for an increase of 1% in T_2 is C_2 (treatment cost for heart disease). How should we allocate resource C, where $C_1 + C_2 = C$, so that life expectancy is maximized? Readers should be able to solve this problem using Monte Carlo techniques after reading Chapter 2.

Algorithm 1.6: Life Expectancy under Competing Risks
Objective: average life expectancy under two potential causes of death.
Input: population size N, single cause life expectancies T_1 and T_2.

$aveLife := 0$
For $i := 1$ **To** N
    Generate t_1 from exponential distribution with hazard rate $1/T_1$.
    Generate t_2 from exponential distribution with hazard rate $1/T_2$.
    $L_i := \min(t_1, t_2)$
    $aveLife := aveLife + L_i/N$
Endfor
Return $aveLife$
§

1.2.9 *Pandemic Disease Modeling*

Endemic disease is a disease that exists permanently in a particular region or population. Malaria is a constant worry in parts of Africa. Epidemic disease refers to an outbreak of disease that attacks many people at about the same time and may spread through one or several communities. Pandemic disease occurs when an epidemic spreads throughout the world. SARS and swine flu (H1N1) are two examples of pandemic diseases.

To model a pandemic disease (e.g., swine flu), let's assume the rate of disease infection is proportional to the number of infected and the number of potentially infected, i.e.,

$$\frac{dn(t)}{dt} = kn(t)(N - n(t) - rt), \tag{1.12}$$

where k is a constant to be determined, N is the overall population size, $n(t)$ is the infected population at time t, and the constant r is the spreading rate of H1N1 vaccine (number of patients who get the vaccine per unit time). In general, (1.12) can be solved using Monte Carlo (Exercise 1.10). However, if the term rt is neglected because no vaccine is available, we can solve (1.12) analytically as follows.

Equation (1.12) can be written as

$$\frac{1}{N - rt}\left(\frac{1}{n(t)} + \frac{1}{N - n(t)}\right) dn(t) = k\, dt. \tag{1.13}$$

Assume at time $t = 0$ there is only one person who carries the disease, i.e., $n(0) = 1$ and define the proportion of the infected population $p(t) = n(t)/N$. Then from (1.13), after integrating, we can obtain the logistic model.

$$p(t) = \frac{e^{kNt}}{1 + e^{kNt}}. \tag{1.14}$$

Suppose you now have the opportunity to have a swine flu vaccine that virtually guarantees you will not get the disease. However, there is a slim chance (probability p_0) of having a side effect that is as serious as swine flu. What should you do? You may want to get the vaccine shot right away if you can. But if you can't you may want to compare the probability p_0 and $p(t)$ at time t and decide to get the shot (if $p(t) > p_0$) or not (if $p(t) \leq p_0$).

Practically, k is unknown; thus (1.14) can be used to assess k, where $p(t) = n(t)/N$ is calculated based on the observed number of infections $n(t)$ at time t.

Considering that $p(t)$ is the overall measure of the infection rate at time t, we may, for our decision making, want to use the instantaneous probability within the unit time interval at time t, i.e., $\frac{dn(t)}{Ndt}$, or the conditional probability (given no disease at time t) of having the infection during the time interval t to L_{exp} (life expectancy):

$$P_c(t) = \int_t^{L_{\text{exp}}} \left[\frac{dn(x)}{Ndx}\right] dx. \qquad (1.15)$$

Substituting (1.12) and $p(t) = n(t)/N$ into (1.15), we have

$$P_c(t) = kN \int_t^{L_{\text{exp}}} p(x)(1 - p(x)) dx. \qquad (1.16)$$

Further substituting (1.16) and carrying out the integral, we obtain the conditional probability of having the infection at time t and beyond:

$$P_c(t) = \frac{1}{1 + e^{kNt}} - \frac{1}{1 + e^{kNL_{\text{exp}}}}. \qquad (1.17)$$

Equation (1.17) can be compared with side-effect probability p_0 to help you decide whether you should get the flu vaccine or not. Clearly, when t gets larger or close to the life expectancy L_{exp}, $P_c(t)$ gets smaller than p_0. In such a case, there is no point in having the flu shot.

However, this is a simple case; if you want to consider regional differences in k and other complications, then Monte Carlo simulation is a simple way to go.

1.2.10   *Random Walk and Integral Equation*

The Laplace partial differential equation has been used to describe many phenomena in physics. It is a basic law governing any potential field $u(x, y)$.

Mathematically, it is written as

$$\begin{cases} \Delta u\,(x,y) = \frac{\partial^2 u}{\partial x^2} + \frac{\partial^2 u}{\partial y^2}, \ (x,y) \in \Omega, \\ u|_S = g\,(S), \end{cases} \tag{1.18}$$

where Ω is a domain in 2D real space and S is the boundary of Ω. The function $g\,(\cdot)$ is given. The goal is to solve for the unknown function $u\,(Q) = u\,(x,y)$ numerically. There are several ways to find $u\,(Q)$, such as finite difference, finite element, or boundary element methods. But here we are going to use the Monte Carlo method to solve the problem. Monte Carlo is efficient here if we are only interested in the potential $u\,(Q)$ at a small set of points Q.

The mathematical basis for the Monte Carlo simulation is described as follows:

Draw a circle C centered at $Q \in \Omega$ with $C \subset \Omega$. Thus we have

$$\begin{aligned} \{S|Q\} &= \{S|Q\} \underset{\varphi}{\cup} \{Q \to C\,(\varphi)\} \\ &= \underset{\varphi}{\cup} \{\{S|Q\}\,\{Q \to C\,(\varphi)\}\} \\ &= \underset{\varphi}{\cup} \{\{S|C\,(\varphi)\}\,\{Q \to C\,(\varphi)\}\}, \end{aligned} \tag{1.19}$$

where $C\,(\varphi)$ is the point on the circle with the parameter angle φ and $\to$ implies the direction of the random walk.

Therefore,

$$P\,\{S|Q\} = \sum_{\varphi} P\,\{Q \to C\,(\varphi)\}\,P\,\{S|C\,(\varphi)\} \tag{1.20}$$

$$\begin{aligned} u\,(Q) &= \int_S g\,(S)\,P\,\{S|Q\} \\ &= \sum_{\varphi} P\,\{Q \to C\,(\varphi)\} \int_S g\,(S)\,P\,\{S|C\,(\varphi)\} \\ &= \frac{1}{2\pi} \int_0^{2\pi} u\,(C\,(\varphi))\,d\varphi \\ &= \frac{1}{m} \sum_{i=1}^{m} u\,(C\,(\varphi_i)) = \tilde{u}_c \end{aligned} \tag{1.21}$$

where φ_i is randomly sampled from uniform distribution $U\,(0, 2\pi)$. If $\varphi_i \notin S$, we can use the average u from another circle C_2 centered at $C\,(\varphi_i) \cdots$ until the boundary is reached or close enough (Figure 1.10).

Based on the result (1.21), we now can construct a random walk algorithm to solve the Laplace problem (Muller, 1956):

Algorithm 1.7: Random Walk-Solving Integral Equation
Objective: return a numerical solution $u(Q)$ for the Laplace problem

(1) Draw the maximum circle C that is centered at Q without crossing the boundary S, i.e., $C \cap S = \phi$.
(2) Generate a random point $Q_1 = 2\pi\xi_1$, ξ_1 from $U(0,1)$; draw the maximum circle C_1 centered at Q_1 such that $C_1 \cap S = \phi$.
(3) Generate a random point $Q_2 = 2\pi\xi_2$, ξ_2 from $U(0,1)$. The process continues until the radius of the maximum circle is smaller than constant $\delta > 0$. Record $g(\Gamma_1)$, where Γ_1 is the closest point on the boundary to the final point of the random walk (in Figure 1.10, $\Gamma_1 = Q_3$).
(4) This finishes a simulation run. Repeat the random walk process n times. The solution at point Q is given by

$$u(Q) \approx \frac{1}{n} \sum_{i=1}^{n} g(\Gamma_i) \tag{1.22}$$

§

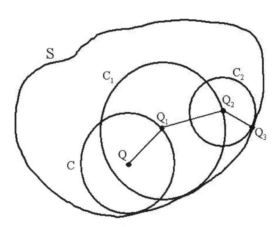

Figure 1.10:   Monte Carlo for the Laplace Problem

For a three or higher dimensional Laplace problem, the Monte Carlo method is similar. There are many other random walk methods (RWM), e.g., RWM based finite difference.

1.2.11 *Financial Index and α Stable Distribution*

Market risks are the prospect of financial losses or gains due to unexpected changes in market prices and rates. Evaluating exposure to such risks is the primary concern of risk management in financial and nonfinancial institutions alike. Until the late 1980s market risks were estimated through gap and duration analysis (interest rates), portfolio theory (securities), sensitivity analysis (derivatives), or "what-if" scenarios. These traditional methods are only applicable to very specific assets and/or based on subjective reasoning (Weron, 2004).

Since the early 1990s a commonly used market risk estimation methodology has been the Value at Risk (VaR). VaR is the percentile defined by

$$\Pr\left(L > \text{VaR}\right) \leq 1 - c \tag{1.23}$$

where $L = -\Delta X\left(\tau\right)$ with $\Delta X\left(\tau\right)$ being the relative change (return) in portfolio value over the time horizon τ. Hence, large values of L correspond to large losses (or large negative returns).

The VaR provides a common consistent measure of risk across different positions and risk factors and takes into account the correlations or dependencies between different risk factors. Artzner et al. (1999) proposed a coherent measure, the Expected Shortfall (ES), also called Expected Tail Loss or Conditional VaR, as the expected value of the losses in excess of VaR:

$$ES = E\left(L|L > \text{VaR}\right). \tag{1.24}$$

The calculations were based on the normality assumption. However, it has long been known that asset returns are not normally distributed. Rather, empirical observations exhibit excess kurtosis (fat tails). The Dow Jones Industrial Average (DJIA) index is a prominent example, where the contrast with the Gaussian law is striking.

An appropriate model is the so-called Stable Distribution (α-stable). It is often argued that financial asset returns are the cumulative outcome of a vast number of pieces of information and individual decisions arriving almost continuously in time (McCulloch, 1996; Rachev and Mittnik, 2000). It seems that the Gaussian distribution should be fine, thanks to the Central Limit Theorem, which states that the sum of a large number of independent, identically distributed variables from a finite-variance distribution will tend to be normally distributed. However, financial asset returns usually have heavier tails. As indicated by Laha and Rohatgi (1979), there are at least two reasons to use α-stable: (1) it is supported by the generalized Central Limit Theorem, which states that stable laws are the only possible limit distributions for properly normalized and centered sums of independent, identically distributed random variables, and (2) α-stable distributions are leptokurtic: since they can accommodate the fat tails and asymmetry, they fit empirical distributions much better.

An α-stable distribution requires four parameters for complete description: an index of stability $\alpha \in (0, 2]$, also called the tail index, tail exponent, or characteristic exponent, a skewness parameter $\beta \in [-1, 1]$, a scale parameter $\sigma > 0$, and a location parameter $\mu \in \mathbb{R}$. The Paretian-Lévy stable or α-stable distributions (Lévy, 1925) don't require a closed form. However, the most popular parameterization of the characteristic function of $X \sim S_\alpha(\sigma, \beta, \mu)$, i.e., an α-stable random variable with parameters α, σ, β, and μ, is given by

$$\ln \phi(t) = \begin{cases} -\sigma^\alpha |t|^\alpha \left(1 - i\beta sign(t) \tan \frac{\pi\alpha}{2}\right) + i\mu t, \ \alpha \neq 1, \\ -\sigma |t| \left(1 + i\beta sign(t) \frac{2}{\pi} \ln(t)\right) + i\mu t, \ \ \alpha = 1. \end{cases} \tag{1.25}$$

The following efficient algorithm for sampling from $S_\alpha(1, \beta, 0)$ was proposed by Chambers, Mallows and Stuck (1976).

Algorithm 1.8: α-Stable (Chambers, Mallows, and Stuck, 1976)

(1) Generate a random variable U uniformly distributed on $(-\frac{\pi}{2}, -\frac{\pi}{2})$ and an independent exponential random variable w with mean 1;
(2) If $\alpha \neq 1$, return

$$X = \left[1 + \left(\beta \tan \frac{\pi\alpha}{2}\right)^2\right]^{\frac{1}{2\alpha}} \frac{\sin(\alpha(U + \xi))}{(\cos u)^{1/\alpha}} \left[\frac{\cos(U - \alpha(U + \xi))}{w}\right]^{\frac{1-\alpha}{\alpha}}, \tag{1.26}$$

otherwise, return

$$X = \frac{2}{\pi} \left\{\left(\frac{\pi}{2} + \beta U\right) \tan U - \beta \ln \left(\frac{\frac{\pi}{2} W \cos U}{\frac{\pi}{2} + \beta U}\right)\right\}. \tag{1.27}$$

§

For sampling from the general α-stable distribution $S_\alpha(\sigma, \beta, \mu)$, we can use the following property: if $X \sim S_\alpha(1, \beta, 0)$, then $Y \sim S_\alpha(\sigma, \beta, \mu)$ can be obtained by variable transform:

$$Y = \begin{cases} \sigma X + \mu, \ \ \ \ \ \ \ \alpha \neq 1, \\ \sigma X + \frac{2}{\pi}\beta\sigma \ln \sigma + \mu, \ \alpha = 1. \end{cases} \tag{1.28}$$

The random numbers generated from $S_\alpha(\sigma, \beta, \mu)$ can be used to study the strategies to maximize gain in stock trading.

1.2.12 *Nonlinear Equation System Solver*

Many problems lead to nonlinear equation systems, which are often impossible to solve analytically. Local linearization approaches are often used, but the methods are not always effective. A Monte Carlo method provides an alternative.

Suppose we have the following system of equations to be solved:

$$f_i(x_1, x_2, ..., x_n) = 0, i = 1, 2, ..., n, \qquad (1.29)$$

where x_i are real and f_i are nonlinear functions.

To find a solution $\boldsymbol{x} = \{x_1, x_2, ..., x_n\}$ to the equation system (1.23), we define an objective function or loss function:

$$L(\boldsymbol{x}) = \sum_{i=1}^{n} f_i^2(\boldsymbol{x}). \qquad (1.30)$$

The vector $\boldsymbol{x}$ will be considered as an approximate solution to (1.23) or (1.24) if it satisfies the following inequality:

$$L(\boldsymbol{x}) < \varepsilon, \qquad (1.31)$$

where $\varepsilon > 0$ is a predefined small positive value. This is a typical classic optimization problem without constraints.

The classic unconstrained optimization problem can formally be presented as finding the set:

$$\Theta^* = \arg\min_{\theta \in \Theta} L(\boldsymbol{\theta}) = \{\boldsymbol{\theta}^* \in \Theta : L(\boldsymbol{\theta}^*) \le L(\boldsymbol{\theta}) \text{ for all } \boldsymbol{\theta} \in \Theta\}, \qquad (1.32)$$

where $L(\boldsymbol{\theta})$ is called the loss function, θ is the p-dimensional vector of parameters that are being adjusted, and $\Theta \in \mathbb{R}^p$. Note that $\boldsymbol{\theta}^*$ may not be unique, i.e., $\boldsymbol{\Theta}^*$ may have more than one element.

For classic optimization (1.32), many algorithms can be used, e.g., Blind Random Search (Algorithm 1.9).

Algorithm 1.9: Blind Random Search
Objective: return an optimal value $\boldsymbol{\theta} \in \Theta^*$ in (1.32)
rejection := **True**
While rejection:
    Generate $\boldsymbol{\theta} \in \Theta$ based on a probability distribution.
    If $L(\boldsymbol{\theta}) < \varepsilon$ **Then** rejection := **False**
Endwhile
Return θ
§

The blind search algorithm is the simplest one, but not very efficient. The next method is to mimic the way a blind man climbs a mountain. He detects the heights nearby using a stick; if he finds a place higher than where he is standing, he steps up to that location. The process continues until he can't find a higher point. In this way, he hopes he can find the peak of the mountain.

Algorithm 1.10: Blind-Man Search for Optima
Objective: return optima

(1) Randomly select a starting point X_0, neighboring length L_0
(2) Randomly search m neighboring points $(X_{0i}, i = 1, ..., m)$,

> If $\theta(X_{0i}) > \theta(X_0)$, then
>> select X_{0i} as a new starting point and go to Step 1.
> If $\theta(X_{0i}) \leq \theta(X_0)$, then continue to search the neighboring points.
> If $i = m$ and $\theta(X_{0i}) \leq \theta(X_0), \forall i \in \{1, 2, ..., m\}$, then
>> change (randomly or not) L_0 and return to Step 1.

(3) If the search criteria have been met, then

> return the final X_{0i} and $\theta(X_{0i})$.

§

This randomized search method allows for searching for global optima, where many deterministic approaches can only find the local optima.

1.2.13 *Stochastic Optimization*

In stochastic optimization, we are dealing with optimization with random noise $\varepsilon(\boldsymbol{\theta})$ in the objective function

$$y(\theta) = L(\boldsymbol{\theta}) + \varepsilon(\boldsymbol{\theta}). \tag{1.33}$$

The noise $\varepsilon(\boldsymbol{\theta})$ is a function of θ. Because of this noise, it fundamentally alters the search or optimization process as illustrated in Figure 1.11.

Stochastic approximation (SA) is a basis for stochastic optimization. Robbins and Monro (1951) introduced SA as a general root-finding method when measurements of the underlying function involve random noise.

If the objective function $L(\theta)$ is known and differentiable, then the optimization can be equivalent to solving the equation

$$\frac{\partial L(\theta)}{\partial \theta} = 0 \tag{1.34}$$

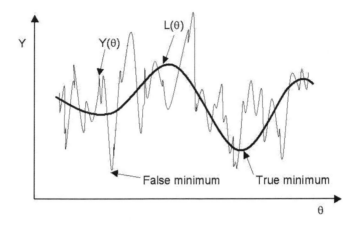

Figure 1.11:   Classic versus Stochastic Optimization

for θ.

The gradient method is based on the formula to obtain the value $\hat{\theta}_{k+1}$ for the $(k+1)^{th}$ iteration from the value $\hat{\theta}_k$ at the kth iteration:

$$\hat{\theta}_{k+1} = \hat{\theta}_k - a_k g\left(\hat{\theta}_k\right), \qquad (1.35)$$

where constant $a_k > 0$ is the step size, and $g\left(\theta\right) = \frac{\partial L(\theta)}{\partial \theta}$.

However, because $g\left(\theta\right)$ is unknown in SA, we use an estimate $\hat{g}\left(\theta\right)$ to replace $g\left(\theta\right)$ in (1.35), which leads to

$$\hat{\theta}_{k+1} = \hat{\theta}_k - a_k \hat{g}\left(\hat{\theta}_k\right), \qquad (1.36)$$

where $\hat{g}$ is estimated using the so-called simultaneous perturbation (SP).

For two-sided SP gradient approximation, this leads to

$$\hat{g}_k\left(\hat{\theta}_k\right) = \begin{bmatrix} \frac{y\left(\hat{\theta}_k + c_k \Delta_k\right) - y\left(\hat{\theta}_k - c_k \Delta_k\right)}{2 c_k \Delta_{k1}} \\ \vdots \\ \frac{y\left(\hat{\theta}_k + c_k \Delta_k\right) - y\left(\hat{\theta}_k - c_k \Delta_k\right)}{2 c_k \Delta_{kp}} \end{bmatrix}. \qquad (1.37)$$

Equation (1.37) provides an optimization algorithm, called SPSA. Because the numerator is the same in all p components of $\hat{g}_k\left(\hat{\theta}_k\right)$, the number of loss measurements needed to estimate the gradient in SPSA is two, regardless of the dimension p.

Applications of SPSA include queuing systems, pattern recognition, industrial quality improvement, aircraft design, simulation-based optimization, bioprocess control, neural network training, chemical process control, fault detection, human-machine interaction, sensor placement and configuration, and vehicle traffic management.

The choice of the distribution for generating the Δ_k is important to the performance of the algorithm. One simple and popular distribution that satisfies the inverse moments condition is the symmetric Bernoulli ± 1 distribution. Two common mean-zero distributions that do not satisfy the inverse moments condition are symmetric uniform and normal with mean zero. The failure of both of these distributions is a consequence of the amount of probability mass near zero (Gentle and Härdle, 2004, p. 170–195)

1.2.14   *Symbolic Regression*

Genetic programming (GP), inspired by biological evolution, is an evolutionary computation (EC) technique that automatically solves problems without requiring the user to know or specify the form or structure of the solution in advance. At the most abstract level GP is a systematic, domain-independent method for getting computers to solve problems automatically starting from a high-level statement of what needs to be done (Oli, Langdon, and McPhee, 2008). The idea of genetic programming is to evolve a population of computer programs. Hopefully, generation by generation, GP stochastically transforms populations of programs into new populations of programs that will effectively solve the problem under consideration. Like evolution in nature, GP has been very successful at developing novel and unexpected ways of solving problems.

Representation: Syntax Tree

To study GP, it is convenient to express programs using syntax trees in GP rather than as lines of code. For example, the programs $(x + y) + 3$, $(y + 1) \times (x/2)$, and $(x/2) + 3$ can be represented by the three syntax trees in Figure 1.12, respectively. The variables and constants in the program (x, y, 1, 2, and 3) are leaves of the tree, called terminals, while the arithmetic operations ($+$, $\times$, and *max*) are internal nodes called functions. The sets of allowed functions and terminals together form the primitive set of a GP system.

Reproduction Mechanism

For the program to evaluate, GP must have the reproduction mechanism to generate new programs or offspring. There are two common ways to generate offspring: crossover and mutation. Crossover is the primary way (about 90% of new generations evolve by crossover, and 10% by mutation) to reduce the chance of chaos because the crossover leads to much similarity between parent and child. Crossover is a selection of a subtree for crossover, whereas mutation randomly generates a subtree to replace a randomly se-

lected subtree from a randomly selected individual. Crossover and mutation
are illustrated in Figure 1.12, where the trees on the left are actually copies
of the parents; their genetic material can freely be used without altering
the original individuals.

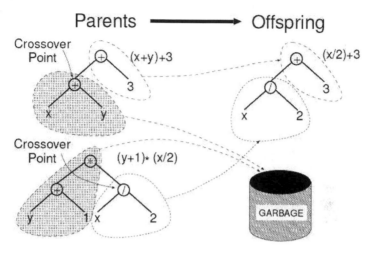

Figure 1.12: Crossover in GP
(Source: Oli et al., 2008)

Survival Fitness

The second mechanism required for program evolution is survival fitness.
There are many possible ways to define the fitness measure. As an example, for the problem of finding a function $g(x)$ to approximate the target
function $f(x)$, it is the mean square error between the two functions.

Algorithm 1.11: Genetic Programming

Objective: return best-fit-individual based GP.
Input generation size M, population size N, and target fitness V_t.
Create an initial population of programs and assess their fitness.
For $i := 1$ **To** M
    For $j := 1$ **To** N
        Determine crossover or mutation operation probabilistically.
        If crossover Then randomly select two trees and cross nodes.
        If mutation Then randomly select one tree and a node.
        Produce an offspring and evaluate its fitness.
    Endfor
If fitness $\geq V_t$ **Then** Exitfor.

Endfor
Return the best-so-far individual
§

An algorithm for genetic programming is presented in Algorithm 1.11 and elaborated as follows.

M is the number of generations, N is the population size for each generation, and V_t is the target fitness. To create an initial population of programs, we use so-called primitives that include a terminal set (leaves) and a function set (nodes). The terminal set typically consists of variables and constants. The function set is driven by the nature of the problem's domain. In a simple numeric problem, for example, the function set may consist of merely the arithmetic functions $(+, -, \times, /)$, but other functions can also be used.

There are two iterative loops: one for generation, and the other for individuals within the generation. Each individual, whether generated by crossover or mutation, will have his fitness assessed. Individuals with lower fitness may be removed from the population. Individuals with higher fitness may have higher probabilities to be selected for generating their offspring for the next generation. The crossover usually operates within the same generation, but theoretically it can be performed between two generations. Fitness (function) can be measured in many ways, for example, in terms of (1) the amount of error between its output and the desired output, (2) the amount of time required to bring a system to a desired target state, (3) the accuracy of the program in recognizing patterns or classifying objects, or (4) the compliance of a structure with user-specified design criteria.

The usual termination criterion is that an individual's fitness should exceed a target value, but could instead be a problem-specific success predicate, or some other criterion. Typically, the single best-so-far individual is then harvested and designated as the result of the run.

Koza (Banzhaf et al., 1998) studied the symbolic regression

$$y = f(x) = \frac{x^2}{2}, \ x \in [0, 1].$$

Using the terminal set: $x \in [-5, 5]$, function set: $+, -, \times$, and protected division $\%$, and 500 individuals in each generation, Koza was able to obtain the best individual (function) f_i in generation i, where $f_0 = \frac{x}{3}$, $f_1 = \frac{x}{6-3x}$, $f_2 = \frac{x}{x(x-4)-1+4/x-(9(x+1)/(5x)+x)/(6-3x)}$, and $f_3 = \frac{x^2}{2}$. Therefore, at generation 3, the correct solution is found. However, as the generation number increases, the best fit function starts to expand again. We will return to this topic in Chapter 13.

1.3 Simulations in Drug Development

1.3.1 *Challenges in the Pharmaceutical Industry*

It is of great concern that the pharmaceutical industry may be undergoing a productivity crisis caused in part by the pragmatic definition of the number of new drugs or new molecular entities (NMEs) approved each year. The number of NMEs and priority review drug approvals have remained relatively flat in the past decades (Figure 1.13). However, the amount of spending in Research and Development has consistently increased yearly from approximately 4B in 1976 to 36B in 2004 based on a 9% inflation adjusted rate for 2002.

Moreover, from 1990 to 1994, 11 new drugs had reached the "top 100 drugs" category in terms of global sales. From 1995 to 1999, ten new approved drugs made it into the "top 100 drugs" category. However, during the period from 2000–2004, only two new approvals broke into the group of top 100 revenue generators. During 2005 to 2007, the FDA approved only half the number of new compounds as it had only a decade before. And fewer than 10% of these newly approved compounds are expected to ultimately generate sales of even $350 million annually (Simon and Pecker, 2003). Five different blockbuster drugs went off-patent in 2006 and more such transitions loom large on the horizon. Price pressures from the public and private sectors have made headlines nationwide. These situations have made the pharmaceutical industry as a whole seem vulnerable in the face of new challenges, new realities regarding drug development, new competition from biotechnology and the emerging world of genomics, and new expectations on the part of consumers and managed care providers (Paich et al., 2009). There are many reasons why this is happening (Woodcock, 2004, Chang, 2007b). Among them is insufficient technology innovation, such as adaptive design and computer simulation.

Traditional drug development is subjective to a large extent, and intuitive decision-making processes are primarily based on individual experiences. Therefore, optimal design is often not achieved. Monte Carlo (MC) is a powerful evaluation tool for development plans in all stages and study designs to support strategic decision making. MC is intuitive and easy to implement with minimal cost and can be done in a short time. The utilities of MC include, but are not limited to (1) sensitivity analysis and risk assessment, (2) estimation of probability of success (power), (3) design evaluation and optimization, (4) cost, time, and risk reduction, (5) clinical development program evaluation and prioritization, (6) trial monitoring and interim prediction of future outcomes, (7) prediction of long-term benefits using short-

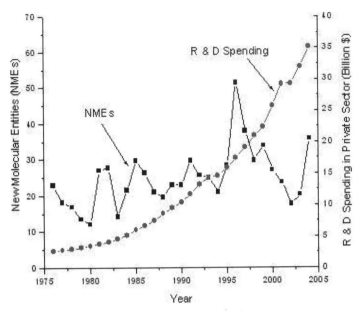

Figure 1.13:   Research and Development Spending and NMEs approved by the FDA
(Data source: Pammolli and Riccaboni, 2007)

term outcomes, (8) validation of trial design and statistical methods, and
(9) streamlining communication among different parties. Within regulatory
bodies, MC can be and has been used for assessing the robustness of results, validating statistical methodology, and predicting long-term benefits
in accelerated approvals. Monte Carlo is often used for power simulation in
hypothesis tests and for selection of the best statistical test method among
several alternatives, but these are just mostly basic applications of Monte
Carlo. Simulation should go well beyond this limited scope, as outlined in
this book.

1.3.2   *Classification of Simulations in Drug Development*

Based on the scope of studies, Monte Carlo simulations can be classified into meta-simulation, macro-simulation, and micro-simulation (Figure
1.14). Meta-simulations target multiple sectors or drug companies. Because
of the nature of competition and collaboration, Monte Carlo can combine
with game and decision theory to solve many problems. The examples of
interest are impact analysis of a technology platform, drug development
globalization, and drug industry partnerships. Macro-simulations deal with
problems involving a single business entity or company. Thus, decision the-

ory, deterministic, Bayesian, and stochastic decision approaches are used in the simulations. Application examples are pipeline optimization, clinical development optimization, and cost-effectiveness analysis across multiple compounds. Micro-simulations concern problems within an Research and Development stage (discovery, preclinical, clinical). Various scientific and statistical approaches can be used. Micro-simulation applications include molecular design and modeling, pharmacokinetic (PK) and pharmacodynamic (PD) modeling and simulation, and classical and adaptive designs.

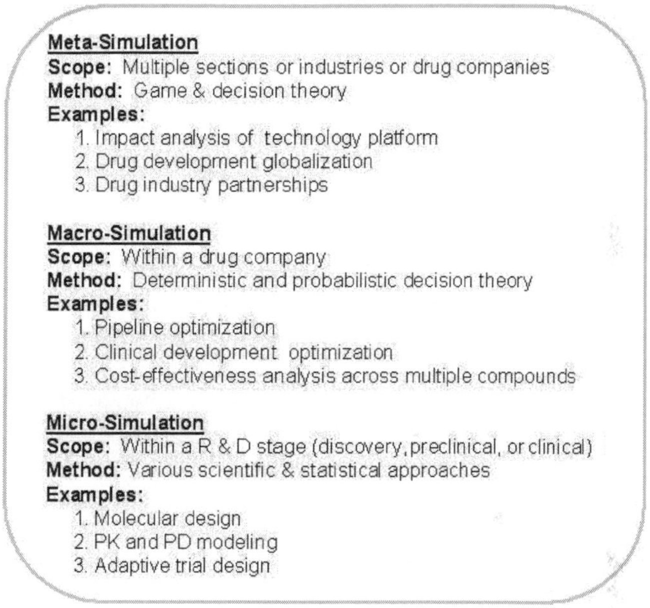

Meta-Simulation
Scope: Multiple sections or industries or drug companies
Method: Game & decision theory
Examples:
    1. Impact analysis of technology platform
    2. Drug development globalization
    3. Drug industry partnerships

Macro-Simulation
Scope: Within a drug company
Method: Deterministic and probabilistic decision theory
Examples:
    1. Pipeline optimization
    2. Clinical development optimization
    3. Cost-effectiveness analysis across multiple compounds

Micro-Simulation
Scope: Within a R & D stage (discovery, preclinical, or clinical)
Method: Various scientific & statistical approaches
Examples:
    1. Molecular design
    2. PK and PD modeling
    3. Adaptive trial design

Figure 1.14: Classification of Simulations in Drug Development

1.4 Summary

Monte Carlo is a simulation technique by means of a computer. Monte Carlo (MC) has been used everywhere, not only in traditional science and engineering, but also in political science, art, music, and bilingual translation. There are various MC methods; some are more complex than others. Building an efficient Monte Carlo model requires abstract thinking skills and the ability to identify similarities between different systems and make analogies. In the Introductory Examples, we discussed how to use a map to mechanically draw random samples and calculate the size of a country.

Then we altered the example slightly and made it into a problem of π calculation by changing the shape of the country into a circular disk. After we deformed the shape into an arbitrary shape, the calculation of the area under curve was equivalent to the definite integral. As a consequence, an MC method for area calculation became an MC for integrals. Since very broad problems can be described mathematically by integrals, MC can be applied to these problems directly. The simple MC algorithm (Algorithm 1.3) for calculating the area or definite integral is justified statistically by the law of large numbers.

We introduced a competing game using the example of finding the fastest route between two locations knowing that other drivers may also have their strategies. We constructed an MC algorithm for solving the problem. To no one's surprise, the pharmaceutical business can be characterized as such a game and we are going to discuss the topic in detail in Chapter 4.

Economic globalization and pandemic disease are two examples using very simple mathematical models for very complex phenomena, one with an infinite population, the other with a finite population. This slight difference leads to two different models, i.e., exponential and logistic. Both are very popular in the modeling and simulation world.

We used percolation as an example to illustrate that MC can be used to simulate the system's chaos for the purpose of preventing that chaos. In contrast, when the failure of a system is inevitable (e.g., death), we employed the competing risks as an example of how we can use MC in health resource allocation and in prolonging our life expectancy.

As with other simulation methods, analogy is the core of pharmaceutical Monte Carlo. In the fish pond example, we showed that two problems lead to virtually an identical modeling and simulation technique: finding the volume of water (continuous media) in the pond and finding the number of fish (discrete in nature) in the pond.

We used Laplace's partial differential equation with a boundary of the first kind to demonstrate how a complex mathematical problem can be easily solved using MC (the random walk method) as outlined in Algorithm 1.7.

In constructing MC, the appropriateness of assumptions is critical and should be checked against observed data whenever possible. In the example of the financial index and the α-stable distribution, we signified that, instead of the normal distribution as suggested by the central limit theorem, the financial data exhibit excessively fat tails, which can be modeled using α-stable distribution. Samples for MC can be generated from the distribution using Algorithm 1.8.

Optimization is a commonly faced problem in our lives. Many problems that appear not to be optimization related can be converted into optimization problems, e.g., solving a system of nonlinear equations. Algorithm 1.10 is an MC algorithm for searching for an optimal value. However, in practice observations often involve random errors such that the optimization goes beyond the classical and becomes stochastic optimization.

In the last but not least important example, symbolic regression, we used the genetic programming method, which is probably the most general MC method. Due to the importance of this MC technology and its great potential uses in the pharmaceutical industry, we will discuss GP in detail in Chapter 13.

In Section 1.3, we addressed the importance of Monte Carlo in drug development and pointed out the utilities of MC in at least eight aspects. To facilitate further discussions, MC methods are classified into three different scopes: meta, macro, and micro levels. As illustrated in Figure 1.14, meta-simulations target multiple drug companies and MC techniques are supported by other methods such game theory. Macro-simulations deal with problems involving a single business entity and are supported by decision theory. Micro-simulations treat problems within an Research and Development stage (discovery, preclinical, or clinical) and here the MC methods are very diverse. We will discuss the MC methods in different stages and aspects of drug development later.

Experience tells us that a wide range of knowledge can help us to make analogies, whereas knowledge in the subject field will help us to formulate the problem and to identify what is important and what is less important for the MC model. Last there is a simple but useful principle: If problem A can be solved using either method B or Monte Carlo C, then method B can be simulated using Monte Carlo algorithm C. For example, if linear equation systems can solve a Laplace problem and the random walk method can solve the same problem, then the random walk method can solve the linear system of equations.

1.5   Exercises

Exercise 1.1: Suppose you are given maps of two countries. Develop an algorithm to compute the ratio of their territories. Efficiency is important to consider in developing your algorithm.

Exercise 1.2: Study the effect of the constant c on the efficiency or convergency rate in Algorithm 1.2.

Exercise 1.3: It is interesting to study how individual micro-motivated behaviors cause different macro consequences, as in the example of the fastest route. Describe how you conduct such a study. Can your strategy be used in market dynamics? If every company's decision on a product is based on sales from the previous year, what will happen?

Exercise 1.4: Study the effect of the initial condition and switching probability (or probabilities in Algorithm 1.4) for the fastest route problem on the overall commuting time of the population and commuting time for each individual.

Exercise 1.5: Use the mark-recapture method to find out the proportion of large fish and small fish (or other kinds of fish).

Exercise 1.6: Study the Monte Carlo algorithm for the mark-recapture method applying the population allowing for migration, birth, and death.

Exercise 1.7: Develop an algorithm for an anisotropic Laplace problem using the random walk method:

$$\begin{cases} \Delta u\,(x,y) = k_x \frac{\partial^2 u}{\partial x^2} + k_y \frac{\partial^2 u}{\partial y^2}, & (x,y) \in \Omega, \\ u|_S = g\,(S), \end{cases}$$

with constants $k_x \neq k_y$.

Exercise 1.8: The time for a random walker to reach a distance of L from his starting point is a power function of L: $t = L^a$. Determine the constant a.

Exercise 1.9: Discussion problem: If we don't know formula (1.8) in the mark-recapture method, can we still discover it through simulation or genetic programming?

Exercise 1.10: Develop a Monte Carlo algorithm to solve differential equation (1.12).

Exercise 1.11: Translating a scientific problem into a Monte Carlo simulation problem requires logical thinking. This exercise, the seven bridge problem, tests your logical reasoning skills.

Problem description: The city of Königsberg in Prussia (now Kaliningrad, Russia) was set on both sides of the Pregel River, and included two large islands which were connected to each other and the mainland by seven bridges (Figure 1.15).

The problem is to find a walk through the city that crosses each bridge once and only once. The islands cannot be reached by any route other than the bridges, and every bridge must be crossed completely. Euler gave an elegant solution to the problem and presented it to the St. Petersburg Academy on August 26, 1735. Solve the problem by reasoning and then convert it to a Monte Carlo problem.

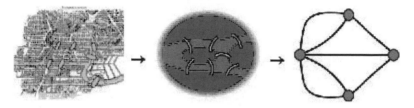

Figure 1.15:   The Konigsberg Seven Bridge Problem (www.wikipedia.org)

Chapter 2

Virtual Sampling Techniques

This chapter will cover the following topics:

- Uniform Random Number Generation
- General Sampling Methods
- Efficiency Improvement in Virtual Sampling
- Sampling Algorithms for Specific Distributions

2.1   Uniform Random Number Generation

To perform simulations, we often need to draw random samples from a certain probability distribution. Typically, the simplest and most important random sampling procedure is sampling from the uniform distribution over $(0, 1)$, denoted by $U(0, 1)$. The computer-generated "random" number is not truly random because the sequence of the numbers is determined by the so-called seed, an initial number. Random variates from other distributions can often be obtained by applying a transformation to uniform variates. There are usually several algorithms available to generate random numbers from a particular distribution. The algorithms differ in speed, accuracy, and the computer memory required.

Definition 2.1   Reduction Model m: For positive integers x and m, the value $a \pmod{m}$ is the remainder (between 0 and $m - 1$) obtained when a is divided by m.

One of the commonly used methods to generate uniform pseudorandom numbers starts with an initial value x_0, called the seed, and then recursively computes successive values $x_n, n \geq 1$, by letting

$$x_n = ax_{n-1} \pmod{m}, \tag{2.1}$$

where a and m are given positive integers. Equation (2.1) means that ax_{n-1} is divided by m and the remainder is taken as the value of x_n. Thus, each x_n is either $0, 1, ...,$ or $m-1$ and the quantity x_n/m is called a pseudorandom number, which is approximately uniformly distributed on $(0, 1)$. This method is called the linear congruential method or multiplicative congruential method. The positive integer a directly impacts the quality of the random deviates. m is the period of the sequence of the random numbers. The number a should be carefully chosen such that it leads to a large m.

Theorem 2.1 *(Period of multiplicative generator) If m is prime, the multiplicative congruential generator $x_n = ax_{n-1} \pmod{m}$, $a \neq 0$, has maximal period $m - 1$ if $a^i \pmod{m}$ for all $i = 1, 2, ..., m - 1$.*

For $m = 2^{31} - 1 = 2147483647$, Park and Miller (1988) have suggested $a = 7^5 = 16807$; other values for a are 7, 39373, 48271, and 69621 among others. Any of these values will generate all of the possible elements of the multiplicative group of integers mod m. This period of m (2147483647) is usually large enough for most simulations.

Although algorithms for random number generation seem fairly simple, there are a number of issues (e.g., period, tail distribution) that must be taken into account when implementing these algorithms in computer programs. See Gentle (1998a) for discussions of this topic.

2.2 General Sampling Methods

2.2.1 Inverse CDF Method

The inverse CDF (cumulative distribution function) method, if available, is a direct method to generate a sample with given distribution.

Theorem 2.2 *Let $\{F(z), a \leq z \leq b\}$ denote a distribution with inverse distribution*

$$F^{-1}(u) = \inf\{z \in [a, b] : F(z) \geq u, 0 \leq u \leq 1\}. \tag{2.2}$$

Let U denote a random variable from the uniform distribution $U(0, 1)$. Then $Z = F^{-1}(U)$ has the c.d.f. F.

The proof is straightforward because $\Pr(Z \leq z) = \Pr(F^{-1}(U) \leq z) = \Pr[U \leq F(z)] = F(z)$. The algorithm for implementing the inverse CDF method is simple (Algorithm 2.1).

Algorithm 2.1: Inverse CDF Method

Objective: generate Z from $\{F(z), a \leq z \leq b\}$ using the inverse CDF method.

Generate U from $U(0,1)$

$Z := F^{-1}(U)$

Return Z

§

The inverse CDF relationship exists between any two continuous (non-singular) random variables. If X is a continuous random variable with CDF F and Y is a continuous random variable with CDF G, then $X = F^{-1}(G(Y))$ over the ranges of positive support. Using this kind of relationship is actually matching percentile points of one distribution F with those of another distribution G.

For example, if $U \sim N(0,1)$, then $Z = F^{-1}(U) = \ln(U) \sim \breve{E}(1)$ (exponential distribution); if $X \sim N(\mu, \sigma^2)$, then $Z = e^X$ has log-normal distribution with p.d.f.

$$f(z) = \frac{1}{\sqrt{2\pi}\sigma z} \exp\left(\frac{-(\ln z - \mu)^2}{2\sigma^2}\right), \ 0 \leq z < \infty. \qquad (2.3)$$

Although the inverse method is simple, the closed form of F^{-1} is not always available. When F does not exist in closed form, the inverse CDF method can be applied by solving the equation $F(x) - u = 0$ numerically.

The inverse CDF method also applies to discrete distributions. Suppose the discrete random variable X has mass points of $m_1 < m_2 < m_3 < ...$ with associated probabilities of $p_1, p_2, p_3, ...$, and the distribution function

$$F(x) = \sum_{m_i \leq x} p_i. \qquad (2.4)$$

To use the inverse CDF method, we first generate a realization u of the uniform random variable U, then deliver the realization of the target distribution as x, where x satisfies the relationship

$$F(x_{(-)}) < u \leq F(x). \qquad (2.5)$$

We leave the algorithm for the inverse CDF method for discrete CDF method as an exercise (*Exercise 2.5*).

2.2.2 *Acceptance–Rejection Method*

The acceptance–rejection method is an elegant method for random number generation. For generating realizations of a random variable X with a p.d.f. $f(x)$, the acceptance-rejection method generates random numbers by using realizations of another random variable Y with a simpler distribution of g. The method is based on the following theorem (Fishman, 2000, p. 171).

Theorem 2.3   *(von Neumann 1996). Let $\{f(z), a \leq z \leq b\}$ denote a p.d.f. with factorization*

$$f(z) = cg(z)h(z), \tag{2.6}$$

where $h(z) \geq 0$, $\int_a^b h(z)\,dz = 1$, $c = \sup_z [f(z)/h(z)]$, $0 \leq g(z) \leq 1$.

Let Z denote a random variable with p.d.f. $\{h(z)\}$ and let U be from $U(0,1)$. If $U \leq g(Z)$, then Z has the p.d.f.$\{f(z)\}$.

Proof.   *The random variables U and Z have the joint p.d.f.*

$$f_{U,Z} = h(z), \; 0 \leq u \leq 1, \; a \leq z \leq b.$$

Then Z has the conditional p.d.f

$$h_Z(z|U \leq g(Z)) = \frac{\int_0^{g(z)} f_{U,Z}(u,z)\,du}{\Pr[U \leq g(Z)]}.$$

Since

$$\int_0^{g(z)} f_{U,Z}(u,z)\,du = h(z)g(z) \;\; and$$

$$\Pr[U \leq g(Z)] = \int_0^b h(z)g(z)\,dz = 1/c,$$

we obtain

$$h_Z(z|U \leq g(Z)) = cg(z)h(z) = f(z). \qquad \square$$

Algorithm 2.2: Acceptance–Rejection Method
Objective: generate a random number from distribution g.
rejection :=**True**
While rejection:
    Generate y from p.d.f. g
    Generate u from $U(0,1)$
    If $u < f(y)/cg(y)$, **Then** rejection := **False**
Endwhile
Return y
§

To gain efficiency, the difference $\varepsilon = cg(x) - f(x) > 0$ should be small for all x. The density g is called the majorizing density and cg is called the majorizing function (Figure 2.1). An important feature of acceptance-rejection is that it can apply directly to multivariate random variables.

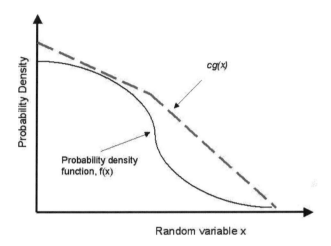

Figure 2.1:   Rejection-Acceptance Method: $cg(x) \geq f(x)$.

2.2.3   *Sampling of Order Statistics*

Let $X_1, ... X_n$ be independent continuous random variables with p.d.f. $f(x)$ or c.d.f. $F(x)$. The order statistic, $X_{(i)}, i = 1, ..., n$, is a random variable defined to be the ith smallest of the set $\{X_1, ..., X_n\}$ such that $X_{(1)} \leq \cdots X_{(i)} \cdots \leq X_{(n)}$. The c.d.f. of the order statistic is given by (Kokoska and Zwillonger, 2000)

$$F_{X_{(i)}}(x) = \Pr\left(X_{(i)} \leq x\right) = \sum_{j=1}^{n} \binom{n}{j} [F(x)]^j [1 - F(x)]^{n-j}. \qquad (2.7)$$

The p.d.f. can be obtained by the derivative of the c.d.f. To draw a sample from an order statistic, the most direct way is to generate x from its c.d.f. $F(x)$ and then sort the observations using a sort algorithm. We will introduce two sorting algorithms: quick-sort and shell-sort, in Chapter 13.

2.2.4   Markov Chain Monte Carlo

A Markov chain $\{X_n\}$ with a countable state space S and transition probability matrix $P \equiv [p_{ij}]$ is said to be irreducible if for any two states i and j the probability of the Markov chain visiting j starting from i is positive, i.e., for some $n \geq 1$, $p_{ij}^{(n)} \equiv P(X_n = j | X_0 = i) > 0$.

Theorem 2.4   *(Law of large numbers for Markov chains) Let $\{X_n\}_{n \geq 0}$ be an irreducible Markov chain with countable states, a transition probability matrix P, and a stationary probability distribution $\pi \equiv (\pi_i : i \in S)$. Then, for any bounded function $h: S \to \mathbb{R}$ and for any initial distribution of X_0*

$$\frac{1}{n} \sum_{i=0}^{n-1} h(X_i) \to \sum_j h(j) \pi_j \qquad (2.8)$$

in probability as $n \to \infty$.

A similar law of large numbers (LLN) holds when the state space S is not countable.

Monte Carlo simulations based on this theorem are called MCMC. For example, to calculate $\sum_j h(j) \pi_j$, we can use an irreducible Markov chain $\{X_i\}$ with state space S and stationary distribution π. Let the stochastic process run sufficiently long. Then the integral of h with respect to π reduces to:

$$\sum_j h(j) \pi_j = \frac{1}{n} \sum_{i=0}^{n-1} h(X_i). \qquad (2.9)$$

A discrete-time Markov chain is the basis for several schemes for generating random numbers, either continuous or discrete, multivariate or univariate. The differences in the various methods using Markov processes come from differences in the transition kernel. To generate variates from an arbitrary distribution $\pi = (\pi_i > 0, i \in \mathcal{L})$ on a finite state space $\mathcal{L} = \{0, 1, ..., v - 1\}$, we use the Metropolis-Hasting method, which is based on Theorem 2.5 (Fishman, 2000, p. 384–385).

Theorem 2.5   *Let P and R denote transition matrices, their elements satisfying*

$$\begin{cases} p_{ij} = \alpha_{ij} r_{ij}, i \neq j \\ p_{ii} = 1 - \sum_{i \neq j} p_{ij}, \end{cases} \qquad (2.10)$$

where $r_{ij} = 0$ if $r_{ji} = 0$,

$$\begin{cases} \alpha_{ij} = \dfrac{t_{ij}}{1 + \pi_i r_{ij} / (\pi_j r_{ji})} & \text{if } r_{ij} > 0 \\ 1 & \text{otherwise,} \end{cases} \qquad (2.11)$$

and $\{t_{ij} = t_{ji}\}$ is chosen to ensure that $0 < \alpha_{ij} \leq 1$ for all $i, j \in \mathcal{L}$ for which r_{ij} and $r_{ji} > 0$. Then

(1) $\boldsymbol{P}$ is reversible; (2) $\boldsymbol{\pi P} = \boldsymbol{\pi}$; (3) If $\boldsymbol{R}$ is irreducible and aperiodic, then so is $\boldsymbol{P}$.

Proof. As a consequence of (2.11) and $t_{ij} = t_{ji}$, $\pi_i \alpha_{ij} r_{ij} = \pi_j \alpha_{ji} r_{ji}$ for $\forall i \neq j$. This establishes reversibility in (1). Recall that detailed balance (reversibility) implies global balance, as in (2). Since $\boldsymbol{P}^k$ has a positive probability of following any k-step path generated by $\boldsymbol{R}^k$, irreducibility and aperiodicity of $\boldsymbol{R}$ also hold for $\boldsymbol{P}$. $\qquad\square$

Algorithm 2.3: Metropolis-Hastings Sampler (for Discrete)

Objective: Generate S_k from $\boldsymbol{P}$ using the Metropolis-Hastings method

Input: initial state $s_0 \in \mathcal{L}$, nominating matrix $\boldsymbol{R}$, procedure for evaluating each α_{ij} and terminal number of steps K.

$S_0 := s_0$

For $m = 1$ **To** K :

> $i := S_{m-1}$
>
> Randomly generate J from p.m.f. $\{r_{ij}, j \in \mathcal{L}\}$
>
> **If** $J = S_{m-1}$ **Then**
>
> > $S_m := S_{m-1}$
>
> **Else**
>
> > Evaluate α_{iJ}
> >
> > Generate u from $U(0, 1)$
> >
> > **If** $u \leq \alpha_{iJ}$ **Then**
> >
> > > $S_m := J$
> >
> > **Else**
> >
> > > $S_m := S_{m-1}$
> >
> > **Endif**
>
> **Endif**

Endfor

Return S_K

§

The MCMC is particularly useful in simulating Bayesian posterior distributions, especially in the Bayesian hierarchical model, where the posteriors are not specified directly. The idea of MCMC is not to directly simulate from the target distribution f, but to simulate an easy Markov chain that has this target density as the density of its stationary distribution. The most popular MCMC is Metropolis-Hastings. Algorithm 2.4 can be used for this purpose, where the number K is sufficiently large so that the Markov process reaches its steady state; r is the acceptance probability.

Algorithm 2.4: Metropolis-Hastings Sampler (for Posterior)

Objective: Generate a sample x_K from posterior density p using the MH method.

Input: posterior density p, proposal density g, terminal number of steps K

Select x_0 in the support of p.

For $i := 1$ **To** $K - 1$

    Generate y from density $g_{Y_{i+1}|Y_i}(y|x_i)$.

    $r := \min\left(1, \frac{p_X(y)g_{Y_{i+1}|Y_i}(x_i|y)}{p_X(x_i)g_{Y_{i+1}|Y_i}(y|x_i)}\right).$

    Generate u from $U(0,1)$

    If $u < r$ **Then**

        $x_{i+1} := y$

    Else

        $x_{i+1} := x_i$

    Endif

Endfor

Return x_K

§

2.2.5 Gibbs Sampling

To generate multivariate $\{x_1, x_2, \ldots, x_m\}$ from a distribution $P(X_1, X_2, \ldots, X_m)$, we can use the Gibbs method when conditional probabilities are available. Specifically, Gibbs sampling is an iterative procedure based on conditional power

$$P(X_i|X_1, \ldots, X_{i-1}, X_{i+1}, \ldots, X_m).$$

The Gibbs method was introduced by Geman and Geman (1984), and further developed by Gelfand and Smith (1990). The convergency criterion used in Algorithm 2.5 is the maximum difference between the two iterations less than a predefined constant $\varepsilon > 0$.

Algorithm 2.5: Gibbs Sampling

Objective: Generate multivariate distribution based on marginal density using the Gibbs method.

Input conditional probabilities

$k := 0$ and choose $x^{(0)} = \left\{x_1^{(0)}, \ldots, x_m^{(0)}\right\}$

rejection := **True**

While rejection:

    For $i := 1$ **To** m

Generate $x_i^{(k+1)}$ based on $P\left(X_i|X_1^{(k)}, ..., X_{i-1}^{(k)}, X_{i+1}^{(k)}, ..., X_m^{(k)}\right)$

$k = k+1$

Endfor

If $\max_i |x_i^{(k+1)} - x_i^{(k)}| < \varepsilon$ **Then**

$x = x^{(k+1)}$

rejection := **False**

Endif

Endwhile

Return x

§

2.2.6   *Sampling from a Distribution in a Simplex*

Consider the simplex

$$\mathcal{L}_n(x) = \left\{ z = (z_1, ..., z_n)^T : z_i \geq 0, i = 1, ..., n; \sum_{i=1}^{n} z_i \leq x, x > 0 \right\}.$$

To generate $\mathbf{Z} = (Z_1, ..., Z_n)^T$ from the uniform distribution in $\mathcal{L}_n(x)$, we can use n order statistics from n samples obtained from the uniform distribution $U(0,1)$.

Algorithm 2.6: Sampling from a Distribution in a Simplex
Objective: generate $\mathbf{Z} = (Z_1, ..., Z_n)^T$ from uniform distribution in $\mathcal{L}_n(x)$.

Input: Dimension n and bound x.

Generate $y_1, ..., y_n$ as the order statistics of n independent draws from $U(0,1)$

$z_1 := xy_1$

For $i := 1$ **To** n

$z_i := x(y_i - y_{i-1})$

Endfor

Return $\{z_1, ... z_n\}$

§

For proof of the algorithm, see Fishman, 2000, p. 232. Note that we can use the inverse c.d.f. method to generate observations from any distribution ϕ in a simplex.

2.2.7   *Sampling from a Distribution on a Hyperellipsoid*

Consider a point $\boldsymbol{Z} = (Z_1, ..., Z_n)^T$ uniformly distributed on the n-dimensional hypersphere

$$\text{ß}_n \left(r \right) = \left\{ \boldsymbol{z} = (z_1, ..., z_n) : z_1^2 + ... + z_n^2 = r^2, r > 0 \right\}.$$

Algorithm 2.7 can be used to generate samples from uniform distribution in $\text{ß}_n \left(r \right)$ (see Fishman, 2000, p. 234, or Tocher, 1963, p. 41).

Algorithm 2.7: Sampling from Uniform Distribution on Hyperellipsoid

Objective: To generate $\boldsymbol{z} = (z_1, ..., z_n)^T$ from the uniform distribution on hyperellipsoid $\text{ß}_n \left(r \right)$.

Input: Dimension n and radius r.

$i := 1$

$w := 0$

For $i := 1$ **To** n

    Generate x_i from $N \left(0, 1 \right)$.

    $w := w + x_i^2$

Endfor

$w := \sqrt{w}$

For $i := 1$ **To** n

    $z_i := r x_i / w$

Endfor

Return $\{z_1, ..., z_n\}$

§

We can use the inverse c.d.f. method to generate observations from any distribution in a hyperellipsoid.

2.3   Efficiency Improvement in Virtual Sampling

2.3.1   *Moments and Variable Transformation*

Moments

The moments of a distribution can be used to check the random numbers generated from an algorithm against the theoretical results. The first three moments are often of interest in validating Monte Carlo algorithms: mean $\mu = E \left(x \right)$; variance $\sigma^2 = E \left((x - \mu)^2 \right)$; skewness $= E \left((x - \mu)^3 \right)$ for p.m.f.; skewness $= E \left((x - \mu)^3 \right) / \sigma^3$.

Variable Transformation

In generating random numbers for a particular distribution, it is sometimes desirable to transfer one variable to another. Suppose random variable $X_1, ..., X_n$ from joint p.d.f. $f(x_1, ..., x_n)$ and $y_i = u_i(x_1, ..., x_n)$ represent a one-to-one transformation from x's to y's with inverse function $x_i = v_i(y_1, ..., y_n)$, $i = 1, ..., n$. Then the joint p.d.f. of Y_i is given by

$$g(y_1, ..., y_n) = f(v_1(y_1, ..., y_n), ..., v_n(y_1, ..., y_n)) |J|$$

where $|J|$ is the determinant of the Jacobian

$$J = \begin{bmatrix} \frac{\partial x_1}{\partial y_1} & \cdots & \frac{\partial x_1}{\partial y_n} \\ \vdots & \ddots & \vdots \\ \frac{\partial x_n}{\partial y_1} & \cdots & \frac{\partial x_n}{\partial y_n} \end{bmatrix}. \tag{2.12}$$

Some simple examples include: if $X \sim f(X; 0, 1)$, then $Y = X\sigma + \mu \sim f(X; \mu, \sigma^2)$, where μ and σ^2 are finite mean and variance. Denote $F(x)$, the c.d.f. of X, then $Y = F^{-1}(X) \sim U(0, 1)$ and $Y = -ln[1 - F(X)] \sim N(0, 1)$; denote $f(x)$, the p.d.f. of X, then $Y = |X| \sim g(Y)$, where

$$g(Y) = \begin{cases} f(Y) + f(-Y), & Y > 0 \\ 0 & \text{otherwise} \end{cases}$$

2.3.2 *Importance Sampling*

Let's discuss a general Monte Carlo method for integration

$$I = \int_{\mathcal{L}} G(\boldsymbol{x}) d\boldsymbol{x} \simeq \sum_{i=1}^{m} \frac{G(\boldsymbol{x}_i)}{f(\boldsymbol{x}_i)}, \tag{2.13}$$

where vector $\boldsymbol{x}_i$ is sampled from p.d.f. $f(\boldsymbol{x}) > 0$ (c.d.f. $F(\boldsymbol{x})$), $\boldsymbol{x} \in \mathcal{L}$.

As a special case, choose the uniform probability density function $f(x) = 1/V$, which leads to

$$\int_{\mathcal{L}} G(\boldsymbol{x}) d\boldsymbol{x} \simeq \frac{V}{m} \sum_{i=1}^{m} G(\boldsymbol{x}_i), \tag{2.14}$$

the method we presented previously in Chapter 1.

Equation (2.13) can be written as Lebesgue-Stieltjes integral

$$I = \int_{\mathcal{L}} \kappa(\boldsymbol{x}) dF(\boldsymbol{x}), \tag{2.15}$$

where the kernel

$$\kappa\left(\boldsymbol{x}\right) = G\left(\boldsymbol{x}\right)/f\left(\boldsymbol{x}\right) \tag{2.16}$$

defines a weighting on $\mathcal{L}$. We call such $\{F\left(x\right), \kappa\left(\boldsymbol{x}\right); x \in\}$ satisfying (2.15) a sampling plan.

The statistical mean, variance, and hypothesis test statistics all can be expressed as integrals.

We now introduce the so-called Important Sampling method to improve the efficiency of the Monte Carlo. The variance I in (2.13) can be written as

$$\sigma_f^2 = \int_{\mathcal{L}} \kappa^2\left(\boldsymbol{x}\right) dF\left(\boldsymbol{x}\right) - I^2$$
$$= \int_{\mathcal{L}} G^2\left(\boldsymbol{x}\right)/f\left(\boldsymbol{x}\right) d\boldsymbol{x} - I^2. \tag{2.17}$$

Therefore, if the distribution function $f(\boldsymbol{x})$ is chosen such that $\frac{G(\boldsymbol{x})}{f(\boldsymbol{x})} = c$ (constant), the variance will be minimized. In other words, more draws are generated at the region where $G(\boldsymbol{x})$ is larger (assume $G(\boldsymbol{x}) > 0$).

Importance sampling can provide significant benefits to improper integrals. For example, to calculate integral

$$I = \int_0^1 x^{\alpha-1} e^{-x} dx, \ 1/2 < \alpha \le 1, \tag{2.18}$$

where the kernel (integrand) is unbounded at $x = 0$, we can use sampling from beta distribution $Be\left(\alpha, 1\right)$ with p.d.f. $f^*\left(x\right) = \alpha x^{\alpha-1}$ and $K^*\left(x\right) = \frac{1}{\alpha}e^{-x}$, so that $K^*\left(x\right)$ is bounded:

$$I = \int_0^1 \frac{1}{\alpha} e^{-x} dx^\alpha, \ 1/2 < \alpha \le 1. \tag{2.19}$$

2.3.3   *Control Variables*

Control variable here refers to a random X variable with known mean μ_x, which can be used to reduce the variance of sampling of another random variance Y by introducing a new variable $W\left(\alpha\right) = Y - \alpha\left(X - \mu_x\right)$. The following theorem provides the basis for the control variable approach.

Theorem 2.6   *(Fishman, 2000, p. 277). Suppose random variable X has a known mean μ_x and variance σ_x^2 and random variable Y has unknown mean μ_y and variance σ_y^2. Then*

(1) $W(\alpha) = Y - \alpha(X - \mu_x)$ *is an unbiased estimator of* μ_y, $\forall \alpha \in (-\infty, \infty)$ *with variance*

$$VarW(\alpha) = \sigma_y^2 - 2\alpha\sigma_{xy} + \alpha^2\sigma_x^2. \tag{2.20}$$

(2) $\alpha^* = \frac{\sigma_{xy}}{\sigma_x^2}$ *minimizes the variance*

$$VarW(\alpha^*) = \min_{\alpha} VarW(\alpha) = \sigma_y^2\left(1 - \rho_{xy}^2\right) \leq VarW(0) = VarY = \sigma_y^2, \tag{2.21}$$

where

$$\rho_{xy} = corr(X, Y) = \frac{\sigma_{xy}}{\sigma_x\sigma_y}. \tag{2.22}$$

Proof. The proof of (1) is straightforward. To prove (2), we notice that function $VarW(\alpha)$ is convex in α, which leads to $\alpha^* = \frac{\sigma_{xy}}{\sigma_x^2}$. Equation (2.22) can be obtained by substitution. $\square$

The efficiency in variance reduction by selecting α^* can be measured by

$$\frac{VarY}{VarW(\alpha^*)} = \frac{VarW(0)}{VarW(\alpha^*)} = \frac{1}{1 - \rho_{xy}^2}, \tag{2.23}$$

which increases as the correlation coefficient ρ_{xy} increases.

2.3.4 *Stratification*

Let $x^{(1)}, ..., x^{(n)}$ be i.i.d. from $F(x)$. Then

$$\bar{I}_n = \frac{1}{n}\sum_{i=1}^{r}\kappa\left(x^{(i)}\right) \tag{2.24}$$

is an unbiased estimator of I.

This directly sampling from $F(x)$ is often not very efficient because of heterogeneity. Stratified sampling is commonly used in variance reduction. Stratification is actually a partition of the set $\mathcal{L}$: $\{\mathcal{L}_1, ..., \mathcal{L}_r\}$ such that $\cup_{i=1}^{r}\mathcal{L}_i = \mathcal{L}$ and $\mathcal{L}_i \cap \mathcal{L}_j = \phi$. Given the partition, the Lebegue-Stieltjes integral can be written as

$$I = \sum_{i=1}^{r}p_i I_i, \tag{2.25}$$

where

$$p_i = \int_{\mathcal{L}_i}dF(x), \quad I_i = \int_{\mathcal{L}_i}\kappa(x)\,dF_{(i)}(x), \quad \text{and } dF_{(i)} = \frac{1}{p_i}dF(x).$$

Let $x^{(1,i)}, ..., x^{(n_i,i)}$ be i.i.d. from stratum i, $\mathcal{L}_i$ for each $i = 1, ..., r$. Then

$$\tilde{I}(n_1, .., n_r) = \sum_{r=1}^{r} \frac{p_i}{n_i} \sum_{j=1}^{n_i} \kappa\left(x^{(j,i)}\right) \qquad (2.26)$$

gives an unbiased estimator of I with variance

$$var\tilde{I}(n_1, ...n_r) = \sum_{i=1}^{r} \frac{p_i^2 \sigma_i^2}{n_i}, \qquad (2.27)$$

where

$$\sigma_i^2 = E\left[\kappa\left(x^{(1,i)}\right) - I_i\right]^2 = \frac{1}{p_i} \int_{\mathcal{L}_i} [\kappa(x) - I_i]^2 \, dF(x), \ 1 \leq i \leq r.$$

For variance reduction, we are interested in the following two questions:
(1) how to choose the partition $\{\mathcal{L}_1, ..., \mathcal{L}_r\}$ and (2) how to determine the
sample size $\{n_1, ..., n_r\}$ in each stratum when $\{\mathcal{L}_1, ..., \mathcal{L}_r\}$ are given and n
is fixed such that $\sum_{i=1}^{r} n_i = n$.

Theorem 2.7   *For fixed $n = n_1 + \cdots n_r$, the sample size assignment*

$$n_i = np_i, \ 1 \leq i \leq r \qquad (2.28)$$

will ensure

$$var\tilde{I}(np_1, ..., np_r) \leq var\bar{I}_n. \qquad (2.29)$$

Proof.

$$var\tilde{I}(np_1, ..., np_r) = \frac{1}{n} \sum_{i=1}^{r} p_i \sigma_i^2$$

$$= \frac{1}{n} \sum_{i=1}^{r} p_i \int [\kappa(x) - I_i]^2 \, dF_{(i)}(x)$$

$$= \frac{1}{n} \sum_{i=1}^{r} p_i \int [(\kappa(x) - I) + (I - I_i)]^2 \, dF_{(i)}(x)$$

$$= var\bar{I}_n - \frac{1}{n} \sum_{i=1}^{r} p_i (I_i - I)^2 \leq var\bar{I}_n.$$

$\square$

This theorem implies that for any partition $\{\mathcal{L}_1, ..., \mathcal{L}_r\}$ of $\mathcal{L}$, the sample
size assignment directed by (2.28) will lead to a variance reduction, whereas
the following theorem provides the most reduction in variance expressed by
(2.27).

Theorem 2.8 *For given stratification* $\{\mathcal{L}_1, ..., \mathcal{L}_r\}$ *of* $\mathcal{L}$ *and integer* n, *the sample size assignment*

$$n_i^* = \frac{n p_i \sigma_i}{\sum_{j=1}^{r} p_j \sigma_j}, \ 1 \leq i \leq r \tag{2.30}$$

will ensure

$$\text{var}\tilde{I}\left(n_1^*, ..., n_r^*\right) = \frac{1}{n}\left(\sum_{i=1}^{r} p_i \sigma_i\right)^2 \leq \text{var}\tilde{I}\left(n_1, ..., n_r\right). \tag{2.31}$$

Proof. Equation (2.30) can be obtained by letting the partial derivative of (2.27) with respect to each n_i be equal to zero. $\square$

2.4 Sampling Algorithms for Specific Distributions

2.4.1 *Uniform Distribution*

The uniform distribution $U(a, b)$ p.d.f. is given by

$$f(x) = \frac{1}{b-a}, \ a \leq x \leq b, \ a < b \in R. \tag{2.32}$$

Table 2.1: $U(a, b)$ Property Table

mean	variance	skewness	mode
$(a+b)/2$	$\frac{(b-a)^2}{12}$	0	

Distribution Relationships:

(1) If $X \sim U(0, 1)$, then $Y = -(lnX)/\lambda \sim \check{E}(\lambda)$ (exponential distribution).
(2) If $X_1 \sim U(0, 1)$ and $X_2 \sim U(0, 1)$ are i.i.d., then $Y = (X_1 + X_2)/2 \sim Tr(0, 0.5, 1)$ (triangular distribution).
(3) If $X \sim U\left(-\frac{\pi}{2}, \frac{\pi}{2}\right)$, then the random variable $Y = tanX \sim Cc(0, 1)$ (Cauchy distribution).
(4) If $U \sim U(0, 1)$, then $X = (b - a)U + a \sim U(a, b)$.

Using Distribution Relationship 4, we can develop an algorithm (Algorithm 2.8) for drawing a sample from $U(a, b)$.

Algorithm 2.8: Uniform Sampler
Objective: generate a random number from $U(a, b)$.
Input: a and b.
Generate u from $U(0, 1)$
$x := (b - a)u + a$

Return x

§

2.4.2 *Triangular Distribution*

The triangular distribution can be obtained from the sum of two uniform distributions.

The triangular distribution $Tr\,(a, c, b)$ p.d.f. is given by

$$f\,(x) = \begin{cases} \frac{2(x-a)}{(b-a)(c-a)}, & a \le x \le c \\ \frac{2(b-x)}{(b-a)(b-c)} & c < x \le b\,, \\ 0 & \text{otherwise} \end{cases} \tag{2.33}$$

where $a < c < b \in R$.

The c.d.f. is given by

$$F\,(x) = \begin{cases} 0 & x < a \\ \frac{(x-a)^2}{(b-a)(c-a)}, & a \le x \le c \\ 1 - \frac{(b-x)^2}{(b-a)(b-c)}, & c < x \le b \\ 1 & x > b. \end{cases} \tag{2.34}$$

The inverse c.d.f. is given by

$$x = F^{-1}\,(u) = \begin{cases} \sqrt{u\,(b-a)\,(c-a)}, & 0 \le u \le \frac{c-a}{b-a} \\ b - \sqrt{(1-u)\,(b-a)\,(b-c)}, & \frac{c-a}{b-a} < u \le 1. \end{cases} \tag{2.35}$$

Table 2.2: $Tr\,(a, c, b)$ Property Table

mean	variance	skewness	mode
$(a + b + c)\,/3$	$\frac{a^2+b^2+c^2-ab-bc-ca}{18}$	$\frac{\sqrt{2}(a+b-2c)(2a-b-c)(a-2b+c)}{5(a^2+b^2+c^2-ab-bc-ca)^{3/2}}$	c

The sampling algorithm for the triangular distribution can be generated using the inverse CDF method as given by Algorithm 2.9.

Algorithm 2.9: Triangular Distribution Sampler
Objective: sampling from $Tr\,(a, c, b)$.
Input: a, b, and c.
Generate u from $U\,(0, 1)$
If $0 \le u \le \frac{c-a}{b-a}$ **Then**
      Return $x := \sqrt{u\,(b-a)\,(c-a)}$
Else
      Return $x := b - \sqrt{(1-u)\,(b-a)\,(b-c)}$
Endif
§

2.4.3 Normal Distribution

The normal distribution $N\left(\mu, \sigma^2\right)$ p.d.f. is given by

$$f\left(x\right) = \frac{1}{\sigma\sqrt{2\pi}} \exp\left(-\frac{\left(x-\mu\right)^2}{2\sigma^2}\right), \ \sigma > 0. \tag{2.36}$$

Table 2.3: $N\left(\mu, \sigma^2\right)$ Property Table

mean	variance	skewness	mode
μ	σ^2	0	μ

Distribution Relationships:

(1) If $X \sim N\left(\mu, \beta\right)$, then variable $Y = \left(X-\mu\right)/\sigma \sim N\left(0, 1\right)$.
(2) If $X \sim N\left(0, 1\right)$, then $Y = e^{\mu+\sigma X} \sim LN\left(\mu, \sigma^2\right)$.
(3) If i.i.d. X_1 and $X_2 \sim N\left(0, 1\right)$, then $Y = X_1/X_2 \sim Cc\left(0, 1\right)$.
(4) A linear combination of independent normal variables has a normal distribution.
(5) If $X_i \sim N\left(0, 1\right)$, then $Y = \sum_{i=1}^{n} X_i^2 \sim \chi^2\left(n\right)$.

We will present an algorithm for sampling from the standard normal distribution using the following theorem developed by Box and Muller (Box and Muller, 1958; Fishman, 2000, p. 190–191; Gentle, 2003, p. 172–173).

Theorem 2.9 *(Box and Muller, 1958). Let U and V denote independent random variables from $U\left(0, 1\right)$ and exponential distribution with the parameter of 1, respectively. Then*

$$X = \sqrt{2V}\cos\left(2\pi U\right)$$

and

$$Y = \sqrt{2V}\sin\left(2\pi U\right)$$

are independent random variables from $N\left(0, 1\right)$.

Proof. *Because*

$$2V = X^2 + Y^2, \ tan\left(2\pi U\right) = Y/X,$$

$$\frac{\partial u}{\partial x} = \frac{-y\cos^2(2\pi u)}{2\pi x^2} = \frac{-y}{4\pi v}, \frac{\partial u}{\partial y} = \frac{\cos^2(2\pi u)}{2\pi x} = \frac{x}{4\pi v},$$

$$\frac{\partial v}{\partial x} = x, \ and \ \frac{\partial v}{\partial y} = y.$$

We have

$$f_{X,Y} = f_{U,V}\left(u\left(x,y\right), v\left(x,y\right)\right)\left|\frac{\partial u}{\partial x}\frac{\partial v}{\partial y} - \frac{\partial u}{\partial y}\frac{\partial v}{\partial x}\right|$$

$$= \frac{1}{2\pi}e^{-(x^2+y^2)/2}, \ -\infty < x, y < \infty. \tag{2.37}$$

We can see that (2.37) gives the p.d.f. requirement of two independent random variables.   □

If we use the inverse CDF method, $V = -\ln U_2$, where U_2 has $U(0,1)$. Algorithm 2.10 is developed for sampling from $N(0,1)$ based on Theorem 2.9.

Algorithm 2.10: Normal Distribution Sampler
Objective: generate a random number from $N(0,1)$.
rejection := **True**
While rejection:
    Generate i.i.d. u_1 and u_2 from $U(-1,1)$
    $r^2 := u_1^2 + u_2^2$.
    If $r^2 < 1$ **Then**
        $x_1 := u_1\sqrt{\frac{-2\ln r^2}{r^2}}$
        $x_2 := u_2\sqrt{\frac{-2\ln r^2}{r^2}}$
        Return $\{x_1, x_2\}$
        rejection := **False**
    Endif
Endwhile
§

2.4.4   *Gamma Distribution*

The p.d.f. for Gamma distribution (Gentle, 2003; Fishman, 2000, p. 193–197) is given by

$$f(x) = \frac{x^{\alpha-1}e^{-x/\beta}}{\Gamma(\alpha)\beta^\alpha} \ \text{for } \alpha, \beta > 0, x \geq 0 \tag{2.38}$$

where $\Gamma(\alpha)$ is the complete gamma function. When $\alpha = 1$ and $\beta = 1/\lambda$ the gamma distribution reduces to the exponential.

Table 2.4: $\Gamma\left(\alpha,\beta\right)$ Property Table

mean	variance	skewness	mode
$\alpha\beta$	$\alpha\beta^2$	$2/\sqrt{\alpha}$	$(\alpha-1)\beta$ for $\alpha \geq 1$

Distribution Relationships:
Let $X \sim G\left(\alpha,\beta\right)$.

(1) If $\alpha = 1$ and $\beta = 1/\lambda$, then $X \sim \breve{E}\left(\lambda\right)$.
(2) If $\alpha = v/2$ and $\beta = 2$, then $X \sim \chi^2\left(v\right)$.
(3) If $\alpha = n$ is an integer, then $X \sim Er\left(\beta,n\right)$.
(4) If $\alpha = v/2$ and $\beta = 1$, then $Y = 2X \sim \chi^2\left(v\right)$.
(5) As $\alpha \to \infty$, X tends to a $N\left(\alpha\beta,\alpha\beta^2\right)$.
(6) If $X_1 \sim G\left(1,\beta_1\right)$ and $X_2 \sim G\left(1,\beta_2\right)$ are independent, then $Y = X_1/\left(X_1+X_2\right) \sim beta\left(\beta_1,\beta_2\right)$.
(7) If $X_1,...,X_n$ are independent and $X_i \sim G\left(\alpha_i,\beta\right)$, then $Y = X_1 + ..., +X_n \sim G\left(\alpha_1 + ... + \alpha_n,\beta\right)$.

An efficient algorithm for values of the shape parameter $\alpha \leq 1$ is the acceptance-rejection method described in Ahrens and Dieter (1974) and modified by Best (1983).

Algorithm 2.11: Ahrens-Dieter-Best's Γ-Distribution Sampler
Objective: Sampling from $\Gamma\left(\alpha,\beta\right)$ distribution for the case $\alpha \leq 1$.
Input α,β
$t := 0.07 + \frac{3}{4}\left(1-\alpha\right)^{1/2}$
$b := 1 + \frac{\alpha}{t}e^{-t}$
rejection := **True**
While rejection:
    Generate i.i.d. u_1 and u_2 from $U\left(0,1\right)$.
    $v := bu_1$.
    If $v \leq 1$ **Then**
        $x := t\sqrt{v}$
        If $u_2 \leq \frac{2-x}{2+x}$ or $u_2 \leq e^{-x}$ **Then** rejection := **False**.
    Else
        $x := -\ln\left(\frac{t(b-v)}{\alpha}\right)$
        $y := \frac{x}{t}$
        $v_2 := u_2\left(\alpha + y\left(1-\alpha\right)\right)$
        If $v_2 \leq 1$ **OR** $u_2 \leq y^{\alpha-1}$ **Then** rejection := **False**.
    Endif
Endwhile
Return βx
§

For the gamma distribution $\Gamma(\alpha, \beta)$ with $\alpha > 1$, Cheng and Feast (1979) use a ratio-of-uniforms method. The efficiency of this algorithm is $O(\alpha^{1/2})$ or more precisely $2\left(\frac{\alpha}{2\pi}\right)^{1/2}$ as $\alpha \to \infty$, so for larger values of α it is less efficient. Cheng and Feast (1980) also developed an acceptance/rejection method that is better for large values of the shape parameter.

Algorithm 2.12: Cheng-Feast's Γ-Distribution Sample
Objective: Generate sample from $\Gamma(\alpha, \beta)$ distribution for the case $\alpha > 1$.
Input: α and β.
$b := \left(\alpha - \frac{1}{6\alpha}\right) / (\alpha - 1)$
rejection := **True**
While rejection:
    Generate i.i.d. u_1 and u_2 from $U(0, 1)$
    $v := bu_2/u_1$
    $v_1 := 2u_1/(\alpha - 1) - 2(1 + 1/(\alpha - 1)) + v + 1/v$
    $v_2 := 2/(\alpha - 1)\ln u_1 - \ln v + v - 1$
    If $v_1 \leq 0$ **OR** $v_2 \leq 0$ **Then**
        $x := (\alpha - 1)\beta v$
        rejection := **False**
    Endif
Endwhile
Return x
§

2.4.5 *Beta Distribution*

Beta distribution $Be(\alpha, \beta)$ p.d.f. is given by (Fishman, 2000, p. 203–206)

$$f(x) = \frac{\Gamma(\alpha + \beta) x^{\alpha-1}(1 - x)^{\beta-1}}{\Gamma(\alpha)\Gamma(\beta)}, \quad \alpha, \beta > 0, \ 0 \leq x \leq 1. \tag{2.39}$$

Table 2.5: $Be(\alpha, \beta)$ Property Table

mean	variance	skewness	mode
$\frac{\alpha}{\alpha+\beta}$	$\frac{\alpha\beta}{(\alpha+\beta)^2(\alpha+\beta+1)}$	$\frac{2(\beta-\alpha)\sqrt{\alpha+\beta+1}}{(\alpha+\beta+2)\sqrt{\alpha\beta}}$	$\frac{\alpha-1}{\alpha+\beta-2}$, for $\alpha, \beta > 1$

Distribution Relationships:

(1) If $X \sim Be(1/2, 1/2)$, then X is an arcsin random variable.
(2) If $X \sim Be(1, 2)$, then $X \sim N(0, 1)$.
(3) As α and β tend to infinity such that α/β is constant, $X \sim Be(\alpha, \beta)$ tends to a standard normal random variable.

(4) If $X_1 \sim G(\alpha, 1)$ and $X_2 \sim G(\beta, 1)$ are independent, then $Y = \frac{X_1}{X_1 + X_2} \sim Be(\alpha, \beta)$.

(5) If $u_1, ..., u_n \sim N(0, 1)$ are i.i.d., with corresponding order statistics $u_{(1)}, ..., u_{(n)}$, then $u_{(k)} \sim Be(k, n - k + 1)$ where $1 \leq k \leq n$.

(6) If $X \sim Be(\alpha, \beta)$, then $Y = 1 - X \sim Be(\beta, \alpha)$.

Distribution relationship (4) provides a way to generate $Be(\alpha, \beta)$ from $G(\alpha, 1)$ and $G(\beta, 1)$. Property (5) reveals how to generate order statistics for any parent distribution for which generation via the inverse transform method applies. Property (6) shows that any development for $\alpha \geq \beta$ applies equally to $\beta \leq \alpha$ by a simple transformation.

Here we describe a method faster than using property (4). There are three algorithms for $max(\alpha, \beta) < 1$ (Atkinson, 1979; Atkinson and Whittaker, 1976), $min(\alpha, \beta) > 1$, and the case of $min(\alpha, \beta) < 1$ (Cheng, 1978), and $max(\alpha, \beta) > 1$ (Cheng, 1978; Fishman, 2000, p. 201–206), respectively.

Algorithm 2.13: Atkinson-Whittaker's Beta Distribution Sampler with $\max(\alpha, \beta) < 1$

Objective: sampling from $Be(\alpha, \beta)$, where $\max(\alpha, \beta) < 1$.

Input: α and β.

$t := 1/ \left[1 + \sqrt{\frac{\beta(1-\beta)}{a(1-\alpha)}} \right]$

$p := \beta t / [\beta t + \alpha(1 - t)]$

rejection := **True**

While rejection:

    Generate u from $U(0, 1)$ and y from exponential $\check{E}(1)$.

    If $u \leq p$ **Then**

        $z := t(u/p)^{1/\alpha}$

        $u_1 := (1 - \beta)(t - z) / (1 - t)$

        $u_2 := (1 - \beta) \ln \left(\frac{1-z}{1-t} \right)$

        If $y \geq u_1$ **OR** $y \geq u_2$ **Then** rejection := False

    Else

        $z := 1 - (1 - t) \left(\frac{1-u}{1-p} \right)^{1/\beta}$

        $v_1 := (1 - \alpha)(z/t - 1)$

        $v_2 := (1 - \alpha) \ln (z/t)$

        If $y \geq v_1$ **OR** $y \geq v_2$ **Then** rejection := False

    Endif

Endwhile

Return z

§

Algorithm 2.14: Cheng's Beta Distribution Sampler with $\min(\alpha, \beta) > 1$

Objective: sampling from $Be\,(\alpha, \beta)$, where $\min(\alpha, \beta) > 1$.

Input: α and β.

$d_1 := \min\,(\alpha, \beta)\,;\; d_2 := \max\,(\alpha, \beta)\,;\; d_3 := d_1 + d_2$

$d_4 := \sqrt{(d_3 - 2)\,/\,(2d_1 d_2 - d_3)}\,;\; d_5 := d_1 + 1/d_4$

rejection := **True**

While rejection:

        Generate i.i.d. u_1 and u_2 from $U\,(0,1)\,$.

        $v := d_4 \ln \left[\frac{u_1}{1 - u_1}\right]$

        $w := d_1 e^v$

        $z_1 := u_1^2 u_2$

        $r := d_5 v - 1.38629436$

        $s := d_1 + r - w$

        If $s + 2.60943791 > 5z_1$ **Then**

            rejection := **False**

        Else

            $t := \ln z_1$

            If $s \geq t$ **Then**

                rejection := **False**

            Else

                If $r + d_3 \ln \left(\frac{d_3}{d_2 + w}\right) \geq T$ **Then** rejection := **False**

            Endif

        Endif

Endwhile

$z := d_2 /\,(d_2 + w)$

If $d_1 = \alpha$ **Then** $z := w /\,(d_2 + w)$

Return z

§

Algorithm 2.15: Cheng's Beta Distribution Sampler with $\min(\alpha, \beta) \leq 1$

Purpose: sampling from $Be\,(\alpha, \beta)$, where $\min(\alpha, \beta) \leq 1$.

Input: α and β.

$d_1 := \max\,(\alpha, \beta)\,; d_2 := \min\,(\alpha, \beta)\,; d_3 := d_1 + d_2;\; d_4 := 1/d_2$

$d_5 := 1 + d_1 - d_2;\; d_6 := \frac{d_5\,(0.0138888889 + 0.0416666667 d_2)}{d_1 d_2 - 0.777777778}$

$d_7 := 0.25 + (0.5 + 0.25/d_5)\,d_2$

rejection := **True**

While rejection:

    Generate i.i.d. u_1 and u_2 from $U\,(0,1)$

        If $u_1 < 0.5$ **Then**

$y_1 := u_1 u_2;\ y_2 := u_1 y_1$
If $0.25 u_2 + y_2 - y_1 \geq d_6$ **Then** rejection := **True**
Else
$\qquad y_2 := u_1^2 u_2$
$\qquad$ **If** $y_2 \leq 0.25$ **Then**
$\qquad\qquad v := d_4 \ln \left(\frac{u_1}{1-u_1} \right);\ w := d_1 e^v$
$\qquad\qquad$ rejection := **False**
$\qquad$ **Endif**
$\qquad$ **If** $y_2 \geq d_7$ **Then** rejecting := **True**
Endif
If rejection = **False Then**
$\qquad v := d_2 \ln \left(\frac{u_1}{1-u_1} \right);\ w := d_1 e^v$
$\qquad v_2 := d_3 \left(\ln \frac{d_3}{d_2 + w} + v \right) - 1.38629436$
$\qquad$ **If** $v_2 \geq \ln y_2$ **Then** rejection := **False**
Endif
Endwhile
$z := d_2 / (d_2 + w)$
If $d_1 = \alpha$ **Then** $z := w / (d_2 + w);$
Return z
§

2.4.6 *Snedecor's F-Distribution*

Snedecor's F-distribution $F(\alpha, \beta)$ p.d.f. is given by (Fishman, 2000, p. 208)

$$f(x) = \frac{(\alpha/\beta)^{\alpha/2}}{B(\alpha/2, \beta/2)} \frac{x^{\alpha/2-1}}{(1 + \alpha x/\beta)^{(\alpha+\beta)/2}}, \quad \alpha, \beta > 0,\ x > 0, \qquad (2.40)$$

where $B(\alpha/2, \beta/2)$ is beta function.

Table 2.6: $F(\alpha, \beta)$ Property Table

mean	$\beta/(\beta-2),\ \beta \geq 3$
variance	$\frac{2\beta^2(\alpha+\beta-2)}{\alpha(\beta-2)^2(\beta-4)},\ \beta \geq 5$
skewness	$\frac{(2\alpha+\beta-2)\sqrt{8(\beta-4)}}{\sqrt{\alpha}(\beta-6)\sqrt{\alpha+\beta-2}},\ \beta \geq 7$
mode	$\frac{\alpha-2}{\alpha}\frac{\beta}{\beta+2},\ \alpha \geq 3$

Distribution Relationships:

(1) If $X \sim F(v_1, v_2)$, then $Y = 1/X \sim F(v_2, v_1)$.
(2) If $X \sim F(v_1, v_2)$, then $Y = v_1 X$ tends to a $\chi^2(v_1)$ as $v_2 \to \infty$.

(3) If X_1 and X_2 are i.i.d. from $F(v, v)$, then $Y = \frac{\sqrt{v}}{2}\left(\sqrt{X_1} - \sqrt{X_2}\right) \sim t(v)$.

(4) If $X \sim F(v_1, v_2)$, then $Y = \frac{v_1 X/v_2}{1+v_1 X/v_2} \sim Be(v_2/2, v_1/2)$.

(5) If $X_1 \sim \Gamma(\alpha/2, 1/2)$ and $X_2 \sim \Gamma(\beta/2, 1/2)$ are independent, then $Z = \frac{\beta X_1}{\alpha X_2} \sim F(\alpha, \beta)$.

(6) If $X \sim Be(\alpha/2, \beta/2)$, then $y = \frac{\beta x}{\alpha(1-x)} \sim F(\alpha, \beta)$.

Properties 5 and 6 allow us to generate F variates easily, as shown in Algorithm 2.16.

Algorithm 2.16: Snedecor's F-distribution Sampler
Objective: generate a random number from $F(\alpha, \beta)$.
Input: α and β.
Generate x from beta distribution $Be(\alpha/2, \beta/2)$.
$y := \frac{\beta x}{\alpha(1-x)} c$
Return y
§

2.4.7   *Chi-Square Distribution*

The chi-square distribution is a special case of the gamma distribution (Gentle, 2003, p. 184), i.e.,

$$\chi^2(v) = \Gamma(v/2, 2).\tag{2.41}$$

Table 2.7: $\chi^2(v)$ Property Table

mean	variance	skewness	mode
v'	$2v$	$2\sqrt{2/v}$	$v - 2, v > 2$

2.4.8   *Student Distribution*

The Student t-distribution $T(v)$ p.d.f. is given by

$$f(x) = \frac{1}{\sqrt{\pi v}} \frac{\Gamma\left(\frac{v+1}{2}\right)}{\Gamma(v/2)} \left(1 + \frac{x^2}{v}\right)^{-(1+v)/2}, \quad v \in N,\ x \in R \tag{2.42}$$

Table 2.8: $T(v)$ Property Table

mean	variance	skewness	mode
$0,\ v \geq 2$	$\frac{v}{v-2},\ v \geq 3$	$0,\ v \geq 4$	0

Distribution Relationships:

(1) If $X \sim t(v)$, then $Y = X^2 \sim F(1, v)$.
(2) If $X \sim t(1)$, then $X \sim Cc(0, 1)$.
(3) If $X \sim t(v)$, then as $v \to \infty$, X tends to $N(0, 1)$.
(4) If $X \sim N(0, 1)$ and $Y \sim \chi^2(\nu)$, then $X/\sqrt{Y} \sim t(v)$.

Property 4 can be used for sampling from the t-distribution (Algorithm 2.17).

Algorithm 2.17: Student t-Distribution Sampler
Objective: sampling from t-distribution
Input: degree of freedom v
Generate x from $N(0, 1)$
Generate y from $\chi^2(v)$
Return $x/\sqrt{y}$
§

Bailey (Bailey, 1994) developed a more efficient algorithm using the rejection polar method, as shown in Algorithm 2.18.

Algorithm 2.18: Bailey's t-Distribution Sampler
Objective: draw a sample from t-distribution $t(v)$.
Input: degree of freedom v
rejection := **True**
While rejection:
  Generate i.i.d. v_1 and v_2 from $U(-1, 1)$.
  $r := v_1^2 + v_2^2$
  If $r < 1$ **Then**
    $x = v_1 \sqrt{\dfrac{v\left(r^{-2/v} - 1\right)}{r}}$
    rejection := **True**
  Endif
Endwhile
Return x
§

2.4.9 *Exponential Distribution*

The exponential distribution $\check{E}(\lambda)$ p.d.f. is given by

$$f(x) = \lambda \exp(-\lambda x), \ \lambda > 0, \ x \geq 0. \tag{2.43}$$

Table 2.9: $\check{E}(\lambda)$ Property Table

mean	variance	skewness	mode
$1/\lambda$	$1/\lambda^2$	2	0

Distribution Relationships:

(1) $\check{E}(1/2) = \chi^2(2)$.

(2) If $X_1, ...X_n \sim \check{E}(\lambda)$ are i.i.d., then $Y = min(X_1, ...X_n) \sim \check{E}(n\lambda)$ and $Y = X_1 + X_2 + ... + X_n \sim Er(1/\lambda, n)$.

(3) If X_1 and $X_2 \sim \check{E}(\lambda)$ are i.i.d., then $Y = X_1 - X_2 \sim Lp(1/\lambda)$ (Laplace distribution).

(4) If X_1 and $X_2 \sim \check{E}(1)$ are i.i.d., then $Y = X_1/(X_1 + X_2) \sim U(0,1)$.

Generating a deviate from an exponential is straightforward using the inverse CDF method, as shown in Algorithm 2.19.

Algorithm 2.19: Exponential Distribution Sampler

Objective: generate a random number from exponential distribution $\check{E}(\lambda)$.

Input: λ

Generate x from $U(0,1)$

Return $-\ln(x)/\lambda$

§

2.4.10 *Weibull Distribution*

Weibull distribution $Wb(\alpha, \beta)$ p.d.f. is given by

$$f(x) = \frac{\alpha}{\beta} x^{\alpha-1} \exp\left(-\frac{x^\alpha}{\beta}\right), \ \alpha, \beta > 0, \ x \geq 0. \tag{2.44}$$

Table 2.10: $Wb(\alpha, \beta)$ Property Table

mean	$\beta^{1/\alpha}\Gamma(1 + 1/\alpha)$
variance	$\beta^{2/\alpha}[\Gamma(1 + 2/\alpha)] - \Gamma^2(1 + 1/\alpha)$
skewness	$\frac{2\Gamma^3(1+1/\alpha)-3\Gamma(1+1/\alpha)\Gamma(1+2/\alpha)+\Gamma(1+3/\alpha)}{[\Gamma(1+2/\alpha)-\Gamma^2(1+1/\alpha)]^{3/2}}$
mode	0

The inverse CDF is given by

$$x = \beta^{1/\alpha}(-\ln u)^{1/\alpha} \sim Wb(\alpha, \beta). \tag{2.45}$$

Distribution Relationships:

(1) Distribution $Wb(1, \beta) = \check{E}(1/\beta)$.
(2) $Wb(2, \beta) = \check{E}(\beta/\sqrt{2})$.

Algorithm 2.20 is an algorithm for generating a random number from a Weibull distribution using the inverse CDF method.

Algorithm 2.20: Weibull Distribution Sampler
Objective: generate a deviate from Weibull distribution $Wb(\alpha, \beta)$.
Input: α and β
Generate u from $N(0, 1)$.
$x = \beta^{1/\alpha}(-\ln u)^{1/\alpha}$
Return x
§

2.4.11 *Inverse Gaussian Distribution*

The inverse Gaussian distribution $IG(\mu, \lambda)$ p.d.f. is given by

$$f(x) = \sqrt{\frac{\lambda}{2\pi}} x^{-3/2} \exp\left(\frac{-\lambda(x - \mu)^2}{2\mu^2 x}\right), \ x > 0. \qquad (2.46)$$

Table 2.11: $IG(\lambda, \mu)$ Property Table

mean	variance	skewness	mode
μ	μ^3/λ	$3\left(\frac{\mu}{\lambda}\right)^{1/2}$	$\mu\left\{\left[1 + \left(\frac{3\mu}{2\lambda}\right)^2\right]^{1/2} - \frac{3\mu}{2\lambda}\right\}$

Distribution Relationships:

(1) The inverse Gaussian distribution with $\mu = 1$ is the Wald distribution.
(2) When $\mu = 1$, the inverse Gaussian distribution becomes the distribution of the first hit in a Brownian motion with positive drift.

Michael and colleagues (Michael, Schucany, and Haas, 1976; Gentle, 2003, p. 193) developed a simple algorithm (Algorithm 2.21) for sampling from the inverse Gaussian distribution.

Algorithm 2.21: Michael-Schucany-Haas's Inverse Gaussian Sampler
Objective: generate a random number from inverse-normal $IG(\mu, \lambda)$.
Input: μ and λ.

Generate v from $N(0,1)$.

$y := \mu + \frac{\mu^2 v^2}{2\lambda} - \frac{\mu}{2\lambda} \left(4\mu\lambda v^2 + \mu^2 v^4 \right)^{1/2}$

If $u \le \frac{\mu}{\mu+y}$ **Then**

$\quad x = y$

Else

$\quad x = \frac{\mu^2}{y}$

Endif

Return x

§

2.4.12 *Laplace Distribution*

The Laplace distribution p.d.f. is given by (Johnson, Kotz, and Balakrishnan, 1995, p. 166)

$$f(x) = \frac{1}{2\lambda} \exp\left(-\frac{|x-\mu|}{\lambda} \right), \ \lambda > 0, \ x \in R. \tag{2.47}$$

The c.d.f. is given by

$$F(x) = \begin{cases} \frac{1}{2} \exp\left(-\frac{\mu-x}{\lambda} \right), & x \le \mu \\ 1 - \frac{1}{2} \exp\left(\frac{\mu-x}{\lambda} \right) & x > \mu \end{cases} \tag{2.48}$$

Table 2.12: $Lp(p)$ Property Table

Mean	Variance	skewness	mode
μ	$2\lambda^2$	0	μ

To generate the random number from the Laplace distribution, we can generate x from the exponential distribution, then change the sign with a probability of 0.5.

Algorithm 2.22: Laplace Distribution Sampler
Objective: sampling from Laplace distribution $Lp(\mu, \lambda)$.
Input: μ and λ.
Generate u from $U(0,1)$.
$y := -\ln(u)/\lambda$
Generate s from Bernoulli distribution $BN(0.5)$
$x = (1-2s)y + \mu$.
Return x
§

2.4.13 *Multivariate Normal Distribution*

Suppose $X = (X_1, ..., X_r)$ has multivariate normal distribution $N(\boldsymbol{\mu}, \boldsymbol{\Sigma})$ with p.d.f. (Fishman, 2000, p. 223)

$$f(x) = \frac{1}{\sqrt{(2\pi)^r |\boldsymbol{\Sigma}|}} \exp\left(\frac{-(\boldsymbol{x} - \boldsymbol{\mu})^T \boldsymbol{\Sigma}^{-1} (\boldsymbol{x} - \boldsymbol{\mu})}{2}\right). \tag{2.49}$$

To generate deviates from $N(\boldsymbol{\mu}, \boldsymbol{\Sigma})$, we can generate deviates $\boldsymbol{Y}$ from standard $N(\boldsymbol{0}, \boldsymbol{1})$ and use variable transform $\boldsymbol{X} = \boldsymbol{c}\boldsymbol{Y} + \boldsymbol{\mu}$ to obtain the desired variates, where c is the unique lower triangular matrix satisfying $\boldsymbol{\Sigma} = \boldsymbol{c}\boldsymbol{c}^T$. A routine for decomposing the matrix can be found elsewhere (e.g., Fishman, 1999, p. 223)

Algorithm 2.23: Multivariate Normal Sampler
Objective: generate deviate from $N(\boldsymbol{\mu}, \boldsymbol{c}\boldsymbol{c}^T)$.
Input $\boldsymbol{\mu}, \boldsymbol{c}, r$.
For $i := 1$ **To** r
    Generate y_i from $N(0, 1)$
    $x_i := \mu_i$
    For $j := 1$ **To** i
        $x_i := x_i + c_{ij} y_j$
    Endfor
Endfor
$\boldsymbol{x} := \{x_1, ..., x_r\}$
Return $\boldsymbol{x}$

2.4.14 *Equal Distribution*

The equal distribution $U_c(n)$ p.m.f. is given by

$$f(x) = \frac{1}{n}, \ x = 1, ..., n. \tag{2.50}$$

Algorithm 2.24 Equal Distribution Sampler
Objective: Generate a random number from $U_c(n)$.
Input: n
Generate u from $U(0, 1)$.
$x := \lfloor n \cdot u \rfloor + 1$
Return x
§

2.4.15   *Binomial Distribution*

Binomial distribution $B(p, n)$ p.m.f. is given by (Fishman, 2000, p. 215–216)

$$f(x) = \binom{n}{x} p^x (1-p)^{n-x}, \ x = 0, 1, ..., n. \tag{2.51}$$

Table 2.13: $B(p, n)$ Property Table

mean	variance	skewness	mode
np	$np(1-p)$	$\dfrac{1-2p}{\sqrt{np(1-p)}}$	$\lfloor (n+1)p \rfloor$

Distribution Relationships:
Let X be a binomial random variable with parameters n and p.

(1) If $n = 1$, then X is a Bernoulli random variable with probability of success p.
(2) As $n \to \infty$ if $np > 5$ and $n(1-p) > 5$, then X is approximately normal with parameters $\mu = np$ and $\sigma^2 = np(1-p)$.
(3) As $n \to \infty$ if $p < 0.1$ and $np < 10$, then X is approximately a Poisson random variable with parameter $\lambda = np$.
(4) Let $X_1, ..., X_k$ be independent, binomial random variables with parameters n_i and p, respectively. The random variable $Y = X_1 + X_2 + ... + X_k$ has a binomial distribution with parameters $n = n_1 + n_2 + ... + n_k$ and p.

The most straightforward method to generate the binomial distribution is to use a sum of Bernoulli distribution random variables. The efficiency of the algorithm is $O(np)$.

Algorithm 2.25 Binomial Distribution Sampler
Objective: generate a random number from binomial distribution $B(p, n)$.
Input: n and p
$x := 0$; $i := 1$
While $i \leq n$:
        Generate u from $U(0, 1)$.
        $x := x + \lfloor u + p \rfloor$
        $i := i + 1$
Endwhile
Return x
§

2.4.16   *Poisson Distribution*

Poisson distribution $Ps(\lambda)$ p.m.f. is given by

$$p(x) = \frac{\lambda^x}{x!} \exp(-\lambda), \ \lambda > 0, \ x = 0, 1, \ldots \tag{2.52}$$

Table 2.14: $Ps(\lambda)$ Property Table

mean	variance	skewness	mode
λ	λ	$1/\sqrt{\lambda}$	λ and $\lambda - 1$ if $\lambda \in N$

Distribution Relationships:
Let X be a Poisson random variable with parameter λ.

(1) As $\lambda \to \infty$, X is approximately normal with parameters $\mu = \lambda$ and $\sigma^2 = \lambda$.
(2) Let $X_1, X_2, \ldots, X_n$ be independent Poisson random variables with parameters λ_i, respectively. The random variable $Y = X_1 + X_2 + \ldots + X_n$ has a Poisson distribution with parameter $\lambda = \lambda_1 + \lambda_2 + \ldots + \lambda_n$.

Algorithm 2.26 is modified based on the algorithm from Fishman (Fishman, 2000, p. 211–212) for a Poisson distribution with $\lambda < 30$.

Algorithm 2.26: Poisson Distribution Sampler ($\lambda < 30$)
Objective: Generate a random number from Poisson distribution $Ps(\lambda)$ ($\lambda < 30$).
Input: λ.
$p := 1; \ N := 0; \ c := exp(-\lambda)$
rejection := **True**
While rejection:
    Generate u from $U(0,1)$.
    $p := pu$
    $N := N + 1$
    If $p < c$, **Then** rejection := **False**
Endwhile
$x = N - 1$
Return x
§

For a Poisson distribution with $\lambda \geq 30$, Atkinson (1979) provided the following algorithm.

Algorithm 2.27: Poisson Distribution Sampler ($\lambda \geq 30$)

Purpose: Sampling from Poisson distribution $Ps(\lambda)$ ($\lambda \geq 30$).

Input: λ

$c := 0.767 - 3.36/\lambda$; $\beta := \pi (3\lambda)^{-1/2}$

$\alpha := \beta\lambda$; $k := \ln c - \lambda - \ln \beta$

rejection := **True**

While rejection:

    Generate u_1 from $U(0,1)$

    $x := [\alpha - \ln((1 - u_1)/u_1)]/\beta$.

    If $x > -1/2$ **Then**

        Generate u_2

        $N := $ **Round**$(x + 0.5)$

        $v := \alpha - \beta x + \ln\left\{u_2/\left[1 + \exp(\alpha - \beta x)^2\right]\right\}$

        If $v \leq k + N \ln \lambda - \ln N!$ **Then** rejection := **False**

    Endif

Endwhile

Return N

§

2.4.17   *Negative Binomial*

The negative binomial $NB(n)$ is used to describe the number of failures, X, before the nth success, in Bernoulli trials with probability of success p. The p.m.f. is given by

$$p(x) = \binom{x + n - 1}{n - 1}(1 - p)^x p^n, \qquad (2.53)$$

where $0 < p < 1$, $n > 0$, $x = 0, 1, ...,$. When n is an integer, the $NB(n)$ is called the Pascal distribution.

Table 2.15: $NB(r)$ Property Table

mean	variance	skewness	mode
$n(1-p)/p$	$\frac{n(1-p)}{p^2}$	$\frac{2-p}{\sqrt{n(1-p)}}$	$\frac{(n-1)p}{1-p}$ and 0 if $n \leq 1$

Distribution Relationships:

Let X be a negative binomial random variable with parameters n and p.

(1) If $n = 1$ then X is a geometric random variable with probability of success p.

(2) As $n \to \infty$ and $p \to 1$ with $n(1-p)$ held constant, X is approximately a Poisson random variable with $\lambda = n(1-p)$.

(3) Let X_i $(i = 1, 2, ..., k)$ be independent negative binomial random variables with parameters n_i and p, respectively. The random variable $Y = X_1 + X_2 + ... + X_k$ has a negative binomial distribution with parameters $n = n_1 + n_2 + ... + n_k$ and p.

Algorithm 2.28 is modified from Algorithm BEGIN (Fishman, 2000, p. 222).

Algorithm 2.28: Negative Binomial Distribution Sampler
Objective: generate a random number from $NB\,(r,p)$.
Input: r and p.
Generate x from $\Gamma\,(r,1)$
Generate y from Poisson $Ps\,(xp/\,(1-p))$
Return y
§

2.4.18 *Geometric Distribution*

The geometric $Ge\,(p)$ p.m.f. is given by

$$p\,(x) = (1-p)\,p^x, \ 0 < p < 1, \ x = 0, 1, ... \tag{2.54}$$

Table 2.16: $Ge\,(p)$ Property Table

mean	variance	skewness	mode
$1/\,(1-p)$	$p/\,(1-p)^2$	$\frac{1+p}{\sqrt{p}}$	1 or 0

Distribution Relationships:
Let $X_1, X_2, ..., X_n$ be independent, identically distributed geometric random variables with parameter p.

(1) The random variable $Y = X_1 + X_2 + ... + X_n$ has a negative binomial distribution with parameters n and p.

(2) The random variable $Y = min(X_1, X_2, ..., X_n)$ has a geometric distribution with parameter p.

Algorithm 2.29 is the same as Algorithm GEO (Fishman, 2000, p.221).

Algorithm 2.29: Geometric Distribution Sampler
Objective: generate a random number from geometric distribution $Ge\,(p)$.

Input: p

$\beta := -1/\ln p$

Generate y from $U\,(0,1)$.

$x := \lfloor \beta \ln y \rfloor$

Return x

§

2.4.19   *Hypergeometric Distribution*

The hypergeometric distribution $HG\,(M,N,n)$ p.m.f. is given by

$$p\,(x) = \frac{\binom{M}{x}\binom{N-M}{n-x}}{\binom{N}{n}}, \quad x = 0,1,...,n, x \leq M, \tag{2.55}$$

where $n - x \leq N - M;\ n, M, N \in \mathbb{N}, 1 \leq n \leq N; 1 \leq M \leq N$.

Table 2.17: $HG\,(M,N,n)$ Property Table

mean	nM/N
variance	$\frac{nM}{N}\left(\frac{N-n}{N-1}\right)\left(1 - \frac{M}{N}\right)$
skewness	$\frac{(N-2M)(N-2n)\sqrt{N-1}}{(N-2)\sqrt{nM(N-M)(N-n)}}$
mode	$\frac{(n+1)(M+1)}{N+2}$

Distribution Relationships:
Let X be a hypergeometric random variable with parameters n, M, and N.

(1) As $N \rightarrow \infty$ if $n/N < 0.1$ then X is approximately a binomial random variable with parameters n and $p = M/N$.
(2) As n, M, and N all tend to infinity, if M/N is small then X has approximately a Poisson distribution with parameter $\lambda = nM/N$.

Kachitvichyanukul and Schmeiser (1985) developed an algorithm (Algorithm 2.30) for sampling from the hypergeometric distribution $HG\,(M,N,n)$. The efficiency of the algorithm is $O\,(n)$.

Algorithm 2.30: Hypergeometric Distribution Sampler
Objective: generate a random number from hypergeometric distribution
$HG\left(M, N, n\right)$, where $M \geq 1, N - M \geq 1$ and $N \geq n \geq 1$
Input: M, N and n
$d_1 := N - n$; $d_2 := \min\left(M, N - M\right)$
$Y := d_2$; $i := n$
While $iY > 0$:

    Generate u from $U\left(0, 1\right)$
    $Y := Y - \lfloor u + \frac{Y}{d_1+i} \rfloor$
    $i := i + 1$
    $Z := d_2 - Y.$
    If $M \leq N - M$ **Then**
        $x := Z$
    Else
        $x := n - Z$
    Endif
Endwhile
Return x
§

2.4.20 *Multinomial Distribution*

The multinomial distribution p.m.f. is given by (Fishman, 2000, p. 225)

$$f\left(x_1, ..., x_r\right) = n! \prod_{i=1}^{r} \frac{p_i^{x_i}}{x_i!}, \tag{2.56}$$

where $0 < p_i < 1$, $\sum_{i=1}^{r} p_i = 1$, integer $x_i \geq 0$, $\sum_{i=1}^{r} x_i = n$.
Note that X_j has the binomial p.m.f.

$$f\left(x_j\right) = \binom{n}{x_j} p_j^{x_j} \left(1 - p_j\right)^{n-x_j}$$

and

$$f\left(x_j | X_1 = x_1, ..., X_{j-1} = x_{j-1}\right) = \binom{n - \eta_j}{x_j} w_j^{x_j} \left(1 - w_j\right)^{n-\eta_j},$$

where $\eta_j = x_1 + \cdots + x_{j-1}$ and $w_j = p_j / \left(1 - p_1 - \cdots - p_{j-1}\right)$, $2 \leq j \leq r$.
This property can be used to develop an algorithm for generating deviates from a multinomial distribution. See Algorithm 2.31.

Algorithm 2.31: Multinomial Distribution Sampler

Objective: generate a deviate random number from a multinomial distribution

Input $n, r, p_1, .., p_r$

$q := 1$; $m := n$; $j := 1$

While $m(r - j + 1) > 0$

    Generate z_j from $B(m, p_j/q)$

    $m := m - x_j$; $q := q - p_j$

    $j := j + 1$

Endwhile

Return $\{x_1, ..., x_{j-1}, 0, ...0\}$

§

2.5   Summary

In this chapter we discussed the most important random variable generation — uniform random number generation. Virtually all random variable generations are based on uniform random number generation. We have particularly studied the multiplicative congruential generator. The quality of random numbers generated is important to the quality of Monte Carlo simulations. One of the most important characteristics is the period, m, of a random number generator, because it determines the ultimate precision we can achieve from a random number generator. If the number of replications in MC exceeds m, the sequence of the random numbers starts to repeat, and precision of the MC can't be improved further by increasing the number of replicates.

We have discussed several general methods for random number generation, including the inverse CDF method, the acceptance-rejection method, the Metropolis-Hasting method, Gibbs sampling, and others. The inverse CDF method is the most direct way to generate variates with a specific distribution, but the inverse function of the CDF must be available. If Inverse-CDF can't be used, then the acceptance-rejection method (ARM) may be a good option. ARM allows for generating variables from a complex distribution using a relatively simple distribution. MCMC is very popular, while the Metropolis-Hasting and Gibbs methods are the two widely used algorithms in MCMC. They can be used to generate complex Bayesian posterior distributions and arbitrary multiple-dimensional distributions. There are other general methods we have not covered, such as the alias method.

We have briefly discussed methods to improve the efficiency of MC methods, including importance sampling, control variable, and stratification.

Finally, we provided an extensive list of algorithms for generating samples from commonly used distributions. These algorithms are very mutual and have been implemented by various software packages such as SAS, ExpDesign Studio, and others. We have also provided the moments of the distributions so that readers can use them to validate their implementations of the algorithms. The massive relationships among various distributions presented in the text are handy and useful. To summarize those relationships, we have copied a figure (Figure 2.2) by Kokoska and Zwillonger (2000).

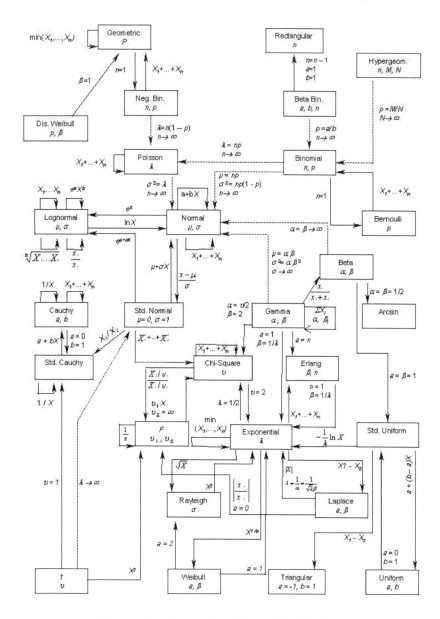

Figure 2.2:   Relationships Among Distributions

2.6   Exercises

Exercise 2.1: Not all random generators implemented in commercial software are good. Devise an algorithm to generate the uniform distribution $U(0,1)$ and use any computer language to implement it. List criteria one could use to check the quality of the random numbers generated by the algorithm and to compare it against a random number generator from a commercial product.

Exercise 2.2: Erlang Distribution
Erlang distribution $Er(\lambda, n)$ has p.d.f.

$$f(x) = \frac{\lambda^n x^{n-1} \exp(-\lambda x)}{(n-1)!}, \ \lambda > 0, \ n \in N, \ x \geq 0.$$

The c.d.f. is given by

$$F(x) = 1 - \sum_{k=0}^{n-1} \frac{e^{-\lambda x} (\lambda x)^k}{k!}$$

Table 2.18: $Er(\lambda, n)$ Property Table

mean	variance	skewness	mode
n/λ	n/λ^2	$2/\sqrt{n}$	$\frac{n-1}{\lambda}, n > 1$

Distribution Relationships:

(1) If X is an Erlang random variable with parameters β and $n = 1$, then X is an exponential random variable with parameter $\lambda = 1/\beta$.
(2) The sum of n independent variates from the exponential distribution with parameter λ is an Erlang (gamma) distribution with parameters λ and n.

From relationship 2, we know that random numbers from $Er(\lambda, n)$ can be computed from the random numbers of $U(0,1)$ using the relationship:

$$Er(\lambda, n) \sim -\frac{1}{\lambda} \ln \Pi_{i=1}^n U_i(0,1).$$

Devise an algorithm for sampling from an Erlang distribution.
Exercise 2.3: Rayleigh Distribution

Rayleigh $Ry(\sigma)$ p.d.f. is given by

$$f(x) = \frac{x}{\sigma^2} \exp\left(-\frac{x^2}{2\sigma^2}\right), \ x \geq 0.$$

Table 2.19: $Ry(\sigma)$ Property Table

mean	variance	skewness	mode
$\sigma\sqrt{\pi/2}$	$\sigma^2\left(2 - \frac{\pi}{2}\right)$	$\frac{(\pi-3)\sqrt{\pi/2}}{(2-\pi/2)^{3/2}}$	σ

Use a relationship between Rayleigh and Weibull distributions to devise an algorithm to generate samples from a Rayleigh distribution.

Exercise 2.4: Pareto Distribution

The Pareto distribution $Pt(\theta, \alpha)$ p.d.f. is given by (Kokoska and Zwillonger, 2000, p. 102)

$$f(x) = \frac{\theta a^\theta}{x^{\theta+1}}, \ \theta, a > 0, \ x \geq a,$$

where are θ and a are the shape and location parameters, respectively.

Table 2.20: $Pt(\theta, \alpha)$ Property Table

mean	$\frac{a\theta}{\theta-1}, \ \theta > 1$
variance	$\frac{a^2\theta}{(\theta-1)^2(\theta-2)}, \ \theta > 2$
skewness	$\frac{2(\theta+1)\sqrt{\theta-2}}{(\theta-3)\sqrt{\theta}}, \ \theta > 3$
mode	a

Use the inverse CDF method to develop an algorithm for generating samples from the Pareto distribution.

Exercise 2.5: Lognormal Distribution

The lognormal distribution $LN(\mu, \sigma^2)$ p.d.f. is given by

$$f(x) = \frac{1}{\sqrt{2\pi}\sigma x} \exp\left(-\frac{(\ln x - \mu)^2}{2\sigma^2}\right).$$

Table 2.21: $LN(\mu, \sigma^2)$ Property Table

mean	variance	skewness	mode
$e^{\mu+\sigma^2/2}$	$e^{2\mu+\sigma^2}\left(e^{\sigma^2} - 1\right)$	$\left(e^{\sigma^2} + 2\right)\sqrt{e^{\sigma^2} - 1}$	$e^{u-\sigma^2}$

Devise an algorithm for generating samples from the lognormal distribution.

Exercise 2.6: Cauchy Distribution

The Cauchy distribution $Cc(\theta, \lambda)$ p.d.f. is given by (Johnson, Kotz, and Balakrishnan, 1994, p. 298–328)

$$f\left(x\right)=\frac{1}{\lambda\pi\left(1+\left(\frac{x-\theta}{\lambda}\right)^{2}\right)},\ \theta\in R,\ \lambda>0,\ x\in R.$$

The c.d.f. is given by

$$F\left(x\right)=\frac{1}{2}+\frac{1}{\pi}\tan^{-1}\left(\frac{x-\theta}{\lambda}\right).$$

Devise an algorithm for generating samples from the Cauchy distribution.

Exercise 2.7: Noncentral F Distribution

Noncentral distributions are often needed in power or sample size calculations.

If X_1 is a noncentral chi-square random variable with noncentrality parameter λ and v_1 degrees of freedom, X_2 is a chi-square random variable with v_2 degrees of freedom, and X_1 and X_2 are statistically independent, then

$$Y=\frac{X_1/v_1}{X_2/v_2}$$

is a noncentral F-distributed random variable with p.d.f.

$$f\left(y\right)=\sum_{k=0}^{\infty}\frac{e^{-\lambda/2}\left(\lambda/2\right)^{k}}{B\left(\frac{v_2}{2},\frac{v_1}{2}+k\right)k!}\left(\frac{v_1}{v_2}\right)^{\frac{v_1}{2}+k}\left(\frac{v_2}{v_2+v_1f}\right)^{\frac{v_1+v_2}{2}+k}y^{v_1/2-1+k},\ y\geq0.$$

Devise two different algorithms for generating the noncentral F-distribution and compare them.

Exercise 2.8: Noncentral t-Distribution

If $Z\sim N\left(\mu,1\right)$ and $X\sim\chi^{2}\left(v\right)$ are independent, then random variable

$$Y=\frac{Z}{\sqrt{X/v}}$$

is a noncentral t-distributed random variable with v degrees of freedom and noncentrality parameter μ.

The p.d.f. is given by

$$f\left(y\right)=\frac{v^{v/2}}{\sqrt{\pi}\Gamma\left(v/2\right)}\frac{e^{-\mu^{2}/2}}{\left(v+y^{2}\right)^{\left(v+1\right)/2}}\sum_{k=0}^{\infty}\Gamma\left(\frac{v+k+1}{2}\right)\frac{\mu^{k}}{k!}\left(\frac{2y^{2}}{v+y^{2}}\right)^{k/2}.$$

Note that the noncentrality parameter of t may be negative. Its square rather than itself is comparable to the noncentrality parameter of the χ^2 or F distribution.

Devise two different algorithms for generating the noncentral t-distribution, implement each one using a computer language, and compare the efficiency of the algorithms.

Exercise 2.9: Devise an algorithm for the inverse c.d.f. method for a discrete probability distribution.

Exercise 2.10: A study population consists of two patient populations with two exponential distributions. Derive the survival distribution for the overall study population and generalize your results to a population consisting of n patient populations with hazard rate λ_i $(i = 1, 2, ..., n)$.

Exercise 2.11: Patients with a progressive disease such as cancer will experience different disease stages. At each stage the patients have different survival distributions. Assume the progression distribution from stage i to $i + 1$ is characterized as an exponential distribution with λ_i. Derive the overall survival distribution for a patient at stage 1. Devise an algorithm for generating samples from such a distribution.

Exercise 2.12: Implement Algorithms 2.16 and 2.24.

Exercise 2.13: Use Monte Carlo to calculate the value of π from the formula $\pi = \frac{4}{\sqrt{2}} \int_0^1 \frac{1+x^2}{1+x^4} dx$.

Exercise 2.14: Use Monte Carlo to calculate the constant $e = \frac{\pi}{2} / \int_0^\infty \frac{\cos x}{1+x^2} dx$.

Chapter 3

Overview of Drug Development

This chapter will cover the following topics:

- Drug Discovery
- Preclinical Development
- Clinical Development

3.1 Introduction

Pharmaceutical research and biotechnology companies are "devoted to inventing medicines that allow patients to live longer, healthier, and more productive lives."

— "Who We Are,"PhRMA, www.phrma.org.

A pharmaceutical or biopharmaceutical company is a commercial business licensed to research, develop, market, and/or distribute drugs, most commonly in the context of healthcare. They are subject to a variety of laws and regulations regarding the patenting, testing, and marketing of drugs, particularly prescription drugs. From its beginnings at the start of the 19th century, the pharmaceutical industry is now one of the most successful and influential, attracting both praise and controversy. Most of today's major pharmaceutical companies were founded in the late 19th and early 20th centuries. Key discoveries of the 1920s and 1930s, such as insulin and penicillin, became mass-manufactured and distributed. Switzerland, Germany, and Italy had particularly strong industries, with the UK and US following suit.

Attempts were made to increase regulation and to limit financial links between pharmaceutical companies and prescribing physicians, some by the relatively new US FDA. Such calls increased in the 1960s after the thalidomide tragedy came to light, in which the use of a new tranquilizer in pregnant women caused severe birth defects. In 1964, the World Medical Association issued its Declaration of Helsinki, which set standards for clinical research and demanded that subjects give their informed consent before enrolling in an experiment. Pharmaceutical companies were then required to prove efficacy in clinical trials before marketing drugs.

The industry remained relatively small until the 1970s when it began to expand at a greater rate. Legislation allowing for strong patents, to cover both the process of manufacture and specific products, came into force in most countries.

Biopharmaceuticals, different from traditional pharmaceuticals, are medical drugs produced using biotechnology. They are usually proteins (including antibodies) or nucleic acids (DNA, RNA, or antisense oligonucleotides) used for therapeutic or in vivo diagnostic purposes, and are produced by means other than direct extraction from a native (nonengineered) biological source. By the mid-1980s, small biotechnology firms were struggling for survival, which led to the formation of mutually beneficial partnerships with large pharmaceutical companies and a host of corporate buyouts of the smaller firms.

Since the early 1990s, drug development cost have increased dramatically, with an unmatched success rate. In 2004 the Food and Drug Administration released the Drug Modernization Act – Innovation/Stagnation: Challenge and Opportunity on the Critical Path to New Medical Products. Pharmaceutical industries seek new and more efficient ways to develop drugs such as genomic and biomarker utilizations, adaptive design, molecular design, and computer simulations.

In the new millennium, drug development is characterized by globalization. In 2006, global spending on prescription drugs topped $600 billion, even as growth slowed somewhat in Europe and North America. Sales of prescription drugs worldwide rose 7% to $600 billion, according to IMS health, a pharmaceutical information and consulting company. The United States still accounts for most, with $250 billion in annual sales. Sales there grew nearly 6%. Emerging markets such as China, Russia, South Korea, and Mexico outpaced the global market, growing a huge 81%.

Drug development is large-length collaboration among people from dozens of disciplines. The entire development process includes multiple stages or phases: from discovery, preclinical, clinical trials, to Phase IV commitment or marketing (Figure 3.1). Interactions with regulatory authorities usually start before Phase I clinical trials. All clinical trial protocols (see later in this chapter) have to be approved by an IRB (investigator review board) and regulatory authorities before clinical trials. It is estimated that, on average, a drug takes 10 to 12 years from initial research to reach the commercialization stage. The cost of this process is estimated to be more than US$500 million.

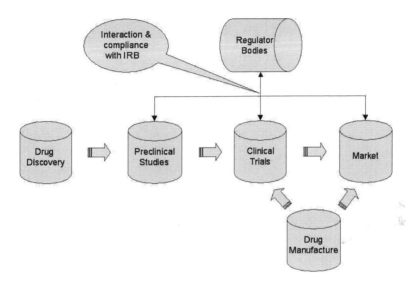

Figure 3.1:   Overview of the Drug Development Processes

3.2   Drug Discovery

Drug discovery involves: (1) identifying and defining medical needs, i.e., an effective prophylactic or therapeutic intervention, (2) research on disease mechanisms, i.e., identifying and validating target (receptors) involved in disease processes, (3) searching for lead compounds that interact with the target, and (4) optimizing the properties of the lead compounds to generate potential drug molecules.

3.2.1   *Target Identification and Validation*

For a drug to work, it has to interact with a disease target in a body to stop its wayward functions. In most situations, it is proteins or receptors that drug molecules are developed to interact with to provide the therapy. The exceptions are in cases such as antisense drugs and gene therapy, where nucleotides and genes, respectively, are targeted. When presented to the target, drug molecules can elicit reactions to switch on or switch off certain biochemical reactions. The main drug targets in the human body can be classified into three categories: enzymes, intracellular receptors, and cell surface receptors. Enzymes are biomolecules that catalyze (i.e., increase the rates of) chemical reactions. Drugs can interact with enzymes to modulate their enzymatic activities. Intracellular receptors are in the cytoplasm or nucleus. Drugs or endogenous ligand molecules have to pass through the cell membrane (a lipid bilayer) to interact with these receptors. The molecules must be hydrophobic or coupled to a hydrophobic carrier to cross the cell membrane. Cell surface receptors are on the cell surface and have an affinity for hydrophilic binding molecules. Signals are transduced from external stimuli to the cytoplasm, and affect cellular pathways via these surface receptors. There are three main superfamilies (groups) of cell surface receptors: C-protein coupled receptors, ion channel receptors, and catalytic receptors using enzymatic activities.

When the action of the drug is to activate or switch on a reaction, the drug is called an 'agonist.' On the other hand, if the drug switches off the reaction, or inhibits or blocks the binding of other agonist components onto the receptor, it is called an 'antagonist.' When the interaction is with an enzyme, the terms 'inducer' and 'inhibitor' are used to denote drugs that activate or deactivate the enzyme. The interactions between drug molecules and targets are desired to be binding-specific. Binding occurs at particular sites in the target molecule, and binding is reversible.

Cells communicate to coordinate biochemical functions within the human body. If the communication system is interrupted or messages are not conveyed fully, our bodily functions can go haywire. For example, if the p53 protein is mutated, cell growth is unchecked and cancer can form. C-protein coupled receptors (CPCRs) represent possibly the most important class of target proteins for drug discovery. They are always involved in signaling from outside to inside the cell. The number of diseases that are caused by a CPCR malfunction is enormous, and therefore it is not surprising that most commonly prescribed medicines act on a CPCE. It is estimated that more than 30% of drugs target this receptor superfamily.

For most diseases, except in the case of trauma and infectious diseases, genetic makeup and variations determine a person's individuality and susceptibility to diseases, pathogens, and drug responses. The current method of drug discovery is to break down the disease process into the cellular and molecular levels such that more specific (fewer side effects) and effective (high therapeutic index) drugs can be discovered and manufactured to intervene or restore the cellular or molecular dysfunction. Among approximately three billion base pairs that make up the DNA module, about 30,000–40,000 genes (DNA segments) encode proteins. Based on these genes, many thousands of proteins are produced. Common drug targets are protein or glycoprotein molecules because proteins are the ingredients for enzymes and receptors, with which drugs interact.

After a potential disease-causing target has been identified, validation is necessary to confirm the functions and effects of the target. Validations are carried out in two ways: *in vitro* laboratory tests, and in vivo disease models using animals. Typically, *in vitro* tests are cell- or tissue-based experiments. The aim is to study the biochemical functions of the target as a result of binding to potential drug ligands. Parameters such as ionic concentrations, enzyme activities, and expression profiles are studied.

For *in vivo* studies, animal models are set up and how the target is involved in the disease is analyzed. One such model is the mouse knockout model. It should be borne in mind, however, that there are differences between humans and animals in terms of gene expression functional characteristics and biochemical reactions. Nevertheless, animal models can provide results that are closer to human results than *in vitro* tests.

3.2.2 *Irrational Approach*

There are two main approaches to discovering small molecule drugs (molecular weights < 500 Da): the irrational approach and the rational approach.

Steps in the traditional irrational approach include: (1) target identification, (2) target purification, and (3) modification of lead compound.

To find lead compounds or potential drug molecules that bind with receptors and modulate disease pathways, thousands of compounds (through natural product collection or laboratory production) are screened using high throughput screening (HTS) or ultra-HTS (UI-ITS). When an interaction happens, it is referred to as 'a hit.' The so-called lead compounds are those that have shown some desired biological activities when tested against assays. However, these activities are not optimized. Modifications to lead compounds are necessary to improve the physicochemical, pharmacokinetic, and toxicological properties for clinical applications.

Following 'hits,' lead compounds are purified using chromatographic techniques and their chemical compositions identified via spectroscopic and chemical means. Structures may be elucidated using X-ray or nuclear magnetic resonance (NMR) methods. Protein purification is a series of processes intended to isolate a single type of protein from a complex mixture. Protein purification is an important step in the characterization of the function, structure, and interactions of the protein of interest.

Further tests are carried out to evaluate the potency and specificity of the lead compounds isolated. This is usually followed up with modifications of the compounds to improve properties through synthesis of variations to the compounds via chemical processes in the laboratory and frequently with modifications to the functional groups. The optimized lead compounds go through many iterative processes to keep improving and optimizing the drug interaction properties to achieve improved potency and efficacy.

Potency is an important concept in drug discovery. It is a measure of drug activity expressed in terms of the amount required to produce an effect of a given intensity. A highly potent drug evokes a larger response at low concentrations. It is proportional to affinity and efficacy. Affinity is the ability of the drug to bind to a receptor. Efficacy is the relationship between receptor occupancy and the ability to initiate a response at the molecular, cellular, tissue, or system level.

After all these exhaustive tests, a few candidates are selected for pre-clinical in vivo studies using animal disease models. Many tests are based on tissue cultures or cell-based assays, as they are less costly and provide results more readily. At the end of this long process is the availability of selected drug candidates with sufficient efficacy and safety for human clinical trials.

3.2.3   *Rational Approach*

The rational approach can be based on the geometric structure of molecules/proteins, the knowledge to identify the genes that are involved in disease pathogenesis, or nanotechnology (nanoMedicime).

Computer-aided molecular design and modeling is the central part of computational chemistry, which uses 3-D structures of compounds in virtual chemical compound libraries to determine the structure–activity relationships (SARs) of ligand-protein receptor binding. The aim of computational chemistry is to perform virtual screening using computer-generated ligands. Libraries of virtual ligands are generated on computers based on certain building blocks or frameworks (scaffolds) of chemical compounds. Methods such as genetic algorithms and genetic programming can be used, which simulate the genetic evolutionary process to produce 'generations' of virtual compounds with new structures that have improved ability to bind the receptor protein, similar to the concept of 'survival of the fittest' in the biological process. See Chapter 13 for more discussion.

Combinatorial chemistry is a laboratory chemistry technique to synthesize a diverse range of compounds through methodical combinations of building block components.

The aim of antisense therapy is to identify the genes that are involved in disease pathogenesis. The strategy for antisense therapy is based on the binding of oligodeoxyribonucleotides to the double helix DNA. This stops gene expression either by restricting the unwinding of the DNA or by preventing the binding of transcription factor complexes to the gene promoter. Another strategy centers on the mRNA. Oligoribonucleotides form a hybrid with the mRNA. Such a duplex formation ties up the mRNA, preventing the encoded translation message from being processed to form the protein.

Although all these seem like elegant ways to stop disease at the source, at the DNA or mRNA level, there are practical problems. First, the antisense drug has to be delivered to the cell interior, and the polar groups of oligonucleotides have problems crossing the cell membrane to enter the cytoplasm and nucleus; second, the oligonucleotides have to bind to the intended gene sequence through hydrogen bonding; third, the drug should not exert toxicities or side effects as a result of the interaction. For these reasons, there have been difficulties in bringing antisense drugs to the market.

3.2.4 *Biologics*

Unlike small molecule drugs (pharmaceuticals), large molecule drugs (biopharmaceuticals) are mainly protein based and similar to natural biological compounds found in the human body or they are fragments that mimic the active part of natural compounds. Today biopharmaceutical discovery is through examining compounds within the human body, for example, hormones or other biological response modifiers, and how they affect the biological process.

Pharmaceuticals are new chemical entities (NCEs) and they are produced (synthesized) in manufacturing plants using techniques based on chemical reactions of reactants. Biopharmaceuticals are made using totally different methods. These protein-based drugs are 'manufactured' in biological systems such as living cells, producing the desired protein molecules in large reaction vessels or by extraction from animal serum.

Biopharmaceuticals are products which are derived using living organisms to produce or modify the structure and/or functioning of plants or animals with a medical or diagnostic use. Biopharmaceuticals are becoming increasingly important because they are more potent and specific, as they are similar to the proteins within the body, and hence are more effective in treating our diseases. There are three major areas in which biopharmaceuticals are used: prophylactic (preventive, as in the case of vaccines), therapeutic (antibodies), and replacement (hormones, growth factors) therapy. Another term that is used for protein-based drugs is biologics.

Vaccines

The basis of vaccination is that administering a small quantity of a vaccine (antigen that has been treated) stimulates the immune system and causes antibodies to be secreted to react against the foreign antigen. Later in life, when we are exposed to the same antigen again, the immune system will evoke a 'memory' response and activate the defense mechanisms by generating antibodies to combat the invading antigen.

In cancer, the immune system does not recognize changes in cancer cells. Cancer vaccines seek to mimic cancer-specific changes by using synthetic peptides to challenge the immune system. When these peptides are taken up by T cells, the immune system is activated. The T cells search for cancer cells with specific markers and proceed to kill them.

Antibodies

The human immune system is a remarkable system for combating foreign substances that invade the body. It protects us from infections by pathogens such as viruses, bacteria, parasites, and fungi. An important aspect of the immune system is the self-nonself recognition function, by means of markers present on a protein called the major histocompatibility complex (MHC). Substances without such markers are discerned and targeted for destruction (Ng, 2005).

This gives rise to autoimmune diseases such as rheumatoid arthritis, diabetes, and multiple sclerosis. However, mistakes can happen occasionally when the immune system responds to the environment, leading to allergies, as in the case of asthma and hay fever.

B cells are produced by the bone marrow. In response to activation of $CD4^+$ T helper cells, B cells proliferate and produce antibodies. The antibodies produced by B cells circulate in the bloodstream and bind to antigens. When this happens, other cells are in turn activated to destroy the antigens.

T cells are lymphocytes produced by the thymus gland. $CD4^+$ (CD positive, helper cells) and $CD8^+$ (CD positive, also called T killer or suppressor cells) are the two types of T cells involved in immune responses. When the APCs present the antigens to $CD4^+$ helper T cells, the secretory function is activated and growth factors such as cytokines are secreted to signal the proliferation of $CD8^+$ killer T cells and B cells. When the $CD8^+$ cells are activated by the APCs, the $CD8^+$ killer T cells directly kill those cells expressing the antigens. Activated B cells produce antibodies, as described above (Ng, 2005).

Cytokines and Hormone Therapies

Cytokines are produced mainly by leukocytes (white blood cells). They are potent polypeptide molecules that regulate the immune and inflammation functions, as well as hemopoiesis (production of blood cells) and wound healing.

Hormones are intercellular messengers. Hormones maintain homeostasis — the balance of biological activities in the body; for example, insulin controls the blood glucose level, epinephrine and norepinephrine mediate response to an external environment, and growth hormone promotes normal healthy growth and development.

Diabetes mellitus occurs when the human body does not produce enough insulin. Production of insulin is triggered when there is a rise in blood sugar, for example, after a meal. Most of our body cells have insulin receptors which bind to the insulin secreted. When the insulin binds to the receptor, other receptors on the cell are activated to absorb sugar (glucose) from the bloodstream into the cell.

When there is insufficient insulin to bind to receptors, the cells are starved because sugar cannot reach the interior to provide energy for vital biological processes. Patients with insulin-dependent diabetes mellitus (IDDM) become unwell when this happens. They depend on insulin injections for survival.

Gene Therapies

Gene therapy is the technology that involves the transfer of normal functional genes to replace genetically faulty ones so that proper control of protein expression and biochemical processes can take place. However, it is challenging to get the normal genes to the intended location using delivery tools or vehicles, called vectors (gene carriers). Whether using the in vitro or in situ method, genes are first loaded onto the vectors, which usually are viruses. Retroviruses are the preferred candidates, as they are efficient vectors for entering humans and replicating their genes within human cells. The hurdle of gene therapy is to overcome our immune and inflammation response toxicity.

Stem Cell Therapies

Stem cell treatment is a cell therapy that introduces new cells into damaged tissue in order to treat a disease or injury. The ability of stem cells to self-renew and give rise to subsequent generations that can differentiate offers a large potential to culture tissues that can replace diseased and damaged tissues in the body, without the risk of rejection. However, cell rejection due to the host's immune system recognizing the cells as foreign has to be overcome to ensure stem cell therapy as a viable treatment.

Bone marrow is the spongy tissue inside the cavities of bones. Bone marrow stem cells grow and divide into the various types of blood cells: white blood cells (leukocytes) that fight infection, red blood cells (erythrocytes) that transport oxygen, and platelets that are the agents for clotting. Patients with leukemia have a condition in which the stem cells in the bone marrow malfunction and produce an excessive number of immature white blood cells, which interferes with normal blood cell production. Bone marrow replacement is often an effective way to treat leukemia patients.

3.2.5 *Nanomedicine*

Nanomedicine is an application of nanotechnology in medical science. Nanotechnologies study features of materials on the scale of nanometers or billionths of a meter. In biology a single human hair is about 80,000 nanometers wide and a red blood cell is about 7,000 nanometers wide. Nanoscale materials often have novel properties related to their high ratio of surface area and quantum effects. Current research and development efforts on nanomedicine are concentrated in six primary categories (The Royal Society, 2004; Tegart, 2003):

(1) Antimicrobial Properties. Investigating nanomaterials with strong antimicrobial properties. Nanocrystalline silver, for example, is already being used for wound treatment.
(2) Biopharmaceutics. Applying nanotechnology to drug delivery system, e.g., using nanomaterial coatings to encapsulate drugs and to serve as functional carriers. Nanomaterial encapsulation could improve the diffusion, degradation, and targeting of a drug.
(3) Implantable Materials. Using nanomaterials to repair and replace damaged or diseased tissues. Nanomaterial implant coatings could increase the adhesion, durability, and lifespan of implants, and nanostructure scaffolds could provide a framework for improved tissue regeneration. Nanomaterial implants could be engineered for biocompatibility with the host environment to minimize side effects and the risk of rejection.
(4) Implantable Devices. Implanting small devices to serve as sensors, fluid injection systems, drug dispensers, pumps and reservoirs, and aids to restore vision and hearing functions. Devices with nanoscale components could monitor environmental conditions, detect specific properties, and deliver appropriate physical, chemical, or pharmaceutical responses.
(5) Diagnostic Tools. Utilizing lab-on-a-chip devices to perform DNA analysis and drug discovery research by reducing the required sample sizes and accelerating the chemical reaction process. Moreover, imaging tech-

nologies such as nanoparticle probes and miniature imaging devices as well as IV imaging agents could promote early detection and diagnosis of disease.

(6) Understanding Basic Life Processes. Using nanoscale devices and materials to learn more about how biological systems self-assemble, self-regulate, and self-destroy at the molecular level. Insights into basic life processes will overlap multiple disciplines and could yield scientific breakthroughs.

3.3 Preclinical Development

3.3.1 *Objectives of Preclinical Development*

Preclinical development is a stage of research that bridges discovery and clinical trials. After a lead compound has been identified, it is subjected to a development process to optimize its properties. The development process includes pharmacological studies of the lead compound to determine its safety and efficacy. Preclinical research includes *in vitro* (in tubes) and *in vivo* (on animals) tests. The research, often called pharmacology study, includes toxicology, pharmacodynamics, and pharmacokinetics. Many iterations are carried out and, at the end of this process, an optimized compound is found and this becomes a potential drug ready for clinical trial in humans.

Two different species are typically used in animal testing. The most commonly used models are murine and canine, although primate and porcine models are also used. The choice of species is based on which will give the best correlation to human trials. Differences in the gut, enzyme activity, circulatory system, or other considerations make certain models more appropriate in terms of the dosage form, site of activity, or noxious metabolites. For example, rodents cannot act as models for antibiotic drugs because the resulting alteration to their intestinal flora causes significant adverse effects. Most studies are performed in larger species such as dogs, pigs, and sheep, which allow for testing in a similar sized model to a human. Some species are used for similarity in specific organs or organ system physiology. Examples are swine for dermatological and coronary stent studies, goats for mammary implant studies, and dogs for gastric studies.

Drug development also extends to formulation and delivery. Most drugs that are administered to patients contain more than just the active pharmaceutical ingredients (the drug molecules that interact with the receptors or enzymes). Other chemical components are often added to improve manufacturing processing, or the stability and bioavailability of drugs. Effective delivery of drugs to target sites is an important factor in optimizing efficacy and reducing side effects.

An ideal drug is *potent*, efficacious, and specific, that is, it must have strong effects on a specific targeted biological pathway and minimal effects on all other pathways, to reduce side effects. *Potency* is the dose required to generate an effect. A potent drug elicits an effect at a low dose. An important concept is so-called *therapeutic index (window)*. The index is defined by the ratio of TD_{50}/ED_{50}, where TD_{50} is the toxic dose for 50% of the population, and ED_{50} is the effective dose for 50% of the population. A high value of the index is preferable. When the index is less than one, the compound cannot be considered as a drug candidate. Another commonly used term is the so-called *standard safety margin* (SSM) defined as

$$SSM = \frac{LD_1 - ED_{99}}{ED_{99}} 100\%$$

where LD_1 is the lethal dose for 1% of the population, and ED_{99} is the effective dose for 99% of the population. Again, a high SSM is desirable.

3.3.2   *Pharmacokinetics*

Pharmacokinetics is often studied in conjunction with pharmacodynamics. Pharmacodynamics explores what a drug does to the body, whereas pharmacokinetics explores what the body does to the drug. Specifically, pharmacokinetics is the study of drug absorption, distribution, metabolism, and excretion (ADME). Absorption is the process of a substance entering the body. Distribution is the dispersion or dissemination of substances throughout the fluids and tissues of the body. Metabolism is the irreversible transformation of parent compounds into daughter metabolites. Excretion is the elimination of the substances from the body. In rare cases, some drugs irreversibly accumulate in a tissue in the body.

Drug Administration (Absorption)

Pharmacokinetic properties of drugs may be affected by elements such as the site of administration and the rate of drug administration. There are several ways to administer a drug, such as oral and intravenous. With intravenous administration, a drug is injected directly into the bloodstream; oral administration requires the drug to be absorbed before it can enter the bloodstream for distribution to target sites, and metabolism may precede distribution to the site of action.

The oral route is the most common way of administering a drug. For a drug to be absorbed into the bloodstream, it has to be soluble in the fluids of our gastrointestinal tract. Drugs are often formulated with excipients (components other than the active drug) to improve manufacturing and dissolution processes. The gastrointestinal tract is lined with epithelial cells, and drugs have to cross the cell membrane. In the stomach, with low pH, drugs that are weak acids are absorbed faster. In the intestine, where pH is high, weak basic drugs are absorbed preferentially.

When a drug is injected (intravenous administration), the entire dose can be considered as being available in the bloodstream to be distributed to the target site. Hence, the dosage can be controlled, unlike with other routes of administration where the bioavailability of the drug is difficult to predict because of complex diffusion processes. Intravenous injection is the normal route for administration of protein-based drugs, as they are likely to be destroyed when taken orally because of the pH conditions in the gastrointestinal tract. The onset of drug action with intravenous injection is quick; therefore it is especially useful for emergency cases, but also potentially the most dangerous. Once a drug is injected, it is almost impossible to remove it.

Distribution

The distribution patterns of a drug from the bloodstream to various tissues depend on a number of factors such as (1) vascularity nature of the tissue, (2) binding of the drug to protein molecules in blood plasma, and (3) drug substance transportation types: perfusion or diffusion of the drug.

Drugs absorbed through the gastrointestinal tract pass into the hepatic portal vein, which drains into the liver. The liver metabolizes the drug and thus reduces the availability of the drug for interaction with receptors. At a certain time after administration, when the rate of drug absorption equals the rate of clearance, it reaches an equilibrium condition called 'steady state.' The area under the concentration curve represents the total amount of drug in the blood, which measures the bioavailability of the drug. Comparison of concentrations in the bloodstream of drugs administered via intravenous injection and the oral route provides information on the bioavailability of the oral drug.

Drug molecules in the blood are transported to tissue until equilibrium is reached. The transporting speed depends on the transportation type: perfusion (fast) and diffusion (slow). Acid drugs usually bind to albumins and basic drugs to glycoproteins. Then, as the drug binds to albumin and proteins in the blood, it becomes less available for distribution to tissues. Last, lipid-soluble drugs can cross the cell membrane more readily than polar drugs and move into the tissues to interact with receptors.

Metabolism

Most drugs are metabolized in the body, though to different extents. Metabolism changes the chemical structures and reduces the pharmacological activity of a new molecular entity (NME). The liver is the major organ for metabolizing drugs, followed by the kidneys. Some drugs also are metabolized in tissue systems.

Two types of biochemical metabolism reactions take place in the liver: (1) Phase I reactions include oxidation, reduction, and hydrolysis, which transform the drugs into metabolites by means of the family of enzymes, cytochrome P-450. They convert lipid-soluble drugs to more water-soluble metabolites. (2) Phase II reactions involve the addition or conjugation of subgroups, such as -OH, -NH, and -SH, to the drug molecules. Enzymes other than P-450 are responsible for these reactions. These reactions give rise to less lipid soluble or more polar molecules that are excreted by the body (Ng, 2005).

Excretion

Drug excretion is the process of discharging medical waste matter from the blood, tissues, or organs. Common routes of excretion are: kidneys, lungs, intestine, colon, and skin. The kidneys are the primary organs for clearing drugs from the body. Water-soluble drugs are usually cleared more quickly than lipid-soluble drugs. Some drugs may be re-absorbed into the intestine and colon and later passed out as solid wastes.

Clearance is a measure of drug elimination from the body without identifying the mechanism or process. Clearance considers the entire body as a drug-eliminating system from which many elimination processes may occur. The clearance of a drug is given by the following expression:

$$CL = \frac{\text{Rate of drug elimination}}{\text{Drug concentration in blood}}$$

In general, drugs that are highly bound to plasma protein have reduced overall drug clearance. Drug elimination is governed mainly by renal and other metabolic processes in the body. When a drug is tightly bound to a protein, only the unbound drug is assumed to be metabolized — restrictively eliminated. In contrast, some drugs may be eliminated even when they are protein bound — nonrestrictively eliminated.

Albumin is a protein (molecular weight about 70k Da) synthesized in the liver, and it is the major component of plasma proteins responsible for reversible drug binding. In the body, albumin is distributed in the plasma and in the extracellular fluids of skin, muscle, and various other tissues. The elimination half-life of albumin is about 18 days. Albumin is responsible for maintaining the osmotic pressure of the blood and for the transport of endogenous and exogenous substances (Shargel et al., 2005).

Pharmocokinetic Analysis Methods

Pharmacokinetic (PK) analysis is traditionally performed by noncompartmental or compartmental methods. Noncompartmental methods estimate exposure to a drug by estimating the area under the curve of a concentration-time curve, whereas compartmental methods estimate the concentration-time curve using kinetic models.

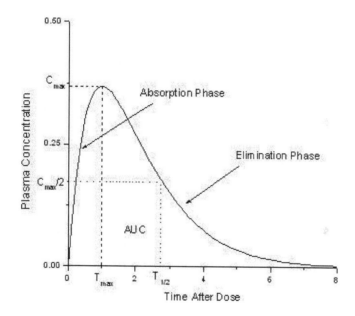

Figure 3.2:   Concentration Curve of Oral Administration

Noncompartmental PK analysis is highly dependent on the estimation of total drug exposure. Total drug exposure is most often estimated by area under the curve (AUC) methods using the trapezoidal rule. In this method, the area estimation is highly dependent on the blood/plasma sampling schedule and the closer the time points are, the closer the trapezoids are to the actual shape of the concentration-time curve. Other important PK parameters include $C_{\max}$ (maximum concentration), $T_{\max}$ (the time to $C_{\max}$), and the half-time $T_{1/2}$ (time to $C_{\max}/2$).

Compartmental PK analysis uses kinetic models to describe and predict the concentration-time curve. The advantage of compartmental over noncompartmental analysis is the ability to predict the concentration at any time. The disadvantage is that the results are model dependent and it is difficult to validate the model. The simplest PK compartmental model is the one-compartmental PK model with oral dose administration and first-order elimination (Figure 3.2). The most complex PK models are based on physiological information, which helps to ease development and validation. Some typical PK parameters of interest are presented in Table 3.1.

Table 3.1: Example of Preclinical PK Parameters

	Dose (mg/kg)		
	20	100	200
$C_{\max}(\mu g/ml)$	99.2 ± 22.3	502 ± 142.2	1261 ± 83
$T_{1/2}\ (hr)$	0.86	0.72	0.67
AUC $(\mu g/hr/ml)$	14.2	83.3	248.1
Clearance $(l/h/kg)$	1.42	1.18	0.82

3.3.3   *Pharmacodynamics*

Pharmacodynamics (PD) is the study of the biochemical and physiological effects of drugs on the body. The mechanisms of most drugs either mimic or inhibit normal physiological processes or inhibit pathological processes in animals. Drug actions can be classified into five main categories: depressing, stimulating, destroying cells (cytotoxic), irritation, and replacing substances.

Many drugs interact with proteins or other macromolecules (e.g., melanin and DNA) to form a so-called drug-protein complex. Most drug-protein bindings are reversible. Unlike free or unbound drug, protein-bound drug can't easily traverse cells or possibly even capillary membranes. A drug in the form of a drug complex is usually pharmacologically inactive. Studies that critically evaluate drug-protein binding are usually performed in vitro using a purified protein such as albumin. Commonly used methods for determining protein binding are equilibrium dialysis and ultrafiltration that uses a semipermeable membrane to separate the protein and protein-bound drug from the free drug.

Kinetics of Protein Binding

According to the occupancy theory in pharmacology, the drug effect depends on (1) binding of the drug to the receptor and drug-induced activation of the receptor, and (2) propagation of this initial receptor activation into the observed pharmacological effect that is proportional to the number of receptor sites occupied by the drug.

The kinetics of reversible drug-protein binding for a protein with one simple binding site can be modeled by the law of mass action, as follows:

$$[P] + [D] = [PD], \tag{3.1}$$

where $[P]$ = protein, $[D]$ = drug, and $[PD]$ = drug-protein complex.

From (3.1), the ratio of the molar concentration of the products and the molar concentration of the reactants is a constant expressed by (assume one binding site per protein molecule)

$$K_a = \frac{[PD]}{[P][D]}. \tag{3.2}$$

The magnitude of K_a indicates the degree of drug-protein binding. To study the binding behavior of drugs, another ratio, r, is used, defined as:

$$r = \frac{[PD]}{[PD] + [P]} \tag{3.3}$$

where $[PD] + [P]$ is the total moles of protein and $[PD]$ is the moles of drug bound.

$$r = \frac{K_a[D]}{1 + K_a[D]}. \tag{3.4}$$

3.3.4   Toxicology

The study of the toxicology of a potential drug is critical in determing the safety of a drug before it is given to humans in clinical trials. Toxicological studies show the functional and morphological effects of the drug, including the mode, site and degree of action, dose relationship, sex differences, latency and progression, and reversibility of these effects.

To study the toxicity of a drug, the maximum tolerable dose and area under the curve are established in rodents and nonrodents. There are two types of toxicity studies: single dose and repeated dose. Single dose acute toxicity testing is conducted for several purposes, including the determination of repeated doses, identification of organs subject to toxicity, and provision of data for starting doses in human clinical trials.

Experiments are carried out on animals, usually on two mammalian species: a rodent (mouse or rat) and a nonrodent (rabbit). Two different routes of administration are studied; one is the intended route for human clinical trials, and the other is intravenous injection. Various characteristics of the animals are monitored, including weights, clinical signs, organ functions, biochemical parameters, and mortality. At the completion of the study, autopsies are performed to analyze the organs, especially the targeted organ for the drug.

Repeated dose chronic toxicity studies are performed on two species of animals, a rodent and nonrodent. The aim is to evaluate the longer-term effects of the drug in animals. Plasma drug concentrations are measured and pharmacokinetic analyses are performed. Vital functions studied include cardiovascular, respiratory, and nervous systems. Animals are retained at the end of the study to check toxicity recovery.

Carcinogenicity studies are performed to identify the tumor-causing potential of a drug. Drugs are administered to rats or rodents continuously for months. Data for hormone levels, growth factors, and tissue enzymatic activities are analyzed after the experiments.

Genotoxicity studies are to determine if the drug compound can induce mutations to genes: assessment of genotoxicity in a bacterial reverse mutation test, detection of chromosomal damage using the in vitro method, and detection of chromosomal damage using rodent hematopoietic cells.

The aim of **reproductive toxicology** studies is to assess the effect of the potential drug on mammalian reproduction. All the stages, from pre-mating through conception, pregnancy and birth, to growth of the offspring, are studied in rats and/or rabbits.

The outcomes of toxicity studies provide a basis for a starting dose for clinical trials in humans. The FDA Guidance — Estimating the Safe Starting Dose in Clinical Trials for Therapeutics in Adult Healthy Volunteers outlines the derivation of the maximum recommended starting dose (MRSD) for a drug to be used in humans for the first time. This MRSD is based on (1) no observed adverse effect level (NOAEL) in animals—the highest dose level that does not produce a significant increase in adverse effects, and (2) conversion of the NOAEL to the human equivalent dose (HED) using the following formula:

$$HED = (\text{animal dose in mg/kg}) \times (\text{animal weight/human weight})^{0.33}$$

3.4   Clinical Development

3.4.1   *Overview of Clinical Development*

After a lead compound passes the preclinical test, the next step is clinical trials. Clinical trials are trials conducted on human subjects in accordance with Good Clinical Practice (GCP) in the US issued by the FDA. Clinical development is a joint effort by different stakeholders, including clinical research scientists, clinical monitors, medical and clinical investigators, physicians, medical liaisons, statisticians, data management professionals, CMC professionals, regulatory affairs professionals, project managers, financial managers, sales managers, and strategic planners. The traditional approach is to divide the development process into stages, from Phase I to Phase IV trials (Figure 3.3). Phase 0 is a new concept recently proposed; it is a mini-trial with micro-doses.

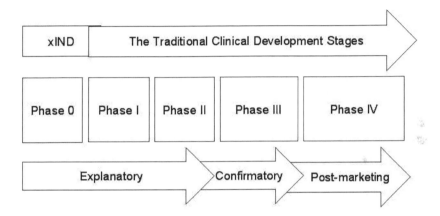

Figure 3.3: Classical Clinical Development Paradigm

However, before we design clinical trials, we have some important upfront work to do, including the clinical development plan (CDP), which is an integrated document to describe the master plan for a compound from Phase I to Phase IV. It is a bird's eye view of the plan for all the sequential trials regarding this compound, starting with verification of medical needs, which is usually done through literature review, consulting with KOLs (key opinion leaders) in the field (Figure 3.4). Key issues may include the size of the target population, the feasibility of running such trials, the key inclusion/exclusion criteria or the target population, major competitors/challenges, and different CDP options. Meanwhile, the commercial and marketing groups of the company start to gather information regarding the size of the target population for different CDP options and return on investment (ROI) through a net present value (NPV) analysis. The company has to evaluate their core competence again their goals and have sensitive risk mitigation plans. After several iterations of this process, the team has to make the decision on market position and deliver a sound CDP.

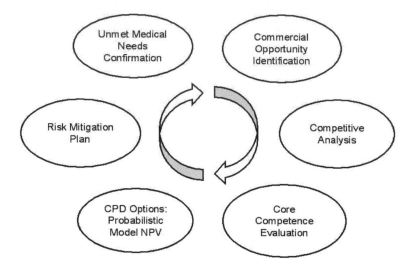

Figure 3.4:   Clinical Development Process

3.4.2   *Classical Clinical Trial Paradigm*

As mentioned earlier, clinical trials are divided into phases chronologically. The size of the trial is increased gradually from Phase 0 to Phase III for patient safety and cost reduction.

Phase 0 Trial

Phase 0 is a recent designation for exploratory, first-in-human trials conducted in accordance with the US Food and Drug Administration's (FDA) 2006 Guidance on Exploratory Investigational New Drug (IND) Studies. The goal is to speed up the development of promising drugs by establishing very early on whether the new molecule entity (NME) behaves in human subjects as predicted from preclinical studies. In a typical Phase 0 trial, single subtherapeutic doses of the study drug are administrated to a small number of subjects to gather preliminary information on pharmacokinetics and pharmacodynamics for the NME.

Therapeutic effects (safety or efficacy) are not expected due to extremely low doses. However, Phase 0 studies can be used to rank drug candidates in order to decide which has the best pharmacokinetic parameters in humans to take forward into further development. They enable go/no-go decisions to be based on relevant human models instead of relying on, traditionally, animal data.

There have been questions raised about whether Phase 0 trials are useful, ethically acceptable, feasible, speed up the drug development process or save money, and whether there is room for improvement. The potential advantages are less time with fewer patients than Phase I trials and providing a quick killer mechanism for ineffective NME, having a Phase 0 trial, the clinical evaluation of new molecular entities can be expedited, and minimize the risk to participants because of the low dose. There are also special concerns: no therapeutic benefit to the participants because of the low dose, and difficulties in patient recruitment. The outcome of Phase 0 trials is usually the PK and PD results; there may be some data on safety too (Figure 3.5).

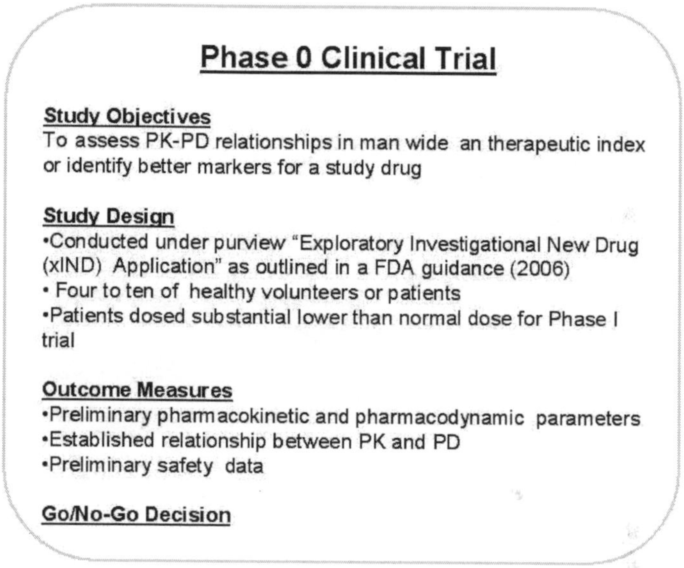

Phase 0 Clinical Trial

Study Objectives
To assess PK-PD relationships in man wide an therapeutic index or identify better markers for a study drug

Study Design
•Conducted under purview "Exploratory Investigational New Drug (xIND) Application" as outlined in a FDA guidance (2006)
• Four to ten of healthy volunteers or patients
•Patients dosed substantial lower than normal dose for Phase I trial

Outcome Measures
•Preliminary pharmacokinetic and pharmacodynamic parameters
•Established relationship between PK and PD
•Preliminary safety data

Go/No-Go Decision

Figure 3.5: Phase 0 Trial (Micro-dosing Trial)

Phase I Trial

Traditionally, Phase I trials are the first stage of testing in human subjects. Normally, a small (6–60) group of healthy volunteers will be selected except in the case of some special diseases such as oncology and HIV. The objective of the trials is to assess the safety, tolerability, pharmacokinetics, and pharmacodynamics of a drug (Figure 3.6). These trials are often conducted in an inpatient clinic, where the subject can be closely monitored. The subject who receives the drug is usually observed until five to several half-lives of the drug have passed. A Phase I trial is often a dose escalation study to determine the appropriate dose for therapeutic use. If the drug is intended to be used for multiple doses, then Phase I trials will include a single ascending dose (SAD) study followed by a multiple ascending dose (MAD) trial.

Phase I Clinical Trial

Study Objectives
• To learn the biological activities of the NCE
• To recommend a dose regimen for the next phase
• To eliminate a bad NCE

Study Design
• Six to dozens of healthy volunteers or patients
• Single ascending dose
• Multiple ascending dose
• Food effect (crossover design)
• Five times the half-life in study duration

Outcome Measures
• Pharmacokinetic parameters
• Pharmacodynamic parameters
• Adverse reaction profile
• Maximum tolerated dose (MTD)

Go/No-Go Decision
Dose window and route of administration established
=> Go for next phase or no-go

Figure 3.6:   Overview of Phase I Clinical Trial

SAD studies are those in which small groups of subjects are given a single dose of the study drug while they are observed for a period of time. If there are no sufficient adverse side effects observed, and the pharmacokinetic data are in line with predicted safe values, the dose is escalated to treat a new group of subjects. This is continued until pre-calculated pharmacokinetic safety levels are reached, or intolerable side effects start showing up. MAD studies are conducted to better understand the pharmacokinetics and pharmacodynamics under multiple doses of the drug. In these studies, a group of patients receives multiple low doses of the drug, while samples (of blood and other fluids) are collected at various time points and analyzed to understand how the drug is processed within the body. The procedure is similar to SAD, but with multiple doses. In addition to SAD and MAD, a study for food effects may also be conducted, which is designed to investigate any differences in absorption of the drug by the body caused by eating before the drug is given. These studies are usually run as crossover studies, with volunteers being given two identical doses of the drug on different occasions, one after fasting, and one after being fed.

Phase II Trial

Once the initial safety of the study drug has been confirmed in Phase I trials, Phase II trials are performed on larger groups (20–300) and are designed to assess how well the drug works, as well as to continue Phase I safety assessments in a larger group of patients (Figure 3.7). In Phase I, we have determined the dose range that will produce some biological effects with tolerable side effects. In Phase II, the dose range will be further identified to the level that it can generate clinical effects but safety issues are still manageable. Therefore, the endpoints are usually clinical endpoints instead of biomarker or PD markers.

Phase II studies are sometimes divided into Phase IIA and Phase IIB. Phase IIA is specifically designed to assess dosing requirements (how much drug should be given), whereas Phase IIB is specifically designed to study efficacy (how well the drug works at the prescribed dose(s)).

Many drug programs are killed in Phase II because the next phase (Phase III) is a huge resource and time commitment. Unless it has shown evidence that the test drug is safe and efficacious enough to warrant for further study, the sponsor won't go forward with a Phase III trial.

Phase III

A Phase III study is usually a randomized controlled multicenter trial on large patient groups (300–10,000) and is aimed at being the definitive assessment of how effective the drug is, in comparison with current 'gold standard' treatment. Because of their size and comparatively long duration, Phase III trials are the most expensive, time-consuming, and difficult trials to design and run (the cost for a typical oncology trial is over $50k per patient). Results from Phase III trials (usually required two) are the basis for drug approval for marketing (Figure 3.8).

Upon completion of Phase III trials, efficacy and safety results are presented in a so-called integrated efficacy summary (IES or ISE), which includes the analysis of all the efficacy data from all trials for the NME, and an integrated safety summary (ISS), which includes all the safety data regarding the NME. These integrated results as well as other documents are organized according to ICH guidance — NDA (New Drug Application) Package Insert — and submitted to the regulatory agency for approval. In the United States, after a 10-month review process, the sponsor will receive a response from the FDA regarding their NDA. The FDA response letter can be of three possible types: (1) approval for marketing the drug, (2) application denied, and (3) incomplete response — request for more information.

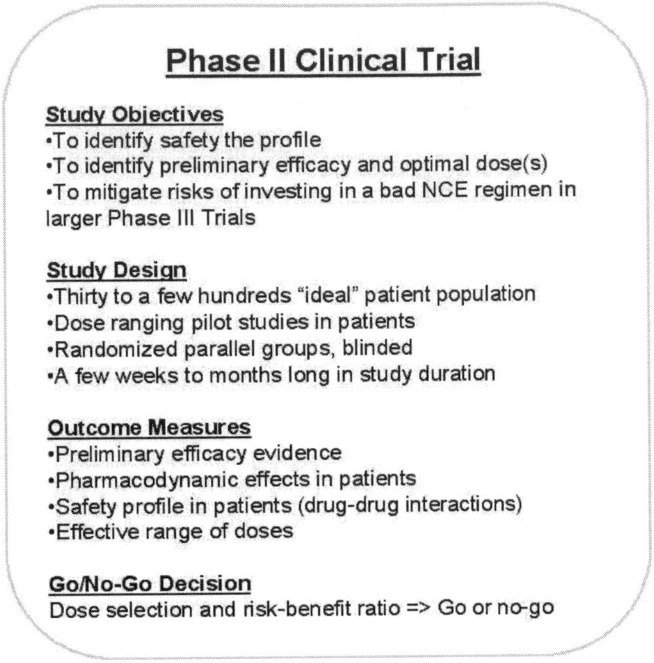

Figure 3.7:   Phase II Clinical Trial

Phase IV Trial

After drug approval, a Phase IV trial may be conducted. A Phase IV trial is sometimes called a post-marketing surveillance trial. Phase IV trials involve safety surveillance (pharmacovigilance) and ongoing technical support of a drug after it receives permission to be sold. Phase IV studies may be required by regulatory authorities because of potential long-term safety concerns or for label extension (e.g., extend the use for the pediatric population). Safety surveillance is designed to detect any rare or long-term adverse effects over a much larger patient population and longer time period than was possible during Phase I–III clinical trials. Harmful effects discovered by Phase IV trials may result in a drug being no longer sold, or restricted to certain uses (Figure 3.9).

3.4.3   *Adaptive Trial Design*

In recent years, the cost drug development increased dramatically, but the success rate of new drug applications (NDAs) remained low. The phamaceu-

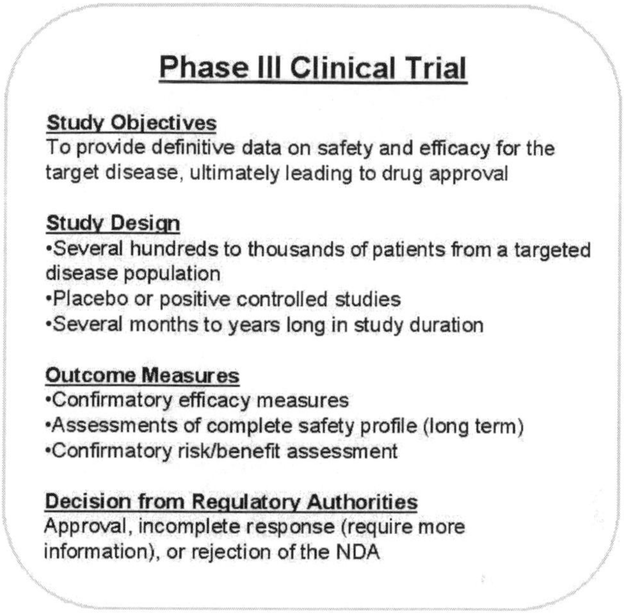

Phase III Clinical Trial

<u>Study Objectives</u>
To provide definitive data on safety and efficacy for the target disease, ultimately leading to drug approval

<u>Study Design</u>
•Several hundreds to thousands of patients from a targeted disease population
•Placebo or positive controlled studies
•Several months to years long in study duration

<u>Outcome Measures</u>
•Confirmatory efficacy measures
•Assessments of complete safety profile (long term)
•Confirmatory risk/benefit assessment

<u>Decision from Regulatory Authorities</u>
Approval, incomplete response (require more information), or rejection of the NDA

Figure 3.8:   Phase III Clinical Trial

tical industry devotes great effort to innovative approaches, especially in adaptive design. An adaptive design is a clinical trial design that allows adaptations or modifications to aspects of the trial after its initiation without undermining the validity and integrity of the trial (Chang 2007b). The adaptation can be based on internal or external information about the trial.

The purposes of adaptive design trials are to increase the probability of success, reduce the cost and the time to market, and deliver the right drug to the right patient.

3.4.4   *Clinical Trial Protocol*

A clinical trial protocol, developed by the sponsor and approved by an investigational review board (an external experts panel) and the FDA, is a document about the trial design and conduct. To protect trial validity and integrity, good clinical practice (GCP) requires that all study investigators adhere to the protocol in conducting the clinical trial.

The protocol describes the scientific rationale, objective(s), endpoints for efficacy and safety evaluations, test drug and its competitor, if any, dose regimen, randomization, assessment schedule, data collection, size of the trial, and statistical considerations. The protocol contains a precise

Figure 3.9:   Phase IV Clinical Trial

study plan for executing the clinical trial, not only to ensure the safety and health of the trial subjects, but also to provide an exact template for trial conduct by investigators to perform the study in a consistent way. This harmonization allows data to be combined collectively through all investigators. The protocol also gives the study monitors as well as the site team of physicians, nurses, and clinic administrators a common reference document for site responsibilities during the trial (www.wikipedia.org).

The format and content of clinical trial protocols sponsored by industries in the United States, European Union, Japan, or Canada should follow the ICH (International Conference on Harmonization) guidelines.

3.5   Summary

Drug development processes are divided into drug discovery, preclinical, and clinical development. A successful development program will lead to drug approval and commercialization.

The objective of drug discovery is to identify and optimize new molecular entities. There are traditional irrational approaches and rational approaches. Pharmaceutical and biotech companies use more and more rational approaches than irrational approaches thanks to advancements in genomics, molecular and systems biology, computational chemistry, and bioinformatics in general. In Chapter 9 (Molecular Design and Simulation) and Chapter 10 (Disease Modeling and Biological Pathway Simulation), we will discuss simulation approaches in drug development, an emerging area in the rational drug discovery paradigm.

When a leading compound is identified and confirmed, further *in vitro* and *in vivo* tests of the NCE will be conducted in the preclinical phase to optimize properties. Preclinical research is often called pharmacology study and includes pharmacokinetics, pharmacodynamics, and toxicology. Pharmacokinetics is the study of drug absorption, distribution, metabolism, and excretion (AMDE). Pharmacodynamics is the study of the biochemical and physiological effects of drugs on the body. In laymen's terms, pharmacokinetics is the study of what the body does to the drug, whereas pharmacodynamics is the study of what a drug does to the body. Toxicological studies explore the functional and morphological effects of the drug, including the mode, site, and degree of action, dose relationship, sex differences, latency and progression, and reversibility of these effects.

Clinical development traditionally includes Phase I to Phase IV clinical trials. Clinical trials are experiments of the test drug conducted on human subjects in accordance with good clinical practice (GCP) in the United States issued by the FDA. Phase I trials are usually conducted on a small group of healthy volunteers. The objectives of a Phase I trial are typically to assess the safety, tolerability, pharmacokinetics, and pharmacodynamics of a drug in humans. Successful Phase I trials will lead to a further test of the NCE in a Phase II trial with an increased sample size to identify the safety profile, preliminary efficacy, and optimal dose range, and to mitigate risks of investing an ineffective NCE on a large scale. If the Phase II results show the test drug is safe and efficacious enough to warrant further study, Phase III trials are launched with the objective of providing definitive trial data regarding the safety and efficacy for the target indication. The size of the populations in the trials, or sample size, should be sufficiently large so that there are adequate probabilities (power) to demonstrate statistical significance if the test drug in fact is effective. Successful Phase III trials lead ultimately to drug approval and commercialization. However, a Phase IV trial sometimes may be conducted as a requirement for conditional regulatory approval or for label extension.

3.6   Exercises

Exercise 3.1: Do a 15-minute verbal presentation to your colleague about drug development with or without Microsoft PowerPoint slides.

Exercise 3.2: How long is a typical drug development cycle and what is the cost? What are the basic differences between pharmaceuticals and biopharmaceuticals (biologics)?

Exercise 3.3: Why are potency and specificity important for an NCE?

Exercise 3.4: What are the mechanisms of most drugs? What are the five main categories of drug actions?

Exercise 3.5: What does therapeutic index measure? Why is a high value of the index desirable? What is the standard safety margin (SSM)? Can an NCE have a high therapeutic index but a low SSM value?

Exercise 3.6: Describe AMDE. What do $C_{\max}$, $t_{\max}$, and $t_{1/2}$ stand for?

Exercise 3.7: Explain the terms carcinogenicity, genotoxicity, and reproductive toxicity.

Exercise 3.8: What is a clinical trial? Why does sample size gradually increase from Phase I to Phase III?

Exercise 3.9: What are the differences between SAD and MAD? What are the differences between Phase IIA and IIB trials?

Exercise 3.10: What is clinical trial protocol? What is it for and what are its key elements? What is the ICH guideline?

Chapter 4

Meta-Simulation for the Pharmaceutical Industry

This chapter will cover the following topics:

- Introduction
- Game Theory Basics
- Pharmaceutical Games
- Prescription Drug Global Pricing

4.1 Introduction

4.1.1 *Characteristics of Meta-Simulation*

Simulation in drug development can be classified into three categories dependent on the subject scales: *meta-simulation*, *macro-simulation*, and *micro-simulation*.

Meta-simulation is a Monte Carlo method that concerns the bird's eye view and its dynamics of the subject field. Meta-simulation in the pharmaceutical industry usually involves more than one independent business entity or company. The granularity of simulation at this meta level is most obvious. Uncertainties in information for building the simulation model are high. Simulation results are quantitative, but the interpretation often leans forward more or less qualitatively. Theoretical approaches such as game theory used in meta-simulation are similar to those used in economics (macroeconomics and microeconomics). Therefore, a brief review of basic concepts of economics and pharmacoeconomics is beneficial.

4.1.2 *Macroeconomics*

Macroeconomics is a branch of economics that deals with the performance, structure, and behavior of a national or regional economy as a whole by using aggregated indicators such as GDP, unemployment rates, and price indices to understand how the whole economy functions. Modeling and simulation are the fundamental tools used to explain the relationship between such factors as national income, output, consumption, unemployment, inflation, savings, investment, international trade, and international finance. The dynamics of macroeconomics involve many entities, including workforce market, household, government, corporation, financial market, commodity market, and foreign, as depicted in Figure 4.1.

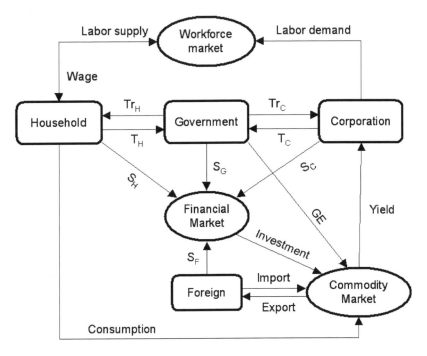

S: Saving, **T**: Tax, **Tr**: Transfer, **GE**: Government expenditures

Figure 4.1:   Circulation in Macroeconomics (www.wikipedia.org)

Classical economists, such as Irving Fisher, assumed that real income and the velocity of money would be static in the short-run; thus a change in price level could only be brought about by a change in money supply. Money supply (M) times the velocity of money (V, how quickly cash is passed from one person to another through a series of transactions) is equivalent to price-level (P) times "quantity of goods and services produced (Q)," i.e.,

$$M \cdot V = P \cdot Q.$$

Until the 1930s, most economic analysis did not separate out individual behavior from aggregate behavior. Starting in the 1950s, macroeconomists developed micro-based models of macroeconomic behavior, such as the consumption function — Keynesianism. The main distinction between the two different approaches is that Keynesian economics focuses on demand and neoclassical economics is based on rational expectations and efficient markets. In the 1970s new classical macroeconomics challenged Keynesians to ground their macroeconomic theory in microeconomics and emphasize monetary policy, such as interest rates and money supply. To the pharmaceutical and health industries, the Keynesian approach is essential methodologically, but policy can also have significant impact. The magnitude of such an impact varies from country to country.

4.1.3 *Microeconomics*

In contrast to macroeconomics, *microeconomics* is primarily focused on the actions of individual agents, such as firms and consumers, and how their behavior determines prices and quantities in specific markets.

Microeconomics studies how households and firms make decisions to allocate limited resources in markets where goods or services are being bought and sold. It also investigates how these decisions on supply-demand chains affect prices. One of the goals of microeconomics is to model market failure (failure to produce efficient results) and describe the conditions needed for perfect competition. An important task of microeconomics is the analysis of market equilibrium. Market equilibrium is reached when quantity demanded is equal to quantity supplied. The equilibrium price (the price for a good at equilibrium) changes whenever the supply or demand curve shifts.

The well-known principle of supply and demand assumes that markets are perfectly competitive (Figure 4.2), i.e., there are many buyers and sellers in the market and none of them has the capacity to significantly influence the prices of goods and services. The demand for various commodities by individuals can be deemed as the outcome of a utility-maximizing process. The interpretation of this relationship between price and quantity demanded of a given good is that the set of choices is the one which makes the consumer happiest.

There are many different approaches to study microeconomics. One of the most widely used is game theory, which will also be used in the rest of the sections in combination with Monte Carlo methods.

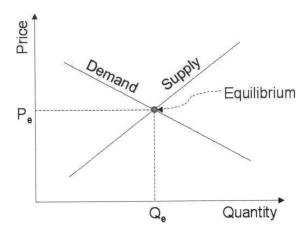

Market equilibrium: When price is established (Pe)
where quantity demanded = quantity supplied.

Figure 4.2:   Market Equilibrium

4.1.4   *Health Economics and Pharmacoeconomics*

Health economics is a branch of economics concerned with issues related to scarcity in the allocation of health and healthcare. Health economics adopts and applies principles and methodologies of economics to healthcare.

Pharmacoeconomics (Walley et al., 2004), a sub-discipline of health economics, refers to the scientific discipline that compares the value of one pharmaceutical drug or drug therapy to another. A pharmacoeconomic study evaluates the cost and effects of a pharmaceutical product. Commonly used approaches in pharmacoeconomic evaluation include *cost-minimization analysis, cost-benefit analysis, cost-effectiveness analysis*, and *cost-utility analysis.* All these analyses are measured in money.

Cost minimization is applied when comparing two drugs of equal efficacy and equal tolerability. Cost-effectiveness analysis compares the relative expenditure (costs) and outcomes (effects) of two or more courses of action. Cost-benefit analysis is used to help appraise, or assess, the case for a project or proposal for guiding decision making. Cost-utility analysis is similar to cost-effectiveness analysis in that there is a defined outcome, and the cost to reach that outcome is measured in money.

Pharmacoeconomics is important to health policy makers and regulatory agencies because pharmacoeconomic studies serve to guide optimal healthcare resource allocation, in a standardized and scientifically grounded manner. Pharmacoeconomics is also interesting to the pharmaceutical industry because pharmacoeconomic studies guide their drug development and allocate more resources for developing cost-effective drugs.

4.1.5 *Profitability of the Pharmaceutical Industry*

As investors, you will be concerned with how profitable the pharmaceutical industry is before you decide to invest. As health policy makers and patients, you may be concerned that high profitability in the industry may lead to unreasonably high drug prices. Indeed, a study shows (Pearlman, 2007) that Big Pharma has consistently been the single most profitable industry of all 47 represented in the Fortune 500 (Figure 4.3).

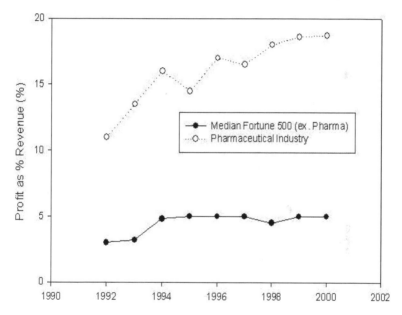

Figure 4.3:   Big Pharma's Relative Profitability
(Data source: Pearlman, 2007)

However, this kind of comparison may not be very informative. As we know, investment in pharmaceutical Research and Development has a high risk. The success rate in the pharmaceutical industry is very low: there are many failures and bankruptcies; only a small proportion of NMEs can make it all the way to marketing. Profitability for successful Big Pharmas is naturally higher. Just like playing the lotteries, if the profitability is calculated based on the winners, it will be much higher than that for the pharmaceutical industry. However, the expected profit of playing the lottery is negative.

To make appropriate drug price policy, it is essential to understand the cost for pharmaceutical Research and Development. Unlike other Research and Development intensive industries, drug companies are allowed to deduct Research and Development expenses for tax purposes and are generously awarded tax credits by governments in nearly all jurisdictions (Pearlman, 2007).

A research study conducted by Tufts University shows the average cost per new drug to be $802M. The study was based on company provided data on a select group of 68 unnamed drugs over a 10 year period. The study included an "opportunity cost," which is defined as the amount a drug manufacturer would have otherwise earned had the money been invested in government bonds. This studied was criticized for its "bias" and inclusion of opportunity loss. Another study performed by Public Citizen (a watchdog group) shows that the average cost is under $400M for drugs approved between 1994 and 2000. When the "me-too" drugs were included, this value dropped to less than $100M (after tax) (Pearlman, 2007).

In my view, first, the cost that includes opportunity-loss provides the bottom line for price determination, i.e., the return on investment in government bonds. Second, calculating the cost for a new drug cannot be simply an aggregation of the cost that is directly related to an NME. In reality, before successfully finding a drug, there were many compound studies that failed. The costs of those studies should be considered in determining the drug price. Third, many biotech and pharmaceutical companies will go out of business before making any drug; those investment losses should also be included in price determination. The estimation of the average cost of $400M for the directly related cost is not very helpful in determining the drug price. We can use the lottery for an analogy again — it is irrational to complain of a lottery winner taking too much profit without considering there are thousands of losers.

A logical approach to calculate the profitability for investment in an industry sector should be the ratio of the total profit of the sector divided by the total amount of investment in the sector, including the investment loss due to bankruptcy in the sector.

If one sector is more profitable than others, there will be more investment moved into the sector in a completely competitive environment. Monopoly by a small group of Big Pharmas may make competition difficult for small new biotech companies, but so far there are still plenty of risk takers willing to invest in the sector despite extremely low success rates. My point is that profitability can be calculated in different ways; extreme caution should be used when interpreting its meaning. Let me elaborate on this by discussing the following two relevant questions:

(1) Does technology innovation make Pharma more profitable?
(2) Dose shortening time-to-market make Pharma more profitable?

The answers to these questions may surprise you.

Drugs must be made available at affordable prices so they are within the financial reach of healthcare services and individuals in need. It is one of the crucial conditions to ensure access to essential drugs (Health Action International, 2000).

A major proportion of the cost in pharmaceutical Research and Development is in the employee compensation. If technology innovations result in more drugs developed in a shorter time, but not a reduced workforce, as has happened in the past 15 years, then the technology innovations will not make Pharma, as a whole, more profitable. This is because the maximum medical cost (as a percentage of individual income S) a person can afford is more or less a fixed number, denoted by p_{max}. Maximum drug sales is $p_{max}SN$, where N is the population size. If the pharmaceutical workforce consists of M full time employees with compensation X per person, then the profit is ($p_{max}SN - MX$) — other costs have been neglected for simplicity, but that does not invalidate the point I am going to make here. Therefore, the smaller the pharmaceutical workforce M is, the bigger the potential profitability will be. Shortening time-to-market can only make that individual drug company more profitable. However, if every company shortens its development time, it will not make any drug company richer — any drug cannot stay on top of the market for long. Nevertheless, due to market competition, technology innovation will greatly impact the redistribution of profitability among pharmaceutical companies, even if it cannot make Pharma more profitable as a whole. This phenomenon is a macro consequence caused by micro-motivated behaviors of individuals or individual companies. This may also partially explain why drug companies have merged frequently in the past decade, i.e., to reduce workforce M. We will discuss more about pharmaceutical partnerships and mergers later in this chapter. We will study the best strategies for individual companies that have different market positions — the queuing game.

4.2   Game Theory Basics

A game is a formal description of a strategic situation. *Game theory* is the formal study of decision making where several players must make choices that potentially affect the interests of the other players. A player is an agent who makes decisions in a game.

Game theory is a distinct and interdisciplinary approach to the study of human behavior. Game theory addresses serious interactions using the metaphor of a game: in these serious interactions, the individual's choice is essentially a choice of a strategy, and the outcome of the interaction depends on the strategies chosen by each of the participants. The significance of game theory is dignified by the three Nobel Prizes: 1994 to Nash, Selten, and Harsanyi, 2005 to Aumann and Schelling, and 2007 to Maskin and Myerson, whose work is largely about game theory.

Most game theories assume three conditions: *common knowledge, perfect information,* and *rationality.* Common knowledge: a fact is common knowledge if all players know it, and know that they all know it, and so on. The structure of the game is often assumed to be common knowledge among the players. Perfect information: a game has perfect information when at any point in time only one player makes a move and knows all the actions that have been made until then. Rationality: a player is said to be rational if he seeks to play in a manner which maximizes his own payoff. It is often assumed that the rationality of all players is common knowledge. A payoff is a number, also called utility, which reflects the desirability of an outcome to a player, for whatever reason. When the outcome is random, payoffs are usually weighted with their associated probabilities. Note that the expected payoff incorporates the player's attitude toward risk.

4.2.1   *Prisoners' Dilemma*

Tucker's Prisoners' Dilemma is one of the most influential examples in economics and social sciences. It is stated like this: two criminals, Bob and John, are captured at the scene. Each has to choose whether or not to confess and implicate the other. If neither man confesses, then both will serve two years. If both confess, they will go to prison for 10 years each. However, if one of them confesses and implicates the other, and the other does not confess, the one who has collaborated with the police will go free, while the other will go to prison for 20 years on the maximum charge.

The strategies offered in this case are: confess or don't confess. The payoffs or penalties are the sentences served. We can express all this in a standard *payoff table* in game theory (Table 4.1).

Table 4.1: The Prisoners' Dilemma

		John	
		confess	don't
Bob	confess	10, 10	0, 20
	don't	20, 0	2, 2

How to solve this game? Assume they both are "rational" and try to minimize the time they spend in jail. Bob might reason as follows: "If John confesses, I will get 20 years if I don't confess and 10 years if I do, so in that case it's best to confess. On the other hand, if John doesn't confess, I will go free if I confess and get 2 years if I don't confess. Therefore, either way, it's better (best) if I confess. John reasons in the same way. Therefore, they both confess and get 10 years. This is the solution or equilibrium for the game.

4.2.2 Extensive Form

An extensive form of a game describes with a tree how a game is played. It depicts the order in which players make moves and the information each player has at each decision point. Figure 4.4 is the extensive form of the prisoners' dilemma.

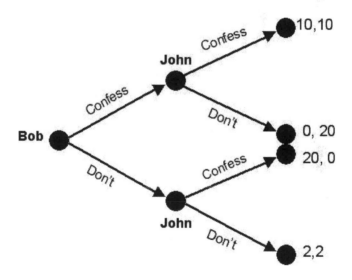

Figure 4.4: Extensive Form of the Prisoners' Game

A game in *strategic form*, also called normal form, is a compact representation of a game, in which players simultaneously choose their strategies. The resulting payoffs are presented in a table with a cell for each strategy combination. Both the extensive form and table form are the normal form of the game.

A *Strategy Tree/Form* (Watson, 2008) has the following properties: (1) every node except the initial node is a successor of the initial node; (2) each node except the initial node has exactly one immediate predecessor; (3) multiple branches extending from the same node have different action labels; (4) each label on a decision node indicates the decision maker and the directed arcs from the node indicate the options provided to the player.

Definition 4.1   Strategy: A strategy is a complete contingent plan for a player in the game.

A typical strategy profile is a vector of strategies $s = (s_1, ...s_n)$, where s_i is the strategy of player i $(i = 1, ..., n)$ and $S = S_1 \times S_2 \times ... \times S_n$ is often used to denote the set of strategy profiles.

A two-person win-lose game can be played on a so-called graph $G = (X, F)$ by stipulating a starting position $x_0 \in X$ and using the following rules:

(1) Player I moves first, starting at x_0.

(2) Players alternate moves.

(3) At position x, the player whose turn it is to move chooses a position $y \in F(x)$.

(4) The player who is confronted with a terminal position at his turn, and thus cannot move, loses.

Definition 4.2   Directed graph: A directed graph is a pair (X, F) where X is a nonempty set of vertices (positions) and F is a function that gives for each $x \in X$ a subset of X, $F(x) \subset X$. For a given $x \in X$, $F(x)$ represents the positions to which a player may move from x (called the followers of x). If $F(x)$ is empty, x is called a terminal position.

A game can often be solved (i.e., how the game will play out) using so-called backward induction.

Definition 4.3   Backward induction: Backward induction is a technique to solve a game of perfect information. It first considers the moves that are the last in the game and determines the best move for the player in each case. Then, taking these as given future actions, it proceeds backwards in time, again determining the best move for the respective player, until the beginning of the game is reached.

4.2.3   *Nash Equilibrium*

In the Prisoners' Dilemma, we have mentioned that {confess, confess} is the equilibrium of the game. We now introduce its formal definition and a relevant term, dominating strategy.

Definition 4.4 Dominating strategy: A strategy dominates another strategy of a player if it always gives a better payoff to that player than other strategies he may take, regardless of what the other players are doing. It weakly dominates the other strategy if it is always at least as good.

Definition 4.5 Dominant strategy equilibrium: If, in a game, each player has a dominant strategy, and each player plays the dominant strategy, then that combination of (dominant) strategies and the corresponding payoffs are said to constitute the dominant strategy equilibrium for that game.

In the Prisoners' Dilemma game, to confess is a dominant strategy, and when both prisoners confess, that is a dominant strategy equilibrium. This is a remarkable result: individual rational action results in both persons being made worse off in terms of their own self-interested purposes. This is what has made the widest impact in modern social science. Just as McCain (McCain, 2009) pointed out: For there are many interactions in the modern world that seem very much like that, from arms races through road congestion and pollution to the depletion of fisheries and the overexploitation of some subsurface water resources. These are all quite different interactions in detail, but are interactions in which (we suppose) individual rational action leads to inferior results for each person, and the Prisoners' Dilemma suggests something of what is going on in each of them.

Among various types of games, a simple and well-studied type of game is the so-called zero-sum game. A zero-sum game is a game in which one player's winnings equal the other player's losses. Bear in mind that the definition requires a zero-sum for every set of strategies (one from each player); if there is even one strategy set for which the sum differs from zero, then the game is not zero-sum.

Definition 4.6 Zero-sum game: If we add up the wins and losses in a game, treating losses as negatives, and we find that the sum is zero for each set of strategies chosen, then the game is a "zero-sum game."

Note that it is mathematically equivalent between "zero-sum" and "constant-sum" for every set of strategies.

Theorem 4.1 *Maximin criterion (von Neumann, 1966): Every two-person zero-sum game has a maximin solution. For a two-person, zero-sum game it is rational for each player to choose the strategy that maximizes the minimum payoff, and the pair of strategies and payoffs such that each player maximizes her minimum payoff is the "solution to the game."*

If we are not considering the thrill of gambling and the pleasure of the social event, gambling can be considered a zero-sum game. However, when we take those rewards into account, even gambling games may not be zero-sum. An important concept in solving a game, whether it is zero-sum or not, is the so-called Nash equilibrium: If there is a set of strategies with the property that no player can benefit by changing her strategy while the other players keep their strategies unchanged, then that set of strategies and the corresponding payoffs constitute the Nash equilibrium. The Nash equilibrium is a pretty simple idea: we have a Nash equilibrium if each participant chooses the best strategy, given the strategy chosen by the other participants.

Definition 4.7   A strategy profile $s \in S$ is a **Nash equilibrium** if and only if $u_i(s_i, s_{-i}) \geq u_i\left(s_i', s_{-i}\right)$ for each $s_i' \in S_i$ and each player i, where s_{-i} is the collective strategies by others.

Any dominant strategy equilibrium is also a Nash equilibrium. The Nash equilibrium is an extension of the concepts of dominant strategy equilibrium and of the maximin solution for zero-sum games.

4.2.4   *Mixed Strategy*

So far we have discussed the *pure game*, where there is no probability involved regarding strategy selection. However, in reality there are other games called mixed strategy where the player's knowledge about strategy selection involves probability distribution. Let's discuss the prisoners' game again.

The Prisoners' Dilemma is very simplified and unrealistic for the following reasons: (1) there are usually more than two players; (2) there can be communication between the players who commit themselves to coordinated strategies; (3) the two prisoners interact only once; repetition of the interactions might lead to quite different results; (4) common knowledge assumptions may not be true in most situations; (5) most strategies in real life are adaptive and adaptations take time and rely on the credibility of the relevant information. Compelling as the reasoning that leads to the dominant strategy equilibrium may be, it is not the only way this problem might be reasoned out. Perhaps it is not really the most rational answer after all; (6) games are carried out on the basis of perceptions, not reality, but reality will adjust the players' perceptions over time; and finally (7) the players' subjective attitudes toward risk, i.e., their risk aversion, will play a critical role in the decision making about strategies.

To elaborate reason 6, each player's action is based on his perception about reality, but not the reality itself. In the prison dilemma, Bob may think this way: "John is 10 years younger and healthier than me; having the same term of sentence implies different losses to him than me; the years of sentence should be weighted." However, John may think differently than what Bob thinks he would think. John may think: "Bob is richer but older; a 10 year could mean the rest of his life. Therefore Bob would be indifferent between sentencing for 10 or 20 years, but he would strongly prefer a 2 year sentence."

We can describe such situations using probability tables to include the information: Bob's perception about probabilistic realities (the joined actions with associated consequences), John's probabilistic actions based on John's view about both the reality and Bob's possible actions. Bob takes the action to maximize his expected payoff. John has similar logical thinking and takes action accordingly.

Definition 4.8 Mixed strategy: If a player in a game chooses among two or more strategies randomly according to specific probabilities, this choice is called a mixed strategy.

The game of matching pennies has a solution in mixed strategies. The game rules are: the two players involved show their pennies at the same time; if both are heads or tails, player A wins; if one is a head and one is a tail, player B wins. In such a game, neither player wants his opponent to know what to show. In other words, they both should randomly choose heads or tails with an equal probability of 0.5.

Definition 4.9 Mixed-strategy Nash equilibrium: Consider a strategy profile $\sigma = (\sigma_1, ..., \sigma_n)$, where $\sigma_i \in S_i$ for each player i. Profile σ is a mixed-strategy Nash equilibrium if and only if $u_i(\sigma_i, \sigma_{-i}) \geq u_i(s'_i, \sigma_{-i})$ for each $s'_i \in S_i$ and each player i. That is, σ_i is a best response to σ_{-i} for every player i.

Theorem 4.2 *(Nash, 1951) Every finite pure or mixed game with a finite number of players and a finite strategy space has at least one Nash equilibrium.*

Definition 4.10 Sequential rationality. An optimal strategy for a player should maximize his or her expected payoff, conditional on every information set at which this player has the move. That is, player i's strategy should specify an optimal action from each player i's information sets, even those that player i does not believe will be treated in the game.

4.2.5 *Game with Multiple Options*

A legendary Chinese horse race problem, known as "Tianji's Horse Race," involving the King of Qi Kingdom and his General Tianji, took place more than 2000 years ago. In the game, the King wanted to race his horses with those of Tianji's. The King and Tianji each selected in turn three horses with different speed classes. The King's horses were labeled K_1, K_2, and K_3; Tianji's horses, T_1, T_2, and T_3. It is common knowledge to both the King and the General that

$$K_1 \succ T_1 \succ K_2 \succ T_2 \succ K_3 \succ T_3, \tag{4.1}$$

where the symbol "$\succ$" denotes the relation "faster than."

In the first sequence of three games, K_1 against T_1, K_2 against T_2, and K_3 against T_3, Tainji lost the games for the obvious reason. However, in the second sequence of games, Tianji took the advice of Sun Bin, a respected philosopher and a military strategist, and used the sequence (T_3, T_1, T_2) because Sun Bin knew the King would use the same sequence (K_1, K_2, K_3) again. This time, Tianji won the race with one loss and two wins.

Let's use modern game theory to analyze the problem. To facilitate the analysis, we can reduce any constant-sum game to a zero-sum game by simply subtracting the constant-sum c from Tianji's payoffs and solve the problem as a zero-sum game in terms of the King's payoffs (Leng and Parlar, 2006). Let's formulate and analyze a sequence of three games with one-unit payoff for the winner.

Player K (or T) makes a decision on the sequence of his horses for the three races. Thus, for each player there are $3! = 6$ horse sequences (strategies): $S_1^K = (K_1, K_2, K_3)$, $S_2^K = (K_1, K_3, K_2)$, $S_3^K = (K_2, K_1, K_3)$, $S_4^K = (K_2, K_3, K_1)$, $S_5^K = (K_3, K_1, K_2)$, and $S_6^K = (K_3, K_2, K_1)$ for the player K and $S_1^T = (T_1, T_2, T_3)$, $S_2^T = (T_1, T_3, T_2)$, $S_3^T = (T_2, T_1, T_3)$, $S_4^T = (T_2, T_3, T_1)$, $S_5^T = (T_3, T_1, T_2)$, and $S_6^T = (T_3, T_2, T_1)$ for player T.

The King's payoff for the sequence S_2^K versus S_1^T is 1 and his payoff for S_3^K versus S_2^T is 0, and so on. The payoff matrix for the King (row player) can be formulated as:

$$A = \begin{bmatrix} 1 & 1 & 1 & 1 & 0 & 1 \\ 1 & 1 & 1 & 1 & 1 & 0 \\ 1 & 0 & 1 & 1 & 1 & 1 \\ 0 & 1 & 1 & 1 & 1 & 1 \\ 1 & 1 & 1 & 0 & 1 & 1 \\ 1 & 1 & 0 & 1 & 1 & 1 \end{bmatrix} \tag{4.2}$$

To solve the problem, we need the following two theorems.

Theorem 4.3 *The Equilibrium Theorem (Ferguson, 1996). Consider a game with $m \times n$ payoff matrix and value V. Let $\boldsymbol{p} = (p_1, ..., p_m)^T$ be any optimal strategy for Player A and $\boldsymbol{q} = (q_1, ..., q_n)^T$ be any optimal strategy* *for Player B. Then*

$$\sum_{j=1}^{n} a_{ij} q_j = V, \quad \text{for all } i \text{ for which } p_i > 0 \qquad (4.3)$$

and

$$\sum_{i=1}^{m} a_{ij} q_i = V, \quad \text{for all } j \text{ for which } q_j > 0. \qquad (4.4)$$

Proof. Suppose there is a k such that $p_k > 0$ and $\sum_{j=1} a_{kj} q_j \neq V$. Then $\sum_{j=1}^{n} a_{kj} q_j < V$. Then

$$V = \sum_{i=1}^{m} p_i \left(\sum_{j=1}^{n} a_{ij} q_j \right) < \sum_{i=1}^{m} p_i V = V. \qquad (4.5)$$

The inequality is strict since it is strict for the kth term of the sum. This contradiction proves the first conclusion. The second conclusion can be proved in a similar way. $\qquad\qquad\square$

Theorem 4.4 *(Dresher, 1961, p. 43). Suppose all pure strategies for each player in a two-person zero-sum matrix game are active (i.e., no dominance or saddle point exists in the game) and the matrix of the game is square and nonsingular. Then a unique optimal mixed strategy for each player can be computed using*

$$q^* = \frac{\left(A' \right)^{-1} 1}{1' A^{-1} 1} \text{ and } p^* = \frac{A^{-1} 1}{1' A^{-1} 1} \qquad (4.6)$$

where $A = \{a_{ij}\}_{n \times n}$ is a nonsingular matrix of the game, $1 = (1, 1, ..., 1)'$ is an $n \times 1$ column vector, and the column vectors q^* and p^* are the optimal mixed strategies for the players with row and column strategies in the matrix game, respectively. The value of the game to the row player using q^* is $u = 1' A^{-1} 1$.

One way of saying this theorem is that Player A searches for a strategy that makes Player B indifferent as to which of the (good) pure strategies to use. Similarly, Player B should play in such a way as to make Player A indifferent among his (good) strategies. This is called the *Principle of Indifference.*

We now can solve the horse-racing problem by substituting matrix A (4.2) into (4.6). The result is the optimal mixed strategy for both the King and Tianji with $p^* = q^* = (1/6, 1/6, 1/6, 1/6, 1/6'6)'$, i.e., equal probability of choosing each of the 6 sequences (pure strategies). The expected value of the game is $u_K = 1'^T A^{-1} 1 = 5/6$ for the King and $u_T = 1 - 5/6 = 1/6$ for Tianji.

For more results about this game, please see the research paper by Leng and Parlar (2006).

4.2.6   Oligopoly Model

We have seen that it is not difficult to find the Nash equilibrium in a matrix game. In fact, computing equilibria of games with infinite strategy space is not difficult. We need only to compute the optimal response mappings for each player and then determine which strategy profiles, if any, satisfy all simultaneously. Let's look into the following duopoly model.

When a drug patent expires, generic versions of the drug can be produced by other companies without paying a penny of royalty. Suppose both the brand drug maker (company B) and a generic drug maker (company G) want to determine the optimal levels of production so that their profit can be maximized. Assume the price is a function of the drug quantities produced. Specifically, the prices for the branded drug and the generic version are $p_B = 1100 - Q_B - 0.8Q_G$ and $p_G = 1000 - 0.8Q_B - Q_G$, respectively (we see there is a slight difference in price between the branded and the generic), where Q_B and Q_G are the quantities produced by companies B and G, respectively. The costs for manufacturing the two versions of the drug are presumably the same, \$100 per unit. Therefore, the net profit for company B is

$$u_B (Q_B, Q_G) = (1100 - Q_B - 0.8Q_G - 100) Q_B \qquad (4.7)$$

and the net profit for company G is

$$u_G (Q_B, Q_G) = (1000 - 0.8Q_B - Q_G - 100) Q_G. \qquad (4.8)$$

To maximize $u_B (Q_B, Q_G)$ in (4.7), take the partial derivative with respect to Q_B, and set it equal to zero

$$1000 - 2Q_B - 0.8Q_G = 0. \qquad (4.9)$$

Similarly, to maximize $u_G (Q_B, Q_G)$, we have

$$900 - 0.8Q_B - 2Q_G = 0. \qquad (4.10)$$

Solving (4.9) and (4.10) for Q_B and Q_G simultaneously, we obtain

$$Q_B = 381 \text{ and } Q_G = 298$$

Therefore, company B should produce 389 units and company G should produce 298 units. However, is this the optimal solution in the sense of a *cooperative game?* The answer is no. We will discuss cooperative games further.

Keep in mind that there are partisan and impartial games. In an impartial game, the set of moves available from any given position is the same for both players, whereas in a partisan game, each player has a different set of possible moves from a given position. Chess is an example of a partisan game. In the real word situations, partisan games are prevalent.

4.2.7 Games with Multiple Equilibria

There are games that have more than one Nash equilibrium point. Here is an example with multiple equilibria. Suppose a biotech company has identified a drug compound that is expected to effectively treat cancer patients with certain genetics or biomarkers. However, there is no commercial screening tool currently available to test the biomarker. Luckily, a diagnostics company has the capability to develop a screening tool. The two companies now face the Go or No-Go decision.

If the biotech company (player A) decides to develop the drug (the Go decision) and the diagnostios company (player B) also decides to develop the screening tool (the Go decision), then if both are approved by the regulatory agency, the drug can be marketed and made available to cancer patients. As a result, the gains for player A and player B are 10 and 5, respectively. If player A chooses "Go" and player B chooses "No-Go," then the drug may be available, but does not have the screening tool to identify the right patients to treat. Therefore, the drug cannot be marketed. In such a case, the payoffs for players A and B are −5 and 0, respectively. Player A has a negative payoff due to the development cost. If player B opts to "Go" and player A opts for "No-Go," then the biomarker patient population can be identified, but no drug is available. Therefore, no one wants to buy the screening tool. The payoffs for A and B are 0 and –3, respectively. If both companies choose "No-Go," then the payoff is zero for both of them. The payoffs are summarized in Table 4.2.

Table 4.2: Payoffs with Multi-Equilibria

		Diagnostics (Player B)	
		Go	No-Go
Biotech	Go	10,5	−5,0
(Player A)	No-Go	0,−3	0,0

There are two Nash equilibria, at the upper left {Go,Go} and the lower right {No-Go, No-Go}. Starting from the upper right, either the column player (B) or the row player (A) will be worse off if he changes strategies unilaterally. Similarly, starting from the lower right, either of the players will be worse off if he changes strategies unilaterally. In either case, they don't want to change unilaterally. In other words, there are two Nash equilibria. However, if communication is allowed so that either of the players can learn immediately when the other player makes a move, then {Go,Go} is the only equilibrium. This is because, under open communication, player A or B is willing to make the first move or Go decision by knowing that the other will immediately follow him and make the same Go decision.

A Nash equilibrium is reached if neither player can be better off by changing strategy unilaterally. However, even though the outcome {No-Go, No-Go} is a Nash equilibrium, it is clearly inferior (Paretian sense, see next section) to {Go, Go}. This illustrates that the game has multiple equilibria, with some equilibria superior to others. It also illustrates the importance of cooperative games: can they make corporative strategies such that they both have better payoffs?

4.2.8   *Cooperative Games*

Games in which the participants cannot make commitments to coordinate their strategies are *noncooperative games*. In a noncooperative game, the rational person's problem is to answer the question "What is the rational choice of a strategy when other players will try to choose their best responses to my strategy?" In contrast, games in which the participants can make commitments to coordinate their strategies are *cooperative games*.

4.2.9   *Pareto Optimum*

In noncooperative games, the solution is from an individual perspective, which often leads to inferior outcomes such as in the Prisoner's Dilemma. It is preferable, in many cases, to define a criterion to rank outcomes for the group of players as a whole. The Pareto criterion is one of this kind: an outcome is better than another if at least one person is better off and no one is worse off. If an outcome cannot be improved upon, i.e., if no one can be made better off without making somebody else worse off, then we say that the outcome is Pareto optimal.

In the real world, a Pareto optimal outcome for a cooperative game is usually not unique or infinite. The set of all Pareto optimal outcomes is called the solution set, which is not very useful in practice. To narrow down the range of possible solutions to a particular price or, more generally, distribution of benefits, is the so-called *bargaining* problem. The range of possible payments might be influenced, and narrowed, by:

- Competitive pressures from other potential suppliers and users
- Perceived fairness
- Bargaining

A group of players who commit themselves to coordinate their strategies is called a coalition. The standard definition of efficient allocation in economics is *Pareto optimality*. In contrast, the allocation is efficient in the Paretian sense if no one can be made better off without making someone else worse off.

An allocation is dominated if some of the members of the coalition can do better for themselves by deserting that coalition for some other coalition.

Definition 4.11 Core: The core of a cooperative game consists of all allocations with the property that no subgroup within the coalition can do better by deserting the coalition.

4.2.10 *Multiple-Player and Queuing Games*

So far our discussions have mainly focused on two-player games. In the real world, there is often a need to consider situations with three or more players. Economic competition and highway congestion are two common examples. When the number of players, N, is larger, we traditionally simplify with some assumptions such as the *representative agent model*, in which we assume that all players are identical, have the same strategy options, and get symmetrical payoffs. We also assume that the payoff to each player depends only on the number of other players who choose each strategy, and not on which agent chooses which strategy. An example of the representative agent model is shown in Figure 4.5, where each investor has to decide whether to invest in inflammation drug or oncology drug development, but the return on investment (ROI) is dependent on the number of investors in the product. In this hypothetical example, at the beginning, the ROI is higher for the oncology drug than for the inflammation drug. When the number of oncology drug investors increases, development gets more expensive and at the same time development of the inflammation drug gets less expensive compared to the oncology drug. Note that when more drugs become available for treating one disease, the chance of having other diseases or dying from other diseases increases. The objective is to maximize the ROI.

Equilibrium is reached at the intersection of the two profit lines in Figure 4.5. From the figure, it is obvious that the first N_c investors will be interested in investing in oncology drugs, but investors who come after will be interested in investing in inflammation drugs.

This is a queuing game, in which multiple players are involved and payoffs are dependent on the order of the player's engagement. Realistically, profit has a probability distribution $f(X, P, N)$, where profit X can be random, and product P and N can be treated as random or fixed factors.

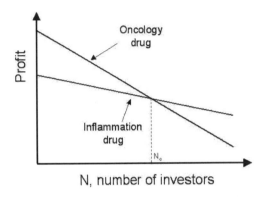

Figure 4.5:   Mechanism of Competition

Here is another example of a queuing game. Suppose there are five customers trying to receive a service. They all want to get the service as early as possible, but at the same time they don't like to stand in line. To quantify, we make the following assumptions that apply to all five players: the gross payoffs and cost of standing depend on the order served as listed in Table 4.3. Net payoffs are the difference between the gross payoff and the cost of standing (Table 4.3).

Table 4.3: Payoff Structures in a Queuing Game

Order served	Gross payoff	Cost of standing	Expected net payoff
1	20	3	17
2	17	3	14
3	14	3	11
4	11	3	8
5	8	3	5

Those who do not stand in line are chosen randomly for service after those who stand in line have been served. Therefore, the expected payoff for anyone not standing in the line is their average gross payoff. The payers' decision on whether to stand in line or not is driven by the maximization of their net payoff. The game can be analyzed as follows:

(1) If no one stands in line, then each person will have an equal probability of being served first, second, ..., and fifth. The expected payoff is $(20+17+14+11+8)/5 = 14$. However, such a case can be improved since an individual can improve his payoff by standing first in line. The net payoff to the person first in line is $(20 - 3) = 17 > 14$, so someone will get up and stand in line.

(2) If no more persons stand in line, the expected payoff is $(17+14+11+8)/4 = 12.5$ for the four remaining. Since the second person in line gets a net payoff of $14 > 12.5$, someone will get up and stand in the second place in line.

(3) This leaves the average payoff at 11 for the three remaining. Since the third person in line gets a net payoff of 11, there may or may not be someone standing in the third place in line. When either two or three persons stand on the line, the Nash equilibrium is reached, i.e., there are two equilibria.

(4) If no one stands in the third place, the game is over; if there is a third person in line, then the remaining two have the expected payoffs of 9.5 for not standing in line and 8 for standing in line. Therefore, no one wants to stand in the fourth place. The game is definitely over.

With two or three people standing in the line, a Nash equilibrium is reached. The total net payoff for queuing is $17+14+11+9.5+9.5 = 61$, which is less than 70 for not queuing at all. We call such a case inefficient queuing. To prevent this happening, the authority (e.g., an airline) can simply ignore the queue and, let's say, pass out lots for order of service at the time of their arrival and no standing in line will be necessary.

We see that earlier standing in line is better. Therefore everyone will rush to the line. However, in reality, the payoff is dependent on how long the person stands in line. Also, both the payoffs and the penalty of standing in line are subjective. To consider these factors in the game, we can use simulations to solve the game (Exercise 4.4).

4.3 Pharmaceutical Games

4.3.1 *Two-Player Pharmaceutical Game*

Suppose two companies are in position to make a decision whether to develop two competitive drugs for anemia — a decrease in the normal number of red blood cells (RBCs) or less than the normal quantity of hemoglobin in the blood. Since hemoglobin (found inside RBCs) normally carries oxygen from the lungs to the tissues, anemia's leading symptoms are nonspecific symptoms of a feeling of weakness, or fatigue, general malaise, and sometimes poor concentration.

The cost (including opportunity loss) for developing such a drug is presumably C_a for company A, and C_b for company B. The probability of success of such an indication for marketing is denoted by p; if the drug gets regulatory approval, gross profit for the successful company is dependent on the success of the other company on the same indication. Assume that the total profit for the two companies is fixed and equals G billion dollars if at least one is successful in developing the drug; if both companies are successful in developing drugs for anemia, they get $G/2$ billion dollars each. If both companies make the Go decision (develop the drug), the expected net profits will be $pG/2 - C_a$ and $pG/2 - C_b$ for companies A and B, respectively. If only one company, say company A, made the Go decision and company B made the No-Go (NG) decision, the net profit for company A is $pG - C_a$ and 0 for company B. Similarly we can calculate the net profits for the other two scenarios and summarize them in Table 4.4.

Table 4.4: Expected Net Profits

		Company B	
		Go	NG
Company	Go	$(0, 0)$	$(0.5, 0)$
A	NG	$(0, 0.5)$	$(0, 0)$

Note: $G = \$10B$, $C_a = C_b = .5$, $p = 0.1$

{Go, Go} is a Nash equilibrium (can you explain why?) with an expected net profit of \$0 for each company. Remember that the values for the parameters in this example more or less reflect the realities in the pharmaceutical industry.

4.3.2 *Mixed n-player Pharmaceutical Game*

We now study an n-player mixed game. In this game, we assume that the total profit is fixed at G billion dollars. Therefore, if k companies successfully developed drugs for an indication, each of them will get a gross profit of G/k.

If $k(> 0)$ of n companies made the Go decision, then the expected payoff for a typical company i is

$$EG_i = pG/k - C_i. \qquad (4.11)$$

We assume $pG - C_i \geq 0$ and $pG/n - C_i \leq 0$ for all $i \in \{1, ..., n\}$ such that (4.11) has a real solution k_i for k, i.e., where $k_i = pG/C_i$. To find an equilibrium, if any, for this game, Algorithm 4.1 can be used to simulate the process. We first notice that no one wants to predecide "Go" or "No-Go"; otherwise he will be in an adverse situation. We suspect a rational player will make Go and No-Go decisions with probability $q_i = k_i/n$ and $1 - q_i$, respectively. The expected payoff of this mixed strategy can be obtained using simulations, where k_i are input parameters. Using simulation results for various combinations of k_i, we can determine the equilibria. In reality, player i doesn't know the $q_j(j \neq i)$, but estimates $q_j(j \neq i)$ using information available to him. This approach is referred to as the Bayesian Game Approach. Algorithm 4.1 allows a player to simulate results with different values of k_i or q_i to optimize his strategy.

Algorithm 4.1: Expected Payoff for Mixed n-Player Game
Input n, $G, p, C_i(i = 1, ..., n), k_i$
$\{AveG_j\} := 0$
For $iRun := 1$ **To** $nRuns$
    $k := 0$
    For $i := 1$ **To** n
        Generate q_i from $U(0, 1)$
        If $q_i \leq k_i/n$ **Then**
            $Go_i := 1$
            Generate p_i from $U(0, 1)$
            $S_i := 0$
            If $p_i \leq p$ **Then**
                $S_i := 1$
                $k := k + 1$
            Endif
        Endif
    Endfor
    For $j := 1$ **To** n
        $G_j := S_j/k - Go_j * C_j$
        $AveG_j := AveG_j + G_j/nRuns$
    Endfor
Endfor
Return $\{AveG_j\}$
§

If the gross profit function is not G/k, but other functions, Algorithm 4.1 can be easily modified to fit the need.

4.3.3 *Bayesian Adaptive Gaming Strategy*

In practice, the payoff is heavily dependent on the order in which the player is engaged in the therapeutic development and is also dependent on the total number (N) of investors involved. Suppose the net payoff for the ith entrant is a random variable with mean $\bar{G}_i(N)$. The payoff for not entering is G (such as buying government bonds). To find the Nash equilibrium for this queuing game, we can use a similar approach as in Section 4.2.10. However, the challenge is that we don't know the total number of investors N at the beginning, hence the net payoffs table (Table 4.5) is difficult to construct. Moreover, not all the game players have the same view of the game; therefore the common knowledge assumption may not hold. Besides, even if all the players have common knowledge, some of them may also be involved in other games; therefore, the potential opportunity loss is different for different players in this game.

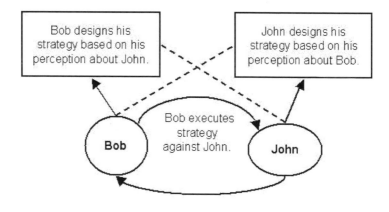

John executes strategy against Bob.

Figure 4.6:   Bayesian Gaming Approach in the Prisoners' Dilemma

Drug development is a sequential game or decision-making problem. Information is accumulated over time and the payoffs change during the game; so do the players' strategies. As a consequence, a person who did not or cannot commit initially may commit himself later and a person who made a commitment earlier may decide to withdraw from the game even if there is a penalty or possibility of retaliation against him. This blurs the distinction we have so carefully set up between cooperative and noncooperative games, but life is like that. Games in which the players can make modifications or change early decisions are called sequential (adaptive) games. The adaptations are based on cumulative information and the Bayesian approach is a natural choice. Note that earlier decisions may prevent the potential opportunist from adapting freely later. We will see this more clearly when we discuss adaptive clinical trial simulations in Chapter 6.

Philosophically speaking, we believe our perceptions do not 100% reflect the semantics, but ironically, we act based on our perceptions instead of the facts because the reality is uncertain (Figure 4.6). However, those perceptions will map closer and closer to the semantics over time — this is the basis for the adaptive game approach.

Adaptations can be justified by: (1) prior knowledge contains uncertainties; (2) there are many possible actions; (3) each action has many possible outcomes; (4) other players' actions are not exactly predictable; (5) knowledge and information may change over time; (6) there is always a traceability involved because any meaningful action has limitations in time and resources.

Table 4.5: Noncooperative Queuing Game

Order of entry	Net payoff for drug
i	$G_i(N)$
No entry	G

In Bayesian adaptive gaming, the players' actions are considered as external dynamics, whereas in Bayesian decision theory, the external environment is nature, which is indifferent about to players' actions.

We now use Bayesian adaptive gaming to solve the problem presented in Table 4.5. We will find the optimal strategy for a player $\wp$ based on his prior knowledge about the number of players involved in the queuing game. We will investigate pure strategies. As an example, we assume $\wp$ has prior knowledge about N, i.e., $N \sim Be(\alpha, \beta)$, which may not be common knowledge to all players. We also assume the principle of asynchronized actions: Other players can only alter their actions against $\wp$'s current strategy after a period of time either because they can't see $\wp's$ strategy immediately or it is not feasible for them to modify the strategy in real time. At the next actionable time, some of the players may change their strategies. However, for a given player $\wp$, the other players' new actions can be considered as a new environment and the game continues.

Algorithm 4.2 is a Monte Carlo algorithm for finding the expected payoff in relation to the order of entering the game. We will study the equilibrium point (the order of entry), at which a player is indifferent regarding whether or not to enter the game. Assume the expected payoff for not being engaged in the game (i.e., engaged in other opportunities) is G. The net gain $G_i(N)$ for the ith entry (the ith player) is a function of N, the total number of players in the game. This function can be as simple as $G_i(N) = G_0/N$, where G_0 is a constant representing the total gain.

Algorithm 4.2: Optimal Entry Probability in the Queuing Game

Objective: return $\{i, AverG_i\}$, the number of investors and average return at equilibrium

 Input nRuns, G

 $\{AveG_i\} := \{0\}$

 For $iRun := 1$ **To** $nRuns$

  Generate N from $Be(\alpha, \beta)$

  For $i := 1$ **To** N

   $aveG_i := aveG_i + G_i(N)$

  Endfor

 Endfor

 Determine i such that $aveG_i \approx G$.

 Return $\{i, AveG_i\}$

 §

4.3.4 *Pharmaceutical Partnerships*

Other than internal development, a firm can acquire necessary resources through partnerships with other stakeholders in the pharmaceutical industry such as Pharma, biotech, CRO, academic, policy maker, and government. Common forms of partnerships include (1) spot market exchanges, (2) contractual agreements/alliances, and (3) mergers/acquisitions (Figure 4.7).

Alliance

An alliance is collaboration between independent organizations, retaining strategic autonomy, or committing resources to a joint activity. Strategic alliances are increasingly important in gaining competitive advantage because through the partnerships, we can obtain needed skills or resources more quickly, reduce asset commitment and increase flexibility, learn from partners, share costs and risks, and build cooperation around a common standard. However, there are risks: (1) adverse selection of partners who may misrepresent their skills, ability, and other resources, (2) moral haz-

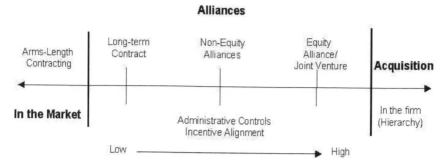

Figure 4.7: Different Partnerships in the Pharmaceutical Industry
(Source: Agarwal, 2008)

ards caused by the partners who may provide lower quality skills and abilities than they had promised, and (3) holdup, where partners exploit the transaction- specific investment made by others in the alliance (Agarwal, 2008).

Cooperative behavior is analyzed by looking at opportunities for profit maximization through "collusion" and incentives for strategic alliances. There are two forms of cooperative strategies: (1) collusive strategies when several firms in an industry cooperate to reduce industry competitiveness, and (2) cooperative agreements and strategic alliances when several firms cooperate but industry competitiveness is not reduced. This form of cooperation can exist among firms within a single industry (e.g., technological alliances) or between firms in different industries (e.g., vertical alliances).

There are several types of collaborative arrangements or strategic alliances: (1) outsourcing, when an organization (or individual) procures services or products from another rather than producing them in-house; (2) licensing, a contractual arrangement that gives an organization the right to use another's intellectual property, typically in exchange for royalties; (3) equity alliances, strategic alliances where partners agree to swap equity; and (4) joint ventures, a particular type of strategic alliance that often establishes a new separate legal entity. Two fundamentally important questions to ask in choosing a partner are (1) what is each party going to bring to the table? and (2) what will each party take from the table? It is preferable that the partner have complementary skills and compatible, but differentiated, goals.

Mergers and Acquisitions

Merger refers to the combination of two entities through mutual negotiation to form a third company, hoping that they have resources and capabilities that together may create a stronger competitive advantage. *Acquisition* refers to acquiring a target company's controlling interest or assets with the intent of using a core competence more effectively by making the acquired firm a subsidiary business within its portfolio. Takeover refers to a type of an acquisition strategy wherein the target firm did not solicit the acquiring firm's bid. Unfortunately, less than 50% of mergers and acquisitions (M & As) are "successful." More than 8 in 10 deals fail to enhance the shareholder value of the acquiring firm.

Case Study: The Xenomouse

Abgenix, Inc. (ABGX), a company specializing in the discovery, development, and manufacture of human therapeutic antibodies, spent seven years and $40 million to produce a genetically engineered mouse that could produce ABX-EGF antibodies that would treat human illnesses. ABX-EGF showed great promise for treating several types of cancer. Abgenix had to decide whether to (Agarwal, 2008):

(1) Pursue the ABX-EGF project as a solo venture (bear all risks and keep all profits)

(2) Use a joint venture with a biotechnology company to complete testing and commercialization (bear moderate risk and split profits)

(3) License ABX-EGF to a pharmaceutical company which would do all further testing and commercialization (bear little risk and receive license royalties)

(4) Be acquired by another company (get all the profit — a percentage of Abgenix's market cap and bear virtually no risk)

What actually happened is that Amgen bought Abgenix for approximately $2.2 billion in cash plus the assumption of debt — all at about an 80% premium to Abgenix' market cap. Amgen benefits in two ways: full ownership of an advanced pipeline product, Panitumumab, and elimination of a royalty from Abgenix sales of Denosumab (formerly AMG 162) — Abgenix's most advanced cancer therapeutic. The purchase adds to Amgen's protein manufacturing capabilities with a 100,000 square foot manufacturing plant in Fremont, California. Abgenix also brings scientific knowledge and assets, such as the ownership and capabilities of the proprietary fully human monoclonal antibody technology, XenoMouse. Amgen also obtains another human antibody for postmenopausal osteoporosis and bone-related cancer indications. The deal also allows Amgen to pick up about $300 million in tax loss to carry forward.

4.4 Prescription Drug Global Pricing

4.4.1 *Prescription Drug Price Policies*

No matter where the analysis results come from or which method, the top priority is the US market, which represents more than the rest of the world (Figure 4.8). The resulting higher price in drug markets has contributed to unregulated drug pricing in the US, according to some scholars (Table 4.6).

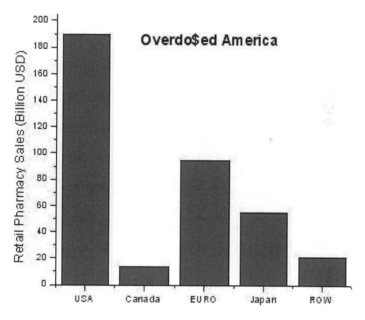

Figure 4.8:   Retail Pharmacy Sales by Region
(Source: Pearlman, 2007)

To study how price policy affects drug development in a nation and different drug policies affect drug development in the world under economic globalization, let's start with the analysis from the document "Prescription Drug Prices in Canada, Europe, and Japan — Prepared by Minority Staff Special Investigations Division Committee on Government Reform U.S. House of Representatives" (www.oversight.house.gov):

The United States is unique among industrialized countries because it is the only country that fails to protect its citizens from discriminatory pricing of prescription drugs. Canada, France, Italy, Germany, Japan, and the United Kingdom all negotiate on behalf of their citizens to obtain lower prices for brand name drugs. As a result, purchasers in these countries pay significantly less for prescription drugs than uninsured senior citizens in the United States.

Drug Pricing in Canada

In Canada, the Patent Medicine Prices Review Board establishes and enforces guidelines that determine the maximum prices at which manufacturers can sell brand-name drugs. Under these guidelines, the introductory prices of "breakthrough" drugs must not exceed the median of the prices of the drugs in other industrialized countries. Prices of patented drugs that do not provide a significant breakthrough in treating diseases must not exceed the maximum price of other drugs that treat the same disease. Once the introductory price is established, subsequent price increases are limited to changes in the Consumer Price Index. The Canadian pricing system results in brand-name drug prices that are an average of 38% lower than prices in the United States.

Drug Pricing in France

The French pricing system allows pharmaceutical companies to sell their products at any price. However, if these companies want the national health care system to reimburse patients for the cost of the drug, the companies must agree to a lower, negotiated price. These negotiated prices and reimbursement rates paid by the healthcare system are based on the therapeutic value of the drug and the price of the drug in other countries. The French pricing system results in brand-name drug prices that are an average of 45% lower than prices in the United States.

Drug Pricing in Germany

Germany has a decentralized national healthcare system, with coverage provided by over 700 insurance funds. With the exception of innovative drugs that have been patented since 1996, pricing is determined by a reference system, with prices for new drugs based upon the prices of existing drugs that provide the same therapeutic benefit. Prices for innovative drugs that were patented after 1995 are not restricted by the government. However, each individual insurance fund can negotiate with pharmaceutical manufacturers on behalf of their covered patients. The German pricing system results in brand-name drug prices that are an average of 35% lower than prices in the United States.

Drug Pricing in Italy

Italy's national healthcare system allows manufacturers to sell their drugs at any price. However, if these drugs are to be eligible for reimbursement under the national healthcare system, pharmaceutical companies must set the price of the drug at a cost that does not exceed a twelve country European average price. The Italian pricing system results in brand-name drug prices that are an average of 48% lower than prices in the United States.

Drug Pricing in the United Kingdom

The National Health Service in the United Kingdom differs from national healthcare providers in other countries because it does not negotiate the prices of individual drugs with manufacturers. Instead, drug companies in the United Kingdom are free to establish their own prices for individual drugs. However, under the country's pharmaceutical laws, the maximum profit that drug manufacturers can earn on sales in the United Kingdom is limited. Companies that set their prices so high that they exceed maximum allowable profit rates must reimburse the government. Allowable profits are based on several factors, including the company's investments in the United Kingdom and the level of long-term risk. Generally, companies are allowed to earn returns of 17% – 21% on capital investments. The pricing system in the United Kingdom results in brand-name drug prices that are an average of 31% lower than prices in the United States.

Drug Pricing in Japan

Japan, like other industrialized countries, has a national healthcare system. The prices paid by this healthcare system are generally determined via a reference system. Prices for new drugs are determined by comparing them with similar drugs that are already on the market. Prices are based upon the safety and effectiveness of the drug; drugs that are shown to be more effective or innovative than existing drugs are priced higher. If there is no comparable drug on the market, the price of the drug is determined by factors such as manufacturing cost and the price of the drug in other countries.

4.4.2 *Drug Pricing Strategy*

In addition to the different drug policies discussed in the previous section, in another study by IMS Health in 2005 (Pammolli and Riccaboni, 2007, p. 183), they listed the branded and generic prices for 30 counties/regions and adjusted for currency exchange rates and parity purchase power (PPP). The data in Table 4.6 are extracted from their table.

The price structure of branded drugs will affect the profitability for pharmaceutical companies. How to maximize the profit within the time period $T_{\max}$ (e.g., 12 years — typically an innovative drug has 20-year patent protection; the time-to-market from the time of patent issued is about 8 years) by determining an appropriate international price structure for a brand drug is of great interest to drug makers. An unreasonably high drug price beyond what consumers can afford is not desired. On the other hand, proportionally low pricing in a country relative to the price in the US will lead to drug importation back to the US at a lower price, i.e., the so-called reimportation or parallel trade. (We will discuss this topic, parallel trade and compulsory licensing, more in Chapter 8 in the context of sequential games for prescription drug commercialization.) Since most countries have stronger controls on drug pricing than the US, in the following Monte Carlo discussion, we assume that the prices for the brand drug are fixed in other countries, but the price in the US is to be determined.

Table 4.6: Related Unit Drug Prices (PPP adjusted), 2004

ID	Country	All products	Generics	Branded
1	USA	100	100	100
2	Canada	71.48	125.12	60.26
3	China	79.26	68.12	95.54
4	French	46.05	108.11	34.98
5	Germany	67.05	122.96	51.56
6	Italy	54.34	123.93	39.20
7	Japan	52.67	77.95	35.91
8	UK	48.73	93.74	39.17

Note: Import/export cost to add x%

We further introduce the following assumptions for the Monte Carlo simulation:

(1) We only study the closed system of the eight countries listed in Table 4.6.

(2) Denote by C_k the fixed policy-price for the brand drug in country k (except the US). For example, $C_2 = 60.26$ for Canada and $C_8 = 39.17$ for the UK as presented in Table 4.6.

(3) The consumption of the drug in country k is a function of the price C_k in the country, i.e., $V_k = V_k(C_k)$.

(4) People always try to buy the drug at the cheapest price. Anyone can import the brand drug from any country for a lower price and sale at the

policy-prices in his country, but he will only do so when there is a profit. For example, based on Table 4.6, Canada may import the brand drug from Japan, but not from China.

(5) The total cost for drug importation or exportation is $C_{ij} > 0$ for the drug between countries i and j $(i \neq j)$ and $C_{ii} = 0$.

(6) There is a future discount r.

(7) The profit of the company is assumed to be proportional to its total drug sales worldwide.

A Monte Carlo simulation algorithm for the problem is presented as follows. The key is to find the cheapest price $C_{\min,i}$ for country i to buy the drug.

Algorithm 4.3: Optimal Drug Pricing Policy
Objective: return optimal price C_{opt} and corresponding sales $S_{\max}$.

Input the number of countries m, $T_{\max}$, $\{V(C_i)\}$, $\{C_{ij}\}$, r, and the set of prices in the US $\{C_1\}$ that you want to try.
For Each $c_1 \in \{C_1\}$
    $S := 0$
    For $t = 1$ **To** $T_{\max}$
        For $i := 1$ **To** m
            $C_{\min,i} := C_i$
            For $j := 1$ **To** m
                $C_{\min,i} = \min(C_{\min,i}, C_j + C_{ij})$
            Endfor
        Endfor
        $S := S + \sum_{i=1}^{m} r^t V(C_{\min,i}) \cdot C_{\min,i}$
    Endfor
    If $S > S_{\max}$ **Then** $C_{opt} = c_1$
    $S_{\max} := \max(S_{\max}, S)$
Endfor
Return $\{C_{opt}, S_{\max}\}$
§

Of course this model is somewhat naive to completely model the dynamics of the prescription drug market worldwide, but more or less reflects the effect of the increasing globalization trend in the drug market.

4.4.3 *Cost Projection of Drug Development*

On the one hand, most "low-hanging fruits" were picked in the early years of drug development; it is much more difficult for pharmaceutical companies to find and develop an effective NCE today than 15 or 20 years ago. On the other hand, advances in science and technology have speeded up prescription drug development. My preliminary analyses indicate some disturbed results, which may suggest a need for a change in the statistical criterion for evaluating the efficacy of a drug. Intuitively, if every new drug is required a minimal Δ_{min} better than the control (the best drug available in the market) in efficacy, then the ith drug to the market will be required to have at least $i\Delta_{min}$ better than placebo. Furthermore, if efficacy response in the placebo is zero and $\Delta_{min} = 10\%$, then the 10th drug for an indication in the market will have a 100% efficacy response. This stringent requirement makes drug development increasingly costly. In fact, only 23% of all NDAs from 1998 to 2002 were innovative drugs and the rest were accounted "me too" drugs (Pearlman, 2007). Those me-too drugs are based on noninferiority criteria. The increasingly popular noninferiority trial is a reflection of regulatory adjustment in response to the increasing challenges in drug development.

In the United States, to gain an NDA approval for marketing, it is usually required to demonstrate a statistical significance. For a given treatment effect and power, the sample size required is inversely proportional to the square of the additional treatment effect (δ) of the NCE over the active control (δ_c). Typically, the pivotal trial sample size is calculated as

$$N = \frac{4(z_{1-\alpha} + z_{1-\beta})^2}{(\delta - \delta_c)^2} \tag{4.12}$$

where δ is the normalized treatment difference, z_t is the $100t$ percentile of the standard normal distribution, $\alpha = 0.025$ is the one-sided significance level (i.e., the type-I error rate permitted), and β is the type-II error or power $= 1 - \beta$.

From (4.12), we can obtain power $(1 - \beta)$:

$$pow := \Phi\left(\frac{\sqrt{N}}{2}(\delta - \delta_c) - z_{1-\alpha}\right). \tag{4.13}$$

Since clinical trials are a major cost in pharmaceutical Research and Development, the total Research and Development cost C can be assumed to be proportional to the sample size $C \propto N$.

We are interested in the trend of the average cost increase over time in drug development, i.e., the cost as a function of i, the order in the sequence of getting FDA approval for a given indication.

To study the problem using the Monte Carlo method, we further assume that: (1) the effect size of NMEs has the standard normal distribution

$\delta \sim N(0,1)$ and we select randomly molecules from this distribution for our Research and Development, and (2) the trials are designed with a power of 80% or $\beta = 0.2$. Under these assumptions, (4.12) becomes

$$N \approx \frac{32}{(\delta - \delta_c)^2}. \tag{4.14}$$

Algorithm 4.4: Drug Development Cost (Normal Endpoint)
Objective: Drug cost over time $\{C_i\}$.
Input: Number of simulations $nRuns$, number of drugs in the sequence m, maximum sample size $N_{\max}$,
Initialize: $\{C_i\} := \{0\}$
For $iRun := 1$ **To** $nRuns$
$\qquad \delta_c = 0$
$\qquad i := 1$
$\qquad$ **While** $i < m$:
$\qquad\qquad$ Generate δ from $N(0,1)$
$\qquad\qquad N := \min(N_{\max}, 32/(\delta - \delta_c)^2)$
$\qquad\qquad pow := \Phi\left(\frac{\sqrt{N}}{2}(\delta - \delta_c) - z_{1-\alpha}\right)$
$\qquad\qquad$ **If** $\delta < \delta_0$ **Then**
$\qquad\qquad\qquad N := 0$
$\qquad\qquad\qquad pow := 0$
$\qquad\qquad$ **Endif**
$\qquad\qquad C_i := C_i + N/nRuns$
$\qquad\qquad$ Generate u from $U(0,1)$
$\qquad\qquad$ **If** $u \leq pow$ **Then**
$\qquad\qquad\qquad i := i + 1$
$\qquad\qquad\qquad \delta_c = \delta$
$\qquad\qquad$ **Endif**
$\qquad$ **Endwhile**
Endfor
Return $\{C_i\}$

4.5   Summary

Meta-simulation is the Monte Carlo method of dealing with the overall dynamics of a subject field. Meta-simulations of the pharmaceutical industry usually involve more than one independent business entity or company. Theoretical approaches such as game theory used for meta-simulation in this book are the same as those in economics.

Pharmacoeconomics is important to health policy makers and regulatory agencies because pharmacoeconomic studies serve to guide optimal healthcare resource allocation, in a standardized and scientifically grounded manner. Pharmacoeconomics is also interesting to the pharmaceutical industry because pharmacoeconomic studies can guide their drug development by allocating more resources to the development of cost-effective drugs.

Profitability calculation in the pharmaceutical industry is controversial. Profitability measures calculated in different ways should be interpreted differently. Due to the highly risky nature of the sector, profit calculated based on the winners (big Pharmas) as the profitability measure for the industry can mislead people. It is irrational to complain about a lottery winner taking too much profit without considering there are thousands of losers.

A game is a formal description of a strategic situation. Game theory is the formal study of decision making where several players must make choices that potentially affect the interests of the other players. A player is an agent who makes decisions in a game.

Most game theories assume three conditions: common knowledge, perfect information, and rationality, but those assumptions may not always apply to the pharmaceutical world.

A game in strategic form, also called normal form, is a compact representation of a game in which players simultaneously choose their strategies. The resulting payoffs are presented in a contingent table with a cell for each strategy combination. An extensive form of a game describes with a tree how a game is played. It depicts the order in which players make moves, and the information each player has at each decision point. Both the extensive form and table form are the normal form of the game.

The zero-sum game is the most widely studied, in which the sum of the wins and losses in a game cancel out each other for each set of strategies chosen. A constant-sum game can be converted into a zero-sum game by subtracting a constant from the payoff.

To solve a game is to find the equilibrium (or equilibria) of the game, e.g., the Nash equilibrium. The Nash equilibrium is a state in which no player wants to move unilaterally.

A player in a game can choose deterministic or probabilistic strategies. If he chooses among two or more strategies randomly according to specific probabilities, this choice is called a mixed strategy. In a game with mixed strategy, sequential rationality is assumed, according to which an optimal strategy for a player should maximize his or her expected payoff.

Games with multiple options or matrix games can be solved using Theorem 4.4, as illustrated with the legendary Chinese horse race problem.

There are games that are partisan or impartial. Impartial oligopoly games can be solved either analytically or numerically through simulations. Partisan games are much more complex but can be solved using Monte Carlo simulation.

A game can have multiple equilibria, but equilibria can change if there is a change in communication and other assumptions, which may lead to a new type of game — a cooperative game. In noncooperative games, the solution is from the individual perspective, which often leads to inferior outcomes such as in the Prisoners' Dilemma. It is preferable, in many cases, to define a criterion to rank outcomes for the group of players as a whole. The Pareto criterion concerns such an optima: an outcome is better than another if at least one person is better off and no one is worse off. If an outcome cannot be improved upon, i.e., if no one can be made better off without making somebody else worse off, then we say that the outcome is Pareto optimal. However, the Pareto optimal outcome for a cooperative game is usually not unique; therefore, it is not very useful unless we narrow down the solution using tools such as bargaining.

A popular game situation in the pharmaceutical world is the queuing game, in which multiple players are involved and payoffs are dependent on the order of the players' engagement.

The assumptions of common knowledge, perfect information, and rationality in game theory are often violated in the pharmaceutical world: people don't have the same perceptions about the game, even if they are given the information. Reasons include, for example, that players may have different views on utility. Therefore, what one player predicts about other players' strategies could be completely different from the reality. In other words, all players play the same game, but each actually plays a different game in his mind. We are often not sure what actions may be taken by other players and we associate a probability distribution to the potential strategies that our opponents may take and adapt as the game plays out. We call this approach Bayesian adaptive gaming.

We have discussed the investment strategy when there are n players in the same therapeutic area and provided the Monte Carlo algorithm. We have analyzed Bayesian noncooperative queuing, provided a Monte Carlo algorithm, and studied the different pharmaceutical partnerships including spot market exchanges, contractual agreements/alliances, and mergers/acquisitions.

Globalization imposes a challenge in prescription drug pricing. After reviewing the prescription drug policies in the United States and other countries in the world, a Monte Carlo algorithm has been devised for optimizing prescription drug policy.

Pharmaceutical investors or ordinary citizens may feel unsettled when they realize that most "low-hanging fruits" were picked in the early years of drug development and drug development has become more challenging and costly, despite advances in science and technology. A Monte Carlo algorithm was devised for cost projection over time for drug development.

Philosophically, the whole world can be viewed as a game and as the macro-consequence caused by micro-motivated individuals. Game theory is a powerful tool to solve the mystery of the world and make it better.

4.6 Exercises

Exercise 4.1: Explain the terms game, strategy, player, zero-sum game, mixed strategy game, matrix game, queuing game, cooperative and non-cooperative games, equilibrium in a game, Nash equilibrium, Pareto optimum, and strategic and extensive forms.

Exercise 4.2: Elaborate the three common assumptions in game theory and discuss the fitness of those assumptions in that situations you.

Exercise 4.3: In the two-player game, assume the probability of success for companies A and B in Section 4.3.1 is dependent on the sample size or the cost, specifically,

$$p_i = p_i(C_i) = \frac{p}{1 + \exp(-C_i)}, \quad i = A \text{ or } B.$$

Find all Nash equilibria using either the analytical or simulation approach.

Exercise 4.4: Change the game in Table 4.4 to a 3-player game and find all Nash equilibria using either the analytical or simulation approach.

Exercise 4.5: Change the sample in Table 4.4 to a 3-player game and payoff $= Gk^\gamma$, where $\gamma = 0.7$ and k is the number of successful drugs. Study the Nash equilibria analytically or using simulation.

Exercise 4.6: Find the Pareto optimal solution set for the following cooperative game (McCain, 2009).

Suppose that Joey has a bicycle. Joey would rather have a game machine than a bicycle, and he could buy a game machine for $80, but Joey doesn't have any money. We express this by saying that Joey values his bicycle at $80. Mikey has $100 and no bicycle, and would rather have a bicycle than anything else he can buy for $100. We express this by saying that Mikey values a bicycle at $100. Analyze the game, construct a 2×2 payoff table, and solve the game. You can make assumptions as necessary.

Exercise 4.7: In Section 4.3.1, Two-Player Pharmaceutical Game, discuss the following cooperative game: the two companies make a strategic alliance, in which they agree to jointly develop a drug for an indication using one of the NMEs; if it is successful, the second NME will not be studied; if it fails, they will bring the second one to the development pipeline.

Exercise 4.8: In Algorithm 4.2, how many players (N) will be involved is a random variable. If we also don't know how many players are already in the game, then what is the optimal mixed strategy to enter the game (i.e., determine the probability p_c, with which the player enters the game)?

Exercise 4.9: Study the existence of Nash equilibria for the queuing game in Table 4.6 using the Monte Carlo method.

Exercise 4.10: Discuss different forms of alliances, their advantages, and disadvantages.

Exercise 4.11: Divide the class into small groups to represent either Abgenix or Amgen. Discuss the pros and cons of the four options in Section 4.3.4. Monte Carlo simulation may be applied to quantify/justify your approach.

Exercise 4.12: The penetration volume V_i in Section 4.4.2 is assumed to be a beta distribution $V_i \sim Be\,(\alpha_i, \beta_i)$, $(i > 1)$, where α_i and/or β_i is a function of the drug price C_i. Develop a Monte Carlo algorithm for finding the optimal pricing policy C_{opt} in the United States.

Exercise 4.13: For binary variables, assume that the proportion of response is $\delta \sim U\,(0,1)$ or beta distribution $Be\,(\alpha, \beta)$. Develop a Monte Carlo algorithm that is similar to Algorithm 4.5 for projecting the cost trend over time for developing a successful drug.

Chapter 5

Macro-Simulation for Pharmaceutical Research and Development

This chapter will cover the following topics:

- Sequential Decision Making
- Markov Decision Process
- Pharmaceutical Decision Process
- Extension of Markov Decision Process

5.1   Sequential Decision Making

5.1.1   *Descriptive and Normative Decisions*

Life is about decisions. You may not be aware that you are making decisions every second, big or small. There are two distinctive decision approaches: descriptive and normative decision theories. Descriptive decision making considers a decision as a specific information processing process; it is a study of the cognitive processes that lead to decisions, for example, the ways humans deal with conflicts or perceive the values of the solutions. Descriptive decision making looks for explanations for the ways individuals or groups of individuals arrive at decisions so that methods can be developed for influencing and guiding the decision process. Normative decision making considers a decision as a rational act of choice under the viable alternatives. It is a mathematical or statistical theory for modeling decision-making processes. Classical decision-making theory and Bayesian decision theory fall into this category. Normative decision making strives to make the optimal decision, given the available information. Hence, it is an optimization approach.

The normative decision approach can be further divided into deterministic and probabilistic approaches. For the deterministic approach, information is considered as completely known, whereas for the probabilistic approach, information is associated with uncertainties or probabilities.

Drug development is a sequence of decision processes. The processes are mixtures of descriptive and normative decisions. It is desirable to move away from the ad hoc descriptive nature toward the normative nature. Probability theory and the Monte Carlo method provide us with powerful tools to achieve this goal.

5.1.2 *Sequential Decision Problem*

A typical *sequential decision problem* concerns a dynamic system or a stochastic process that is characterized by a sequence of states $s_0, s_1, s_2...$ at times $t = 0, 1, 2, ...$. The motion or process can be controlled by choosing a sequence of actions $a_0, a_1, a_2...$ at the times $t = 0, 1, 2, ...$. There is a cost c_t associated with action a_t. The goal is to find a policy (a sequence of actions/decisions) or strategy that minimizes the sum of these costs.

In principle, the state s_t and the corresponding action at time t can be vectors, but for simplicity, we assume s_t is a one-dimension scale. We further assume the immediate cost c_t is only dependent on the current state s_t and the action taken a_t, i.e.,

$$c_t = K(s_t, a_t, t), \tag{5.1}$$

where inclusion of time t in the cost function K is for the purpose of convenience (see below).

We use function L to define a law of motion for the dynamic system:

$$s_{t+1} = L(s_t, a_t, t). \tag{5.2}$$

This law implies that the transition of the system from one state to the next state is independent of earlier states.

The decision problem is to choose the sequence of actions $\{a_1, ..., a_{T-1}\}$ to minimize the total cost over a given period T:

$$\min_{a_1,...,a_{T-1}} c_0 + c_1 + \cdots + c_{T-1}, \tag{5.3}$$

subject to conditions (5.1) and (5.2).

Thanks to mathematical induction, we realize that if $c_0 + c_1 + \cdots + c_{t-1}$ is minimized at any discrete time point t, we need only concern ourselves with minimizing the total future cost:

$$c_t + c_{t+1} + \cdots + c_{T-1}. \tag{5.4}$$

Having said that, we imply that choice of present and future actions will not affect the past — the principle of optimality to be discussed in the next section. This reduced problem (5.4) involves the actions $a_t, a_{t+1}, ... a_{T+1}$ with only $n = T - t$ decision variables.

5.1.3   Backwards Induction

Bellman's Optimality Principle: An optimal policy has the property that, whatever the initial state and initial decision are, the remaining decisions must constitute an optimal policy with regard to the state resulting from the first decision.

Bellman introduced this principle (Bellman, 1957). Bather (2000) justified it with the following arguments: suppose that the remaining decisions do not constitute an optimal policy as the principle claims. Then, starting at s_0, the policy determines a_0 and hence s_1, but the total future cost $c_0 + c_1 + \cdots + c_{T-1}$ is not minimized. In other words, by changing the remaining decisions, this future cost can be reduced. However, any such changes can be included in the policy $a_0, a_1, .., a_{T-1}$ for the whole period, which shows that the original policy cannot be optimal. This is the required contradiction.

Another point worth noting is that an optimal policy may not exist; it may be that the minimum total cost cannot be attained exactly. To include this situation, we provide the following definition of minimization of future cost.

Definition 5.1   For any state s and positive integer $n = T - t$, the future cost is given by

$$\tilde{K}_n(s) = \inf_{a_t, a_{t+1}, ..., a_{T-1}} (c_t + c_{t+1} + ..., + c_{T-1}), \qquad (5.5)$$

where $s_t = s, s_{t+1} = L(s, a_t, T - n)$ and so on.

This notation shows that the relevant variables are n and s. We are going to show you how backwards induction works.

At each stage in the argument, we consider a typical transition from s to $s' = L(s, a, T - n)$ generated by choosing the action a. For simplicity, assume that there is an optimal action in every case and denote this by $a = \tilde{a}_n(s)$. Let's start with the last cost c_{T-1}, where $n = 1$ and $t = T - 1$. For this last state, there is only a single cost term $c_{T-1} = K(s, a, T - 1)$ and we have the infima

$$\tilde{K}_1(s) = \inf_a K(s, a, T - 1). \qquad (5.6)$$

After obtaining $\tilde{K}_1(s)$, we can proceed to the second to the last case for $n = 2$. There are two actions involved this time, but one of them is already determined and one is left to be optimized. Thus, for any initial state s and action a, the total cost is

$$K(s, a, T - 1) + \tilde{K}_1(s'), \tag{5.7}$$

where $s' = L(s, a, T - 2)$. Hence

$$\tilde{K}_2(s) = \inf_a \left\{ K(s, a, T - 2) + \tilde{K}_1(L(s, a, T - 2)) \right\}. \tag{5.8}$$

Recursively, we can determine $\tilde{K}_n$ in terms of $\tilde{K}_{n-1}$ by using the following equation:

$$\tilde{K}_n(s) = \inf_a \left\{ K(s, a, T - n) + \tilde{K}_{n-1}(L(s, a, T - n)) \right\}. \tag{5.9}$$

The solution for the sequential decision problem is $\{\tilde{a}_1, ..., \tilde{a}_n\}$. This backwards induction method converts an n-parameter $(a_1, ..., a_n)$ optimization problem to a sequence of n optimization problems with single parameter action a. It dramatically improves computational efficiency. As an example, if a grid search is used, the computational effort will be reduced from $O(m^n)$ to $O(nm)$.

Note that optimal actions do not always exist and the decision functions may not be properly determined. Strictly speaking, in such cases there is no optimal policy, but policies can be found to approximate the required infimum of the total cost.

So far we have discussed the deterministic decision problem. However, there are many situations where the transition from one state to another is probabilistically related to an action. To study such a decision problem, we are going to introduce the so-called Markov decision process.

5.2 Markov Decision Process

5.2.1 *Markov Chain*

The simplest and most widely studied stochastic process is the Markov chain, named after Andrey Markov, in which the probability of transiting from one state to the next state does not depend on how the agent got to the current state. Formally, the Markov chain is defined by

(1) A set of states S

Transition probability: $T : S \times S \to [0, 1]$

$$T\left(s, s'\right) = \Pr\left(s_{t+1} = s' | s_t = s\right),$$

(2) Initial state distribution $P_0 : S \to [0, 1]$

$$P_0\left(s\right) = \Pr\left(s_0 = s\right),$$

and

(3) The transition probability from state i to state j is given by

$$P_{ij} = \prod_{k=i}^{j-1} T\left(s_k, s_{k+1}\right).$$

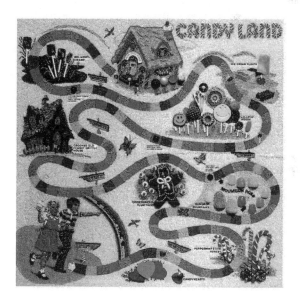

Figure 5.1: Candyland Game — A Markov Chain

A simple example is the Candyland game (Figure 5.1). In the game, two players roll the dice in turns to determine the number of steps they should move ahead. The person who arrives at the destination first wins. Obviously, the probability of moving from one position to another position is fully determined by the current position and independent of how the person got to the current position.

Example 5.1

As we discussed early in Chapter 3, clinical trials are often conducted in sequences from Phase I to Phase III. Sufficiently positive results from a phase set off the next phase trial and promising Phase III results will trigger the company to submit an NDA to the FDA for marketing approval. Results from earlier phases other than the immediate phase play only a minor role in the decision process. Such a decision process can be modeled by a Markov chain (Figure 5.2).

Research (Pammolli and Riccaboni, 2007, p. 116) shows that average success rates are around 50%, 30%, 40% for Phase I, II, and III trials, respectively. Based on these rates, transition probabilities are 0.5 from Phase I to Phase II (probability of No-Go is $P_{11} = 0.5$) and 0.3 from Phase II to Phase III (probability of no-Go is $P_{22} = 0.7$). There are about 40% Phase III trials that finally get approval for marketing (probability of failure is $P_{33} = 0.6$).

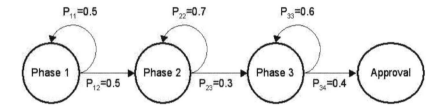

Figure 5.2:   Markov Chain for Clinical Trials and Approval

The transition probability matrix for the clinical trial processes in Figure 5.2 can be written as

$$[T] = \begin{bmatrix} 0.5 & 0.5 & 0.15 & 0.06 \\ 0 & 0.7 & 0.3 & 0.12 \\ 0 & 0 & 0.6 & 0.4 \\ 0 & 0 & 0 & 0.6 \end{bmatrix}.$$

From the transition probability matrix, we know that the probability move from Phase I to Phase III is 15% and to approval is 6%; the probability from Phase II to NDA approval is 0.12. However, no one will use the naive transition probabilities to make "Go, No-Go" decisions. Instead, results from clinical trials have to be considered in the decision-making process. In the Bayesian approach, the naive probability is the prior probability $P(A)$, which will be combined with observed data $P(B|A)$ to calculate the posterior probability $P(A|B)$ using Bayes' law:

$$P(A|B) = \frac{P(B|A)P(A)}{P(B)}.$$

Since each step moving forward in drug development is one step closer to success, it can be considered as a reward in the process. When a Markov process is attached to rewards, it becomes a *Markov decision process* (MDP).

5.2.2 *Markov Decision Process*

A Markov decision process is similar to a Markov chain, but there are also actions and utilities (rewards or gains, see Figure 5.3). MDPs provide a powerful mathematical framework for modeling the decision-making process in situations where outcomes are partly random and partly under the control of the decision maker. MDPs are useful in studying a wide range of optimization problems solved via dynamic programming and reinforcement learning. Since the 1950s when MDP was first known (Bellman 1957a; Howard, 1960), it has been widely used in robotics, automated control, economics, business management, nursing systems, and manufacturing (Gosavi, 2003; Bertsekas, 1995; Van Nunen, 1976).

There are two types of MDPs, finite and infinite horizon problems (Powell, 2007, p. 53–56). In the finite horizon problem, the transition probabilities (from state s at time t to state s' at time $t+1$) vary over time, i.e.,

$$T(s, a, s') = \Pr(s_{t+1} = s'|s_t = s, a_t = a), \tag{5.10}$$

whereas in the infinite MDP problem, the system reaches steady state and the transition probability is only dependent on the two states and the action taken a, but independent of the time when the transition occurs. Thus the transition probability can be simplified as

$$T(s, a, s') = \Pr(s'|s, a). \tag{5.11}$$

In the rest of this chapter, we will discuss infinite MDPs only.

Let's denote a dynamic system (Figure 5.3) which moves over states $s_i \in S, i = 1, 2, ..., N$ and the motion is controlled by choosing a sequence of actions $a_i \in A, i = 1, 2, ...N$. There is a net numerical gain (immediate reward or cost) $g_i(\alpha_i)$ associated with each action a_i. The goal is to find a policy (strategy) which maximizes the total expected gain. This problem can be formalized as a Markov decision process.

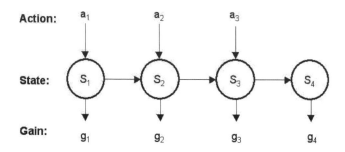

Figure 5.3:   Dynamic System and Sequential Decision Making

An infinite horizon Markov decision process is a 4-tuple of four elements $\{S, A, \Pr(S, A), g(S, A)\}$ with the following properties:

(1) Finite (N) set of states S

(2) Set of actions A (can be conditioned on the state s)

(3) Policy/strategy/action rule — action mapping to state s

(4) Discount rate for future rewards $0 < \gamma < 1$.

(5) Immediate reward (utility or gain function) $g : S \times A \to \Re$

$g(s, a)$ = immediate fixed reward by reaching the state s and taking action a.

(6) Transition model (dynamics) $T : S \times A \times S \to [0, 1]$

$T(s, a, s')$ = probability of going from s to s' under action a.

$$T(s, a, s') = \Pr(s'|s, a_i = a).$$

(7) The goal is to find a policy $\pi^* = \{a_i^*, i = 1, ..., N\}$ that maximizes the total expected reward over the course of motion, which is subject to some initial conditions and other constraints, if any. Note that a often associates with state s. We may write a_s for action at state s.

Here are examples of the Markov decision process in clinical trials (Figure 5.2):

(1) s_1 = Drug discovery phase, s_2 = Preclinical phase, s_3 = Clinical development phase, and s_4 = Regulatory approval and marketing. a_i represent the general decision rule or action rule for moving from the ith phase to the next phase in drug development.

(2) s_1 = Preclinical phase, s_i = the ith phase clinical trial $(i = 1, 2, 3)$, and a_i has a similar meaning as in (1).

(3) s_1 = initiation of a clinical trial, s_i = interim and the final analyses for the $(i - 1)^{th}$ phase trial $(i = 2, 3, 4)$; actions are the stopping and adaptive rules (see details in Chapter 6).

An example of an MDP from an anonymous university lecture handout about undergraduates' career options is presented in Figure 5.4, where r is the reward and the person's initial state is U or unemployed. The rewards and transitional probabilities, or even the model itself, may vary from individual to individual, but the model has well illustrated the fact that many decision problems we are facing in our life journey can be modeled by MDPs. The determination of the transition probabilities between the states $\{U, I, G, A\}$ are dependent on our actions toward the goals.

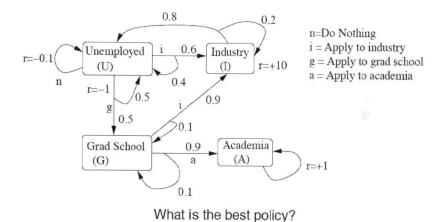

What is the best policy?

Figure 5.4:   Career Options

5.2.3   *Dynamic Programming*

In Section 5.1.3, we introduced Bellman's optimality principle in dealing with a deterministic sequential decision problem: an optimal policy has the property that, whatever the initial state and initial decision are, the remaining decisions must constitute an optimal policy with regard to the state resulting from the first decision. This principle is applied to the stochastic decision problem here, but the optimal policy regards the expected gain (loss) as opposed to loss in the deterministic case.

Computationally, stochastic decision problems are usually solved using so-called Bellman equations:

$$V(s) = \max_{a_s \in A} \left(g(s, a) + \gamma \sum_{s' \in S} \Pr(s'|s, a_s) \cdot V(s') \right). \qquad (5.12)$$

The optimal policy $\pi^* = \{a_1^*, a_2^*, ..., a_N^*\}$ for the MDP is a vector whose components are defined by

$$a_s^* = \arg\max_{a_s} \left\{ g(s, a_s) + \gamma \sum_{s' \in S} \Pr(s'|s, a_s) \cdot V(s') \right\}. \tag{5.13}$$

Equation (5.12) can be written in matrix form:

$$\boldsymbol{V}_\pi = \boldsymbol{g}_\pi + \gamma \boldsymbol{P}_\pi \boldsymbol{V}_\pi. \tag{5.14}$$

The solution to (5.14) can be written in a matrix form:

$$\boldsymbol{V}_\pi = (\boldsymbol{I} - \gamma \boldsymbol{P}_\pi)^{-1} \boldsymbol{g}_\pi. \tag{5.15}$$

The standard family of algorithms to calculate the policy requires storage for two arrays indexed by state: value V, which contains real values, and policy π, which contains actions. The Bellman equations can be used to develop the dynamic programming (a backwards induction algorithm). The iteration is going from the last state to the first state (Algorithm 5.1).

Algorithm 5.1: Dynamic programming for Markov decision problem (value iteration, Bellman, 1957b, Powell, 2007)

Objective: return the optimal policy and expected total rewards (a^*, V^*).

Input precision ε.

$V_0(s) := 0 \; \forall s \in S$.

$i := 1$

$\varepsilon_i := 2\varepsilon$

While $\varepsilon_i > \varepsilon$:

    For Each $s \in S$ compute

        $V_i(s) := \max_{a_s \in A} \left(g(s, a_s) + \gamma \sum_{s' \in S} \Pr(s'|s, a_s) \cdot V_{i-1}(s') \right)$

    Endfor

    $\pi^* :=$ solution vector for action rule a to equation (5.12)

    $\varepsilon_i := \max_s \|V_i(s) - V_{i-1}(s)\|$

    $V^* = V_i(s)$

    $i := i + 1$

Endwhile

Return (a^*, V^*)

§

Although we have not included the necessary maximization algorithm in Algorithm 5.1, there are many effective algorithms for finding the single-parameter optimization problem $\max_x f(x)$, where $f(x) < \infty$. See, e.g., Algorithms 1.9 and 1.10.

Convergence is always a concern in simulation. The following theorem addresses the convergence rate of the value iteration algorithm (Powell, 2007).

Theorem 5.1 *Suppose the value iteration Algorithm 5.1 with stopping parameter ε terminates at iteration n with value function $\boldsymbol{V}_{n+1}$, then*

$$||\boldsymbol{V}_{n+1} - \boldsymbol{V}^*|| \leq \varepsilon/2,$$

where $\boldsymbol{V}^*$ is the optimal value.

Furthermore, let π^ε be the policy that we terminate with, and let $\boldsymbol{V}_{\pi_\varepsilon}$ be the value of this policy. Then

$$||\boldsymbol{V}_{\pi_\varepsilon} - \boldsymbol{V}^*|| \leq \varepsilon.$$

The proof of the theorem can be found Powell's book (Powell, 2007, p. 79–80).

The solution to a Markov decision process can be expressed as a policy π, a function from states to actions such that for a given policy, the action for each state is fixed and the MDP behaves just like a Markov chain. Therefore, in addition to the value iteration approach, there is also the policy iteration approach, in which finite numbers of policies (strategies) are identifiable and denoted by

$$\pi_i(s, a), i = 1, ..., m. \tag{5.16}$$

The Bellman equation for evaluating policy $\pi(s, a)$ is given by

$$V(s) = \max_a \pi(s, a) \left\{ g(s, a_s) + \gamma \sum_{s' \in S} \Pr(s'|s, a_s) \cdot V_{s'} \right\}. \tag{5.17}$$

Algorithm 5.2: Dynamic programming for Markov decision problem (policy iteration, Howard, 1960, Powell, 2007)

    Objective: calculate optimal policy using policy iteration

    Input precision ε, and policy set $\pi = \{\pi_1, ..., \pi_n\}$

    Select a initial policy π_0

    For $i := 0$ **To** n

        Compute transition probability matrix $\boldsymbol{P}_{\pi_i}$ for policy π_i

        Compute gain vector $\boldsymbol{g}_{\pi_i}$ for policy π_i

Let $v_{i+1} :=$ the solution to equation

$$(\boldsymbol{I} - \gamma \boldsymbol{P}_{\pi_i})v = \boldsymbol{g}_{\pi_i}.$$

Find a policy $\boldsymbol{\pi}_{i+1}$, whose action elements are defined by

$$a_{s,i+1}^* = \arg\max_{a_s} \left(g\left(s, a_s\right), \gamma P_\pi v_{i+1} \right).$$

This requires computing an action for each state s.

If $a_{s,i}^* = a_{s,i-1}^*$ for all state s **Then**

　　$\pi^* = \pi_{i+1}$

　　Exitfor

　Endif

Endfor

Return π^*

§

The procedure-wise difference between value iteration and policy iteration is that in value iteration, we find the maximum expected reward for a given state and then loop over all states, whereas in policy iteration, for a given policy, we calculate the total expected reward from all states and then loop over all possible policies.

In general, either value iteration or policy iteration can solve the problem, but their efficiency will depend on particular situations: If there are lots of actions or if there is already a fair policy, choose policy iteration. If there are few actions, acyclic networks, use value iteration. It is also possible to use a mix of value iteration and policy iteration (Van Nunen, 1976; Puterman and Shin 1978). Another commonly used method for solving the problem is linear programming.

5.3   Pharmaceutial Decision Process

5.3.1   *MDP for a Clinical Development Program*

The success of a pharmaceutical company depends on integrating scientific, clinical, regulatory, and marketing approaches to the development and commercialization of therapies. Clinical development program design offers several important benefits (Pharsight.com): (1) eliminate unnecessary or redundant clinical trials used for internal decision making; (2) identify and address critical path issues that could delay development timeliness; (3) ensure that clinical programs focus quickly and unambiguously on key attributes of the compound.

Monte Carlo simulations can provide a rational basis for decision making and help in optimizing the compound's regulatory strategy and determining its commercial position and value. Simulation of the clinical development program (CDP) can increase confidence in decision making and help to define and track critical success factors and their uncertainties.

Let's study how to model a clinical development program using the Markov decision process.

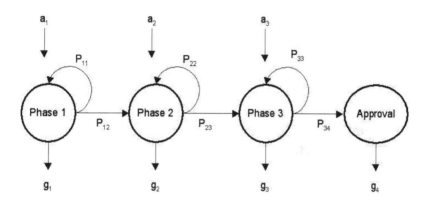

Figure 5.5:   Markov Decision Process for Clinical Trials

A typical drug development program including Phase I to Phase III clinical trials is conducted in sequence. At the end of each phase the decision is made regarding whether to stop the program (the "No-Go" decision) or carry on to the next phase (the "Go" decision). Each action is associated with an estimated net gain (Figure 5.5). Formally it can be modeled by the following MDP:

(1) A finite set of states S
    For the case in Figure 5.5, the state space is given by
    $S = \{$Phase I, Phase II, Phase III, NDA approval$\}$.
(2) A set of actions A_s (state-dependent action space)
    The choice of action set can be $A_s = \{$Go, No-Go$\}$ and/or sample size n_i for the ith phase.
(3) Action rules:
    The action rule or decision rule is typically a set of values, $A_i = \{a_{ij}, j = 1, 2, ...m, i = 1, 2, 3\}$, where a_{ij} can be a set of sample size options $(j = 1, ..., m)$ for the ith phase trial, or $A_i = [a_{\min}, a_{\max}]$ as the range of cutpoint for "Go, No-Go" decision making. The action space can also be a vector, e.g., corresponding to efficacy and safety require-

ments or corresponding to a point estimate and confidence interval of a parameter (or p-value).

The goal is to find the optimal policy $A_i^* = \{a_{1*}, a_{2*}, a_{3*}\}$ that maximizes the expected gain.

(4) A discount factor for future rewards $0 < \gamma \leq 1$.

(5) Immediate reward

In the simplest case, the immediate reward $g_i (a_i = a)$ or $g_i (a)$ for simplicity at the ith state (phase) can be a cost c_{i+1} and a reward of NDA approval or value of out-licensing of the NME.

(6) Transition dynamics $T : S \times A \times S \to [0, 1]$

The transition probability of going from the ith phase to the $(i + 1)^{th}$ phase is a function of action rule A_i written as

$$T (s_i, a, s_{i+1}) = \Pr (s_{i+1} | s_i, A_i). \tag{5.18}$$

We now use a numerical example to illustrate the process.

Example 5.2: Optimal Sample Size for Trials in a Clinical Development Plan

Suppose the CDP team wants to develop a clinical development program for a disease indication, which includes Phase I to III trials (see Figure 5.8). Phase I is a single arm toxicity study; Phase II and III trials are two-group efficacy studies with two parallel groups. One common and important question is how to determine the optimal sample size for each trial so that the success or the expected overall gain for the CDP is maximized. Let's build, step by step, a Markov decision process for this problem.

(1) State space

$$S = \{\text{Phase I, Phase II, Phase III, NDA approval}\}$$

(2) Action space

In practice, there are limits for sample size. For simplicity, assume the limits (i.e., the action space) are independent of state (the phase):

$$A = \{10, ..., 1000\}.$$

(3) Discount rate

Based on typical trial durations, assume the discount rate

$$\gamma = 0.95.$$

(4) Immediate reward and cost

In calculating immediate gains in Phase I to III trials, the costs are approximately proportional to the corresponding sample size. After approval for marketing there is a commercial/advertising cost. The net gains (cost) for Phases I to III can be written as a function of sample size or simply the sample size:

$$g_i(n_i) = n_i, i = 1, 2, 3 \tag{5.19}$$

and the net gain for marketing the drug, less commercial cost, is assumed to be $g_4 = 10000$.

(5) Decision rules and transition probabilities

Assume the decision rule for the Phase I trial is that if the toxicity rate $r_1 \leq \eta_1 = 0.2$, the study will continue to Phase II; otherwise it will stop. The decision rules for Phase II are based on a hypothesis test for treatment difference a in efficacy. Specifically, if the one-sided p-value for the test $p_2 \leq \eta_2 = 0.1$, the study will continue and a Phase III trial will be launched; otherwise, the study will stop after Phase II. Similar to Phase II, Phase III is a parallel two-group active-control trial. The decision rules are: if the one-sided p-value for the efficacy testing $p_3 < \eta_3 = 0.025$, the drug will be approved for marketing; otherwise the NDA will fail.

From these decision rules, we can determine the transition probabilities. The transition probability from Phase I to Phase II can be calculated using binomial distribution (see Chapter 2)

$$p_{12}(n_1) = \sum_{i=0}^{\lfloor \eta_1 n_1 \rfloor} B(i; p_0, n_1) = \sum_{i=0}^{\lfloor \eta_1 n_1 \rfloor} \binom{n_1}{i} p_0^i (1 - p_0)^{n_1 - i}, \tag{5.20}$$

where p_0 is the toxicity rate of the NME, $B(\cdot; \cdot, \cdot)$ is the binomial p.m.f., and the floor function $\lfloor x \rfloor$ gives the integer part of x.

The transition probability p_{23} from Phase II to Phase III is the power of the hypothesis test in the Phase II trial at the one-sided alpha level of 0.1, i.e.,

$$p_{23}(n_2) = \Phi\left(\frac{\sqrt{n_2}}{2}\delta - z_{1-\eta_2}\right) \tag{5.21}$$

where δ is the normalized treatment difference, and Φ is the standard normal c.d.f. See Chapter 6 for more about power for clinical trial designs.

Similarly, the transition probability from Phase III to NDA approval is given by

$$p_{34}(n_3) = \Phi\left(\frac{\sqrt{n_3}}{2}\delta - z_{1-\eta_3}\right). \tag{5.22}$$

Note that there is no repeated trial, even though p_{ii} in Figure 5.8 seems to represent a transition loop. Keep in mind that in this simple case each state has only one immediately proceeding state. The rest of the transition probabilities can be easily calculated as follows:

$$p_{11} = 1 - p_{12}, \tag{5.23}$$
$$p_{22} = 1 - p_{23},$$
$$p_{33} = 1 - p_{34}.$$

(6) Dynamic programming

We are now ready to use dynamic programming to solve this problem. Start with Bellman's equation:

$$\begin{cases} V_4 = g_4 \\ V_i = \max_{n_i \in A} \left\{ g_i\left(n_i\right) + \gamma p_{i,i+1}\left(n_i\right) V_{i+1} \right\}, i = 3, 2, 1. \end{cases} \tag{5.24}$$

Note that, compared to (5.12), there is no summation $\sum$ in (5.24). This is because for the MDP in Figure 5.5, there is only one state leading in and one coming out.

(7) Monte Carlo algorithm

The value iteration algorithm, Algorithm 5.1, can be directly used.

Example 5.3: In Example 5.2, we were only concerned with the optimization of sample size, but in practice, it is also important to optimize the cutpoints $\{\eta_1, \eta_2, \eta_3\}$ simultaneously. Let's build an MDP for the decision problem:

(1) State space

$$S = \{\text{Phase I, Phase II, Phase III, NDA approval}\}.$$

(2) Action space

$$A_i = \boldsymbol{u}_i \times \boldsymbol{v}_i, \tag{5.25}$$

where the sample-size space and cutpoint space are given, respectively, by

$$\boldsymbol{u}_i = \{n_{i,\min}, ..., n_{i,\max}\} \text{ and } \boldsymbol{v}_i = [\eta_{i,\min}, \eta_{i,\max}], i = 1, 2, 3.$$

(3) Discount rate

Let $\gamma = 1$ for simplicity.

(4) Immediate reward and cost

$$g_i(a_i) = c_{0i} + n_i, i = 1, 2, 3, \tag{5.26}$$

where c_{0i} is constant.

The net gain for marketing the drug less commercial costs is assumed to be a linear function of the normalized treatment effect δ:

$$g_4 = g_0 + b\delta,$$

where g_0 and b are constants.

(5) Decision rules and transition probabilities

Assume the decision rules are similar to those in Example 5.2 and specified as follows

Phase I: if the observed toxicity rate $r_1 \leq \eta_1$, the study will continue to Phase II; otherwise it will stop.

Phase II: if the one-sided p-value for the efficacy test $p_2 \leq \eta_2$, launch a Phase III trial; otherwise, stop.

Phase III: if the one-sided p-value for the efficacy test $p_3 < 0.025$ (0.025 is a regulatory requirement for approval, and therefore is not considered a variable), the drug will be approved for marketing; otherwise the NDA will fail.

Expressions for the transition probabilities are the same as in Example 5.2, but for clarity, we rewrite p_{ij} as a function of both sample size n_i and the cutpoint η_i.

$$p_{12}(n_1, \eta_1) = \sum_{i=0}^{\lfloor \eta_1 n_1 \rfloor} B(i; p_0, n_1), \tag{5.27}$$

where p_0 is the toxicity rate of the NME.

The transition probability p_{23} from Phase II to Phase III is the power of the hypothesis test in the Phase II trial, i.e.,

$$p_{23}(n_2, \eta_2) = \Phi\left(\frac{\sqrt{n_2}}{2}\delta - z_{1-\eta_2}\right) \tag{5.28}$$

where δ is the normalized treatment difference, and Φ is the standard normal c.d.f.

Similarly, the transition probability from Phase III to approval is given by

$$p_{34}(n_3) = \Phi\left(\frac{\sqrt{n_3}}{2}\delta - z_{1-0.025}\right). \tag{5.29}$$

The rest of the transition probabilities can be calculated using (5.23).

(6) Dynamic programming

We are now ready to use dynamic programming to solve this problem. Start with Bellman's equation:

$$\begin{cases} V_4 = g_4 \\ V_i = \max_{n_i \in u_i, \eta_i \in v_i} \{g_i(n_i) + p_{i,i+1}(n_i) V_{i+1}\}, i = 3, 2, 1. \end{cases} \quad (5.30)$$

(7) Monte Carlo algorithm

Algorithm 5.1 can be used with consideration of the initial condition $s(t = 0) = s_0$, the financial, time, patient population, and other constraints.

Example 5.4:

So far, we have not considered the action rules (policy) that consider efficacy and safety jointly. In most realistic settings, they have to be considered simultaneously at some point, e.g., in Phase II and Phase III trials. The key is to construct the transition probabilities using the policy with efficacy and safety components.

Let's first consider the situation in which efficacy and safety are independent. The action rules are specified as follows (refer to Figure 5.8).

For the Phase I trial, if the observed toxicity rate $r_1 \leq \eta_{11}$, a Phase II trial will be launched with sample size n_2; for the Phase II trial, if the observed toxicity rate $r_2 \leq \eta_{21}$ and the p-value for the efficacy test $p_2 < \eta_{22}$, a Phase III trial will be initiated with sample size n_3. Drug approval for marketing requires observed toxicity rate $r_3 \leq \eta_{31}$ and one-sided p-value $p_3 < 0.025$. Based on these action rules, the transition probabilities can now be calculated using the following formulations:

$$p_{12}(n_1) = \sum_{i=0}^{\lfloor \eta_1 n_1 \rfloor} B(i; p_0, n_1) = \sum_{i=0}^{\lfloor \eta_1 n_1 \rfloor} \binom{n_1}{i} p_0^i (1 - p_0)^{n_1 - i}, \quad (5.31)$$

$$p_{23}(n_2) = \Phi\left(\frac{\sqrt{n_2}}{2}\delta - z_{1-\eta_2}\right) \sum_{i=0}^{\lfloor \eta_2 n_2 \rfloor} B(i; p_0, n_2) \quad (5.32)$$

$$p_{34}(n_3) = \Phi\left(\frac{\sqrt{n_3}}{2}\delta - z_{1-\eta_3}\right) \sum_{i=0}^{\lfloor \eta_3 n_3 \rfloor} B(i; p_0, n_3). \quad (5.33)$$

In these formulations, we have assumed that toxicity and efficacy are independent responses in any given patient with a given dose, which is often reasonable — we know that it is not necessary that a patient with high efficacy will have high toxicity. We should not confuse this with the common concept that efficacy and toxicity are correlated in the sense that an increase in dosage will likely increase both efficacy and toxicity for the same patient.

Note that we have not considered the efficacy criterion in the action rule for Phase I trial. The reason is that in an early phase trial, there are usually no observable clinical efficacy endpoints. In such a case, we have to use the partial observable Markov decision process (POMDP), as discussed in the next section. When considering the biomaker in the Monte Carlo simulation, data have to be generated with some joint probability distributions using the techniques presented in Chapter 2, Virtual Sampling Techniques.

Example 5.5:

We now consider another common situation, i.e., multiple optional paths in a clinical development plan (Figure 5.6). One path is to follow the traditional paradigm: single ascending dose (SAD) study → dose finding study (DFS) → pivotal Phase III studies (PPS) → NDA approval. The second path is an innovative approach with adaptive design: SAD → adaptive seamless trial (AST) → NDA approval. The adaptive seamless trial combines the DFS and PPS as a single (seamless) trial.

Let's build an MDP for this problem:

The power of a trial is dependent on the true but unknown treatment effect; therefore, the transition probabilities will be estimated from the data available at the decision point. Consequently, the same transition probability (e.g., from Phase II to Phase III) may have different values when it is calculated at the end of Phase I and the end of Phase II.

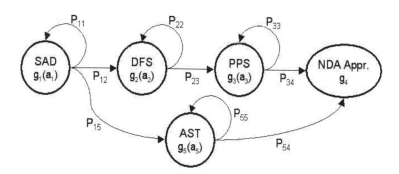

Figure 5.6:   Clinical Development Options

(1) State space

$$S = \{\text{SAD, DFS, PPS, NDA approval, AST}\}$$

(2) Action space

$$A_i = \boldsymbol{u}_i \times \boldsymbol{v}_i, \tag{5.34}$$

where the sample-size space and cutpoint space are given, respectively, by

$$\boldsymbol{u}_i = \{n_{i,\min}, ..., n_{i,\max}\} \text{ and } \boldsymbol{v}_i = [\eta_{i,\min}, \eta_{i,\max}], i = 1, 2, 3, 5$$

where $\eta_{3,\min} = \eta_{3,\max}$.

(3) Discount rate

Let $\gamma = 1$ for simplicity.

(4) Immediate reward and cost

$$\begin{cases} g_i(a_i) = c_{0i} + n_i, i = 1, 2, 3, 5 \\ g_4 = g_0 + b\delta. \end{cases} \tag{5.35}$$

The net gain can also be a random function.

(5) Decision rules and transition probabilities

Assume the decision rules are similar to those in Example 5.3, i.e.,

Phase I: if the observed toxicity rate r_1 is bounded within $\eta_1 < r_1 \le \eta_5$, the Phase II trial will start; if $r_1 \le \eta_1$, the adaptive trial will initiate; otherwise it will stop. (Questions to students: What will happen to the decision rules if $\eta_1 = \eta_5$? What will happen if $\eta_1 < 0$?)

Phase II: if the one-sided p-value for the efficacy test $p_2 \le \eta_2$, launch a Phase III trial; otherwise, stop.

Phase III: if the one-sided p-value for the efficacy test $p_3 < 0.025$, the drug will be approved for marketing; otherwise the NDA will fail.

Expressions for the transition probabilities are

$$p_{12}(n_1, \eta_1, \eta_5) = \sum_{i = \lfloor \eta_1 n_1 \rfloor + 1}^{\lfloor \eta_5 n_1 \rfloor} B(i; p_0, n_1), \tag{5.36}$$

$$p_{15}(n_1, \eta_1) = \sum_{i=0}^{\lfloor \eta_1 n_1 \rfloor} B(i; p_0, n_1), \tag{5.37}$$

$$p_{23}(n_2, \eta_2) = \Phi\left(\frac{\sqrt{n_2}}{2}\delta - z_{1-\eta_2}\right), \tag{5.38}$$

and

$$p_{34}(n_3) = \Phi\left(\frac{\sqrt{n_3}}{2}\delta - z_{1-0.025}\right). \tag{5.39}$$

The transition probability p_{54} is the power of the adaptive trial (see Chapter 6) and simulation is required to calculate power for a given sample size. However, at the macro-simulation level, an approximation based on the corresponding classical design can be used. In this case, we can write

$$p_{54} \approx \zeta p_{34}(n_3),$$

where coefficient ζ varies from adaptive design to adaptive design, but for two-group trials, it is about 0.9.

The rest of the transition probabilities are straightforward calculations.

Other possible decision rules at Phase I that can be used are choosing transition probabilities p_{12} and p_{15} based the expected Q-value (net gain) of the traditional approach (Q_T) and the innovation approach (Q_I). There are two common ways: (1) if $Q_T < Q_I$, set $p_{12} = 0$; otherwise $p_{15} = 0$. (2) Choose the probability proportional to the corresponding Q-value, i.e., $\frac{p_{12}}{p_{15}} = \frac{Q_T}{Q_I}$. Therefore, $p_{12} = \frac{Q_T}{Q_T + Q_I}(1 - p_{11})$.

(6) Dynamic programming

We are now ready to use dynamic programming to solve this problem. Start with Bellman's equation:

$$
\begin{cases}
V_4 = g_4 \\
V_5 = \max\limits_{n_5 \in \boldsymbol{u}_5, \eta_5 \in \boldsymbol{v}_5} \{g_5(n_5) + p_{5,4}(n_4) V_4\} \\
V_i = \max\limits_{n_i \in \boldsymbol{u}_i, \eta_i \in \boldsymbol{v}_i} \{g_i(n_i) + p_{i,i+1}(n_i) V_{i+1}\}, i = 3, 2 \\
V_1 = \max\limits_{n_1 \in \boldsymbol{u}_1, \eta_1 \in \boldsymbol{v}_1} \{g_1(n_1) + p_{1,2}(n_1) V_2 + p_{1,5}(n_1) V_5\}
\end{cases}
\tag{5.40}
$$

5.3.2 *Markov Decision Tree and Out-Licensing*

So far we have not considered the value of adaptive design, which may shorten the development time or time-to-market, which is a significant factor driving the CDP. If an adaptive trial shortens the time-to-market, the value can be reflected in the gain g_4 from drug marketing in Example 5.4. Thus the gain g_4 in Figure 5.6 becomes path dependent. To solve this problem, we can convert the stochastic decision problem (no longer the Markov decision process) to a stochastic decision tree (SDT). In a stochastic decision tree, there can be several paths out from a decision node, but only one parent decision node from which the path comes in. Furthermore, each state in a stochastic decision tree can at most be visited once. Figure 5.7 is an SDT converted from Figure 5.6 in Example 5.5.

After the conversion, the transition probabilities can be calculated sim-

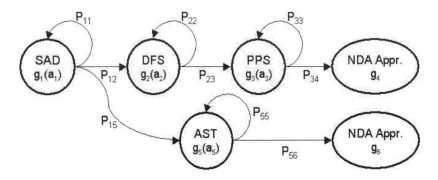

Figure 5.7:   MDP Conversion to Stochastic Decision Tree

ilarly as in an MDP. The expected net gain for each path can easily calculated using the transition probability $p_{ij}(a_i)$ and the net gains g_i associated
with that path. Note that a stochastic decision tree is a simple MDP with
a single path in for each decision node. However, when converting to SDT
from MDP, the total number of paths in a stochastic decision tree will grow
very fast. If each node has $k = 2$ action-lines connected and the tree has
$m = 4$ layers of nodes, there will be $n = 2^4 = 16$ possible paths to reach
the end-nodes. If $k = 3, m = 6, n = 3^6 = 729$; if $k = 6, m = 14, n = 6^{14} =$
$78,364,164,096$. The computational time quickly becomes overwhelming
or inractable.

Example 5.6

In this example, we consider the option of out-licensing an NME at a
certain stage (e.g., the end of the Phase II trial) or a joint venture (share
risk and profit) after a promising result from Phase II. This option is often
considered when an internal resource is limited, as discussed in Chapter 4.
the MDP for including out-licensing (OL) and joint venture (JV) options
in the CDP in Example 5.2 is plotted in Figure 5.8.

From various examples in this section so far, we can see that action rules
are a critical element to the MDP. They affect the transitional probabilities
because action rules often include a statement about state space and action
space. We can simplify the steps for building an MDP as follows (assume
the discount rate $\gamma = 1$).

(1) Draw an MDP diagram (see, e.g., Figure 5.8)

(2) Specify a family of action (decision) rules

A family of decision rules or a policy is a collection of options for choosing different decision rules. In the previous several examples, "if $p_3 < 0.025$,
drug approved" is an action rule, whereas "if $p_2 < \eta_2$, launch a Phase III

trial" is a family of action rules because each value of η_2 determines an action rule. For this reason, the goal of using an MDP is to determine an optimal action rule for each state.

Note that a family of action rules doesn't have to be a simple smooth function; it is often expressed using a combination of several equations such as in Example 5.4.

The expected gain from OL is dependent on the results at stage 2, i.e., $g_5(a_2)$. The net gain (cost) $g_6 (a_6) > g_3 (a_3)$ because of risk sharing, and $g_7 < g_4$ because of profit sharing by JV.

(3) Determine the transition probabilities

The transition probabilities are determined by the action rules, and numerical values are usually obtained through Monte Carlo simulation.

(4) Apply dynamic programming algorithms

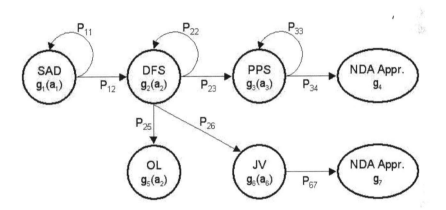

SAD = single ascending, DFS = Dose finding study, OL = out-licensing, JV = Joint venture, PPS = Pivotal phase 3 study

Figure 5.8: MDP with Out-Licensing and Joint Venture

5.3.3 *Research and Development Portfolio Optimization*

Most pharmaceutical research efforts have focused on four major disease areas: central nervous system, cancer, cardiovascular, and infectious disease. Increasingly, it will have to search for products in poorly understood and more complex therapeutic areas such as autoimmune diseases and genitourinary conditions (Bernard, 2002; Hu, et al. 2007). The increasing failure rate and cost in Pharma Research and Development (5000 patients per NDA based on data from 1999 to 2003 — Mathieu, 2003) alert pharmaceutical companies to be extremely cautious in their decision making. They have to carefully evaluate their core competency, technological advantages, competitive barriers, and financial resources before committing to develop a drug to fulfill unmet needs. They have to weigh their options carefully from the perspectives of market potential, patent, intellectual property portfolio, competitive forces and regulatory status, and core competencies, and build their Research and Development portfolio accordingly.

In this regard, many new technologies can be used in conjunction with traditional methods to accelerate the Research and Development process and reduce the cost. From this perspective, computer simulation can play a significant role and the following example illustrates how.

Example 5.7

Suppose a biotech company has identified two leading compounds (NME-1 and NME-2) from drug discovery and preclinical studies. However, due to financial constraints, the management team proposed the following strategy for evaluations: If the NME-1 Phase I or Phase II trial failed, we consider launching NME-2 trials. If Phase I and II trials are successful but NME-1 Phase III fails, the sponsor doesn't have enough cash to invest in NME-1 clinical trials and NME-2 will be considered for out-licensing. However, if Phase III is successful for drug marketing, we consider investigating NME-2 in clinical trials. Other options such as a joint venture are not considered for simplicity. This strategy is plotted as an MDP in Figure 5.9.

What the working team needs to do is to develop an MDP with specific action rules that optimize the MDP and evaluate the maximum expected net gain and variations of the gain (for students: Why is the variation also an important factor to consider for the biotech company?).

Example 5.8: Risk Aversion and Pick-Winner Strategy

Risk aversion is a concept in economics, finance, and psychology related to the behavior of consumers and investors under uncertainty. Risk aversion is the reluctance of a person to accept a bargain with an uncertain payoff rather than another bargain with more certain, but possibly lower, expected payoff. This concept is also applicable to the pharmaceutical industry. Risk aversion is measured as the additional marginal reward required for an investor to accept additional risk, which is measured as the standard deviation of the return on investment.

Risk aversion is reflected in the diversity of the pharmaceutical portfolio. With multiple leading NMEs in the drug discovery and preclinical pipeline,

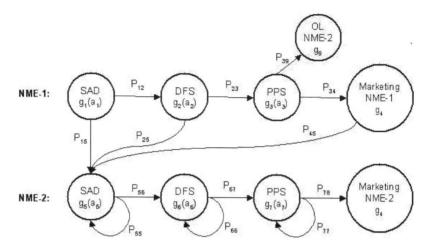

SAD = single ascending, DFS = Dose finding study, OL = out-licensing,
JV = Joint venture, PPS = Pivotal phase 3 study

Figure 5.9:   CDP with Multiple-Indication Options

an optimal strategy to pick the winners and carry them forward to clinical development is critically important. We can do this by means of an MDP. Suppose there are n leading NMEs identified. If n is relatively small, we can launch all n NMEs at the same time. In the development process (preclinical to Phase III trials), an MDP can be used to tune the decision rule of picking the winner so that the gain is optimized. If n is large, a subset of the NMEs can be tested first, and losers (bad NMEs) are dropped over time in the development process. Then more NMEs can be tested later in development.

There are many criteria (i.e., decision rules) that can be used for picking the winners. For example, pick the safest m_0 out of n NMEs, based on observed toxicity rate (aggregated toxicity rate from multiple components) in preclincal, for further testing in Phase I; pick m_1 best responses out of m_0 NMEs in Phase I and carry on to the Phase II trial; the criteria for the best response can be measured by some utility index that consists of safety and efficacy biomarkers. After a set of decision rules is formed, the corresponding transition probabilities can be constructed as well as gain/reward functions. Next, the optimal policy can be found using the dynamic programming algorithm (Algorithm 5.1) to maximize the gain or success.

5.4   Extension of the Markov Decision Process

5.4.1   *Q-Learning*

We have seen, in the previous examples, extensions of the MDP: (1) the reward may be a function of the action as well as the state, $g(s, a)$; (2) the reward may be a function of the resulting state as well as the action and state, $g(s, a, s')$; or (3) the action space may be different at each state, so that it is A_s rather than A. These extensions only complicate the notation, but make no real difference to the problem or the solution method. In this section we will discuss several important extensions that are demanded by practice.

The MDPs we discussed so far have known transition probabilities so that calculation can be carried out. What if the probability is unknown or too complicated and becomes intractable? In our previous examples for clinical development, the transition probabilities and consequently the expected overall gain are heavily dependent on the toxicity rate p_0 and normalized treatment effect δ, the two unknown parameters. If the assumptions about the two parameters change, the overall expected gain will change. In other words, the optimal action rules will depend on the assumptions around the parameters. To solve this dilemma, there are several methods available including Q-learning and bayesian stochastic decision process (BSDP). We are going to discuss the methods in the next sections.

Q-Learning (Watkins, 1989; Sutton and Barto, 1998; Gosavi, 2003) is a form of model-free reinforcement learning. It is a forwards induction and an asynchronous dynamic programming. The power of reinforcement learning lies in its ability to solve the Markov decision process without computing the transition probabilities that are needed in value and policy iteration.

The key algorithm in Q-learning is the recursive formulation for the Q-value:

$$Q_i = \begin{cases} (1 - \alpha_i)Q_{i-1}(s, a) + \alpha_i [g_i + \gamma V_{i-1}(s_i')] & \text{if } s = s_i, \ a = a_i \\ Q_{i-1}(s, a), \text{ otherwise,} \end{cases} \quad (5.41)$$

where the learning rate $0 \leq \alpha_i < 1$ is a constant chosen and

$$V_{i-1}(s_i') = \max_b \{Q_{i-1}(s', b)\}. \quad (5.42)$$

The convergence of Q-learning is ensured by the following theorem (Watkins and Dayan, 1992).

Theorem 5.2   *Let $Q^*(s, a)$ be the reward corresponding to the optimal policy and $\alpha_n^i(s, a)$ be the learning rate at the ith time that action a is* *associated with state s. Given bounded rewards $|g_n| \leq G$, learning rates $0 \leq \alpha_n < 1$, and*

$$\sum_{i=1}^{\infty} \alpha_n^i(s,a) = \infty, \quad \sum_{i=1}^{\infty} \left[\alpha_n^i(s,a)\right]^2 < \infty, \quad \forall s,a, \qquad (5.43)$$

then $Q_n(s,a) \to Q^*(s,a)$ as $n \to \infty$, $\forall s, a$, with probability 1.

Q-learning is feasible for the situation where many repetitive experiments, such as robotics studies, are conducted. For example, a Robotic Floor Cleaner (an automatic vacuum machine) can learn from every step in the cleaning process using an MDP. However, for a clinical trial, the usefulness of Q-learning is limited due to the limitation in the number of clinical trials for a therapeutic indication or an NME in the short term, but it can be useful in the long run.

5.4.2 *Bayesian Learning Process*

In Bayesian inference, a prior probability distribution, often called simply the prior, is a probability distribution representing knowledge or belief about an unknown quantity prior, that is, before any directly related data have been observed. A prior is related to individual experiences and those experiences are at least remotely related to the current problem and serve as the basis for the individual's prior.

Denote prior distribution $\pi(\theta)$, and sample distribution $f(x|\theta)$. The following are four basic Bayesian elements:

(1) The joint distribution of (θ, x) given by

$$\varphi(\theta, x) = f(x|\theta)\pi(\theta), \qquad (5.44)$$

(2) The marginal distribution of x given by

$$m(x) = \int \varphi(\theta, x)\, d\theta = \int f(x|\theta)\pi(\theta)\, d\theta, \qquad (5.45)$$

(3) The posterior distribution of θ given by Bayes' formula

$$\pi(\theta|x) = \frac{f(x|\theta)\pi(\theta)}{m(x)}, \quad \text{and} \qquad (5.46)$$

(4) The predictive probability distribution given by

$$P(y|x) = \int P(x|y, \theta)\pi(\theta|x)\, d\theta. \qquad (5.47)$$

Example 5.9: Beta Posterior Distribution

Assume that $X \sim Bin(n, p)$ and $p \sim Beta(\alpha, \beta)$.

The sample distribution is given by

$$f(x|p) = \binom{n}{x} p^x (1-p)^{n-x}, \quad x = 0, 1, ..., n. \tag{5.48}$$

The prior about the parameter p is given by

$$\pi(p) = \frac{1}{B(\alpha, \beta)} p^{\alpha-1} (1-p)^{\beta-1}, \quad 0 \le p \le 1, \tag{5.49}$$

where beta function $B(\alpha, \beta) = \frac{\Gamma(\alpha)\Gamma(\beta)}{\Gamma(\alpha+\beta)}$.

The joint and marginal distributions can be written as

$$\varphi(p, x) = \frac{\binom{n}{x}}{B(\alpha, \beta)} p^{\alpha+x-1} (1-p)^{n-x+\beta-1} \tag{5.50}$$

and

$$m(x) = \frac{\binom{n}{x}}{B(\alpha, \beta)} B(\alpha + x, n - x + \beta), \tag{5.51}$$

respectively.

Therefore, the posterior distribution is given by

$$\pi(p|x) = \frac{p^{\alpha+x-1} (1-p)^{n-x+\beta-1}}{B(\alpha + x, \beta + n - x)} = Beta(\alpha + x, \beta + n - x). \tag{5.52}$$

Example 5.10: Normal Posterior Distribution

Assume that $X \sim N(\theta, \sigma^2/n)$ and $\theta \sim N(\mu, \sigma^2/n_0)$.

The posterior distribution can be written as

$$\pi(\theta|X) \propto f(X|\theta) \pi(\theta) \tag{5.53}$$

or

$$\pi(\theta|X) = Ce^{-\frac{(X-\theta)^2 n}{2\sigma^2}} e^{-\frac{(\theta-\mu)^2 n_0}{2\sigma^2}}, \tag{5.54}$$

where C is a normalization constant.

We immediately recognize that posterior (5.54) is the normal distribution $N\left(\frac{n_0\mu+nX}{n_0+n}, \frac{\sigma^2}{n_0+n}\right)$.

Conjugate Family of Distributions

A family F of probability distribution on Θ is said to be conjugate (or closed under sampling) if, for every $\pi \in F$, the posterior distribution $\pi(\theta|x)$ also belongs to F.

The main interest of conjugacy becomes more apparent when F is as small as possible and parameterized. When F is parameterized, switching from prior to posterior distribution is reduced to an updating of the corresponding parameters. This is a main reason why conjugate priors are so popular, as the posterior distributions are always computable, at least to a certain extent.

The conjugate prior approach, which was originated by Raiffa and Schlaifer (1961), can be partially justified through an invariance reasoning. Updating the model should not be radical, e.g., only the values of the parameters, not the model or function itself, are updated. On the other hand, the conjugate model approach is not appreciated in the long run because it does not allow for correcting the model itself (not the parameters in the predefined model) when it is found to be unfitt. Commonly used conjugate families are presented in Table 5.1.

Table 5.1: Commonly Used Conjugate Families

Model $f(x|\theta)$	Prior $\pi(\theta)$	Posterior $\pi(\theta|x)$
Normal $N\left(\theta, \sigma^2\right)$	$N\left(\mu, \tau^2\right)$	$N\left(\frac{\sigma^2\mu+\tau^2 x}{\sigma^2+\tau^2}, \frac{\sigma^2\tau^2}{\sigma^2+\tau^2},\right)$
Poisson $P(\theta)$	$G(\alpha, \beta)$	$G(\alpha+x, \beta+1)$
Gamma $G(\nu, \theta)$	$G(\alpha, \beta)$	$G(\alpha+\nu, \beta+x)$
Binomial $Bin(n, \theta)$	$Beta(\alpha, \beta)$	$Beta(\alpha+x, \beta+n-x)$
Neg. Bin $NB(m, \theta)$	$Beta(\alpha, \beta)$	$Beta(\alpha+m, \beta+x)$

Bayesian Q-Learning

When the Bayesian learning paradigm is applied to the uncertainty of the Q-value, it becomes Bayesian Q-learning (Dearden, Friedman, and Russell, 1998).

5.4.3 *Bayesian Decision Theory*

The theory focuses on instrumental rationality, that is, on reasoning about how people can best achieve their desires in light of their beliefs. Decisions take place under three conditions: certainty (outcomes of actions are certain), risk (outcomes are not certain but their probabilities are known), and uncertainty (probabilities of outcomes are unknown).

In decision theory, statistical models involve three spaces: the observation space X, the parameter space Θ, and the action space A. Actions are guided by a decision rule $\delta(x)$. An action $\alpha \in A$ always has an associated consequence characterized by the so-called loss function $L(\theta, a)$. In hypothesis testing, the action space is $A = \{\text{accept; reject}\}$.

Because it is usually impossible to uniformly minimize the loss $L(\theta, a)$, in the frequentist paradigm, the decision rule δ is determined such that it minimizes the following average loss:

$$R(\theta, \delta) = \int_X L(\theta, \delta(\boldsymbol{x})) f(\boldsymbol{x}|\theta) d\boldsymbol{x}. \qquad (5.55)$$

The rule $a = \delta(\boldsymbol{x})$ is often called an estimator in estimation problems. Common examples of loss function are *squared error loss* (SEL), $L(\theta, a) = (\theta - a)^2$, *absolute loss*, $L(\theta, a) = |\theta - \alpha|$, the $0-1$ *loss*, $L(\theta, a) = \mathbf{1}(|\alpha - \theta|)$, etc.

By averaging (5.55) over a range of θ for a given prior $\pi(\theta)$, we can obtain:

$$r(\pi, \delta) = \int_\Theta \int_X L(\theta, \delta(\boldsymbol{x})) f(\boldsymbol{x}|\theta) \pi(\theta) d\mathbf{x} d\theta. \qquad (5.56)$$

Theorem 5.3   *Bayesian expected loss is the expectation of the loss function with respect to the posterior measure, i.e.,*

$$\rho(\delta(\boldsymbol{x}), \pi) = \int_\Theta L(\theta, \delta(\boldsymbol{x})) \pi(\theta|\boldsymbol{x}) d\theta \qquad (5.57)$$

An action $a^* = \delta^*(\boldsymbol{x})$ that minimizes the posterior expected loss is called a Bayes action.

The two notions (5.56) and (5.57) are equivalent in the sense that they lead to the same decision.

5.4.4   *Bayesian Stochastic Decision Process*

So far we have assumed that the parameters of an NME, such as the toxicity rate and treatment effect, more precisely the toxicity and efficacy response characteristics, are known. In reality, the transition probability $\Pr(s'|s, a; \delta)$ is not a fixed function; rather, it is dependent on the cumulative information about δ and others. In Bayesian terms, there is a need to differentiate the prior and posterior distributions. We rewrite the transition probability $\Pr(s'|s, a; \delta)$ to include the parameter δ (normalized treatment effect) to stress the δ dependency of the transition probability. In the frequentist paradigm, the parameter δ is an unknown but fixed number. However, people make decisions based on knowledge (estimate) about δ, not δ itself, because the true value of δ is unknown.

Because $\Pr(s'|s, a; \delta)$ and δ is updated based on cumulative data from previous states, the stochastic process is usually not stationary or Markovian any more. This implies that the backwards induction algorithm cannot be applied. However, an approximate solution is to use posterior distribution in Bellman's equation. That is,

$$V(s) = \max_{a_s \in A} \left(g(s, a) + \gamma E \sum_{s' \in S} \Pr\left(s'|s, a_s; \tilde{\delta}_s\right) \cdot V(s') \right), \qquad (5.58)$$

where $\tilde{\delta}_s$ is the posterior estimate of δ at stage s and E denotes the expectation taken with respect to the posterior distribution of $\tilde{\delta}_s$.

We can see that the Bayesian stochastic decision process (BSDP) is similar to the MPD except for the calculation of the transition probability. In the MDP, parameter δ is a fixed number, whereas in the BSDP, the posterior $\tilde{\delta}_s$ is used in the probability calculation.

For Example 5.2, the p_{12} for the BSDP will be the same as the MPD, where the prior toxicity rate p_0 is used. For $p_{23}(n_2)$ is also the same for the two methods, where the prior effect size $\delta = \delta_0$ is used. However, the calculation for $p_{34}(n_3)$ is different for the BSDP than for the MDP. For the BSDP, the transition probability is given by

$$p_{34}(n_3) = \Phi\left(\frac{\sqrt{n_3}}{2}\tilde{\delta}_3 - z_{1-n_3} \right), \qquad (5.59)$$

where the posterior

$$\tilde{\delta}_3 \sim N\left(\frac{n_0 \delta_0 + n_2 \hat{\delta}_2}{n_0 + n_2}, \frac{1}{n_0 + n_2} \right). \qquad (5.60)$$

Note that δ_0 and n_0 are prior (normalized mean treatment effect) and sample size; $\hat{\delta}_2$ is the observed treatment effect (normalized) in the Phase II trial.

We can see that the calculation of the BSDP is much more intensive due to both the calculation of the posterior distribution and the expectation. Approximations may be used to reduce the computational burden, e.g.,

$$V(s) = \max_{a_s \in A} \left(g(s, a) + \gamma \sum_{s' \in S} \int \Pr(s'|s, a_s; \delta) \pi(\delta) \cdot V(s') \right), \qquad (5.61)$$

where $\pi(\delta)$ is the prior distribution.

Algorithm 5.3: Bayesian Stochastic Decision Process
Objective: Optimization with the Bayesian stochastic decision process
While precision$>\varepsilon$:

Record the current path and best path with maximum $V(s)$.
Calculate the posterior distribution of the model parameters
Calculate p_{ij} based on action and posterior parameters
Use Bayesian Bellman equation (5.58) for value iteration
Stop if the predefined precision ε is reached.
Endwhile
§

Object-oriented simulation software such as ExtentSim provides a powerful tool for simulation where statistical models can be built into each object. Simulations using such a tool are intuitive and can solve many simulation problems, but they usually have low computational efficiency.

5.4.5   *One-Step Forward Approach*

One of the popular approaches in robotics is to let the agent randomly choose an action with the selection probability proportional to the potential gain from each action. The idea behind this approach is to modify the randomization probability gradually in such a way that when our initial judgment about expected gains is wrong, the action will be corrected over time. However, this approach is effective only when the same experiments can be repeated many times. We will use this concept in designing adaptive trials, i.e., response-randomization trials, in Chapter 6.

In dealing with the computational complexity, we can use the one-step forward approach with the following transition probability:

$$p_{ij} = \frac{g_j}{\sum_k g_k},   (5.62)$$

where the summation is performed over all nodes that can be reached by one-step forward from node i.

In the Monte Carlo simulation, this formulation can be used iteratively until all p_{ij} are not changing any more. Theoretical studies are needed for this approach.

5.4.6   *Partially Observable Markov Decision Processes*

So far we have assumed the state s is known at the time when action is to be taken; otherwise policy $\pi(s)$ cannot be calculated. However, in the early stage of drug development, the clinical effects of an NME are usually not directly observable; instead, observations are made on biomarkers, which supposedly have a correlation with the definitive clinical endpoint. This leads to the so-called partially observable Markov process (POMDP).

A POMDP is a generalization of a Markov decision process. In robotics, a POMDP models an agent decision process in which it is assumed that the system dynamics are determined by an MDP, but the agent cannot directly observe the underlying state. Instead, it must infer a distribution over the state based on a model of the world and some local observations. The framework originated in the operations research community, and has spread into artificial intelligence, automated planning communities, and the pharmaceutical industry (Lee, Chang, and Whitemore, 2008).

In some cases in early drug development, the efficacy of an NME is not completely observable. In such a case, the motion is modeled by a hidden Markov chain (HMC). Table 5.2 summarizes the differences between MC, MDP, POMDP, and HM with respect to the state observability and motion controllability.

Table 5.2: Comparison of Stochastic Processes

Markov Models		Transition Controllable?	
		Yes	No
State Observable?	Yes	MDP	MC
	No	POMDP	HMC

Recall that the Markov chain has three properties: (1) a set of states S, (2) transition probabilities: $T(s, s') = P(s_{t+1} = \acute{s} | s_t = s)$, and (3) the starting distribution $P_0(s) = P(s_0 = s)$. For a HMC, two additional properties are required: (1) set of observations Z, and (2) observation probabilities: $O(s, z) = P(z_t = z | s_t = s)$, where s is not observable.

The computations of a POMDP are too complex to cover here without significantly increasing the chapter.

Case Study 5.1: Classical and Adaptive CDPs for CABG patients

In coronary heart disease (CHD), the coronary arteries become clogged with calcium and fatty deposits. Plaques narrow the arteries that carry blood to the heart muscle and can cause ischemic heart disease (too little blood and oxygen reaching the heart muscle). Coronary artery bypass graft (CABG) surgery is a treatment option for ischemic heart disease. CABG surgery is used to create new routes for blood to flow around the narrowed and blocked arteries so that the heart muscle will receive needed oxygen and nutrients. According to the American Heart Association, 427,000 CABG surgeries were performed in the United States in 2004.

The problem is that during a heart bypass procedure, a substance called complement is activated by the body. This complement activation causes an inflammation that can lead to side effects such as chest pain, heart attacks, stroke, heart failure, impairment of memory, language, and motor skills, or death.

A test drug XYZ was brought to the development phase in company A; it was expected to block complement activation and thus reduce side effects. Meanwhile another company B was at the stage of designing a Phase II trial for their test compound ABC for the same indication. The concern for company A was that at the time of designing a Phase III trial for XYZ, ABC could be approved for marketing so that company A would not only lose time and the majority of the market, but also would be required to run an active-control trial (using ABC as the control), instead of a placebo-control trial. As a result, the required Phase III trial for XYZ would be much larger and more costly. During brainstorming, the CDP team in company A proposed another option: using a seamless adaptive design that combines the Phase II and Phase III trials as a single trial such that when the competitor starts its Phase III trial, company A will start the seamless Phase II–III trial. With that strategy, company A would be able to catch up and conduct the placebo-controlled trial since no drug would have been approved for marketing yet. The team summarized their comparisons between the classical and adaptive approaches as follows:

The classical design with separated Phase II and III trials is economically infeasible: (1) potential third in class position, (2) pivotal trial would be noninferior to ABC with a larger sample size, and (3) disadvantages in the US market would not be fully offset by the market gains in the EU which would potentially be realized by the classical CDP paradigm.

Seamless adaptive design is preferable: (1) large combined trial, protracted recruitment period, (2) short treatment period, good timing for registration in the US, and (3) placebo-controlled trial with reduced cost.

5.5   Summary

There are two distinctive decision approaches: descriptive and normative decision theories. Descriptive decision making is a study of the cognitive processes that lead to decisions. Normative decision making considers a decision as a rational act of choice under the viable alternatives using mathematical or statistical modeling techniques. The normative decision approach can be further divided into deterministic and probabilistic approaches. For the deterministic approach, information is considered as completely known, whereas for the probabilistic approach, information is associated with uncertainties or probabilities.

Drug development is a sequence of decision processes. The processes are a mixture of intuitive (descriptive) and normative decisions. We have studied the normative decision approach with the goal of moving (gradually) the decision process in drug development from basically an intuitive approach to essentially a normative approach.

Many problems in our life can be viewed as sequential decision processes to find an optimal solution, either minimizing loss or maximizing gain. The optimum can be obtained using a backwards induction algorithm derived from Bellman's optimality principle. This principle states that an optimal policy has the property that, whatever the initial state and initial decision are, the remaining decisions must constitute an optimal policy with regard to the state resulting from the first decision.

There are two commonly used backwards induction algorithms: value iteration and policy iteration. In addition, there is also an approach of combining the two algorithms.

The deterministic sequential design process is not very practical in drug development without the inclusion of probabilities in the model. The Markov decision process (MDP) is an extension of the Markov chain, in which actions and rewards are attached to the MC states. An MDP can have a finite or infinite horizon. In a finite horizon MPD, the transition probabilities are time dependent, whereas in an infinite horizon MPD, the system has reached its steady state and the transition probabilities are independent of time. An MDP for an infinite horizon problem is defined as follows.

An infinite horizon Markov decision process is a 4-tuple of four elements $\{S, A, \Pr(S, A), g(S, A)\}$ with the following properties:

(1) Finite (N) set of states S
(2) Set of actions A (can be conditioned on state s)
(3) Decision rules
(4) Immediate reward $g(s, a)$, $a \in A$ and $s \in S$
(5) Transition probabilities from state s to s' with action a:

$$T(s, a, s') = \Pr(s'|s, a_i = a).$$

The goal is to find a set of decision rules or a policy $\pi^* = \{a_i^*, i = 1, ..., N\}$ that maximizes the total expected reward.

The commonly used method to solve the MDP is the backwards induction (5.12) with value or policy iterations as presented in Algorithms 5.1 and 5.2.

MDPs can be used in clinical development planning, as illustrated in

Examples 5.2–5.6. A major task in the application of an MDP to a CDP is the calculation of transition probabilities, which is often based on power calculations in clinical trials with respect to various decision (stopping and adaptive) rules.

An MDP can also be used in pharmaceutical Research and Development portfolio optimization, where more than one NME is considered, as illustrated in Examples 5.7 and 5.8.

One of the challenges in the application of the MDP in drug development is that the transition probability is dependent on model parameters (e.g., treatment effect) that are unknown. Different estimation procedures of the parameters can be used, but they are not very convincing. Alternatively, Q-learning, Bayesian Q-learning, and the one-step forward approach can be used. All these methods are forward induction methods as opposed to backward induction methods based on the Bellman optimality principle.

The second challenge is that in the early stage of drug development, the definitive clinical endpoint, such as survival, usually can't be measured, but assessments on certain biomarker, may be done, which can be used to serve as a marker for the clinical endpoint. In such a case, the partial observable Markov decision process can be used.

5.6   Exercises

Exercise 5.1: Give two problems in your life that can be modeled using the Markov decision process.

Exercise 5.2: Solve the Markov decision problem for the career options in Figure 5.4 by maximizing the total reward. The initial state is U (unemployed). Hint: You can use Monte Carlo simulation or construct the transition probability matrix and the equation system to be solved deterministically.

Exercise 5.3: Develop computer pseudocode for the MDP in Example 5.2.

Exercise 5.4: In Example 5.2, assume the sample size at each phase is determined, but you are asked to determine the optimal cutpoints $\{\eta_1, \eta_2, \eta_3\}$ to maximize the expected overall gain for the CDP. Develop an MDP for this problem.

Exercise 5.5: In Example 5.4, consider a model with bi-logistic model (safety & efficacy), where parameters for safety and efficacy have a joint distribution. Develop computer pseudocode for the CDP problem.

Exercise 5.6: Formulation (5.40) provides a backwards induction algorithm for the multi-path CDP problem; develop a computer pseudocode based on (5.40).

Exercise 5.7: Figure 5.10 can represent different models depending on how p_{15} and p_{25} are defined. Can you elaborate these models?

Exercise 5.8: In Example 5.8, suppose there are $n = 10$ NMEs in the preclinical pipeline; formulate an MDP for the problem using a pick-winner strategy. Make additional assumptions as necessary.

Exercise 5.9: Figure 5.10 represents the actual success rates of different phases of clinical trials. Success is defined as the launch of the next phase with the exception of Phase III. Success of the Phase III trial means NDA approval. Discuss how to use this prior in your CDP modeling and simulation.

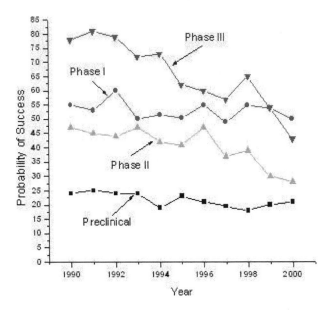

Figure 5.10:   Success Rates of Clinical Trials
(Source: Pammolli and Riccaboni, 2007, p. 116)

Exercise 5.10: In early drug development phases, because a definitive endpoint (DE) is not available, a biomarker (BM) is often used to predict treatment effect on the definitive endpoint. Study the validity of this approach using the following artificial data. If your conclusion is negative, do you support the idea of a POMDP for the same problems?

Table 5.3: Artificial Data for Biomarker Study

Trt=1	BM	1	2	3	4	5	6	7
	DE	1	2	3	4	5	6	7
Trt=2	BM	3	4	5	6	7	8	9
	DE	1	2	3	4	5	6	7

Hint: Plot the relationship between the biomarker and the definitive endpoint for each of the two treatment groups and compare the two lines.

Exercise 5.11: For Case Study 5.1, study the cost or sample size needed for both the classical and adaptive CDP approaches.

Hint: You may need to read the next chapter before you can complete this assignment. The primary endpoint is assumed to be all cause mortality and 30-day MI. Find additional information you need from other sources or make sensible assumptions as needed.

Chapter 6

Clinical Trial Simulation (CTS)

This chapter will cover the following topics:

- Classical Trial Simulation
- Adaptive Trial Simulation

6.1 Classical Trial Simulation

6.1.1 *Types of Trial Designs*

There are several ways to classify trial design. We can classify trials into exploratory and confirmatory trials; noninferiority, superiority, equivalence, and dose-response trials; parallel, crossover, and factorial designs; or classical and adaptive trials. The definitions of most of the terms can be found in the FDA guidance (FDA, 1988) and summarized as follows.

Exploratory Trial

The rationale and design of confirmatory trials nearly always rests on earlier clinical work carried out in a series of exploratory studies. Like all clinical trials, these exploratory studies should have clear and precise objectives. However, in contrast to confirmatory trials, their objectives may not always lead to simple tests of pre-defined hypotheses. In addition, exploratory trials may sometimes require a more flexible approach to design so that changes can be made in response to accumulating results. Their analysis may entail data exploration; tests of hypotheses may be carried out, but the choice of hypothesis may be data dependent. Such trials cannot be the basis of the formal proof of efficacy, although they may contribute to the total body of relevant evidence. Any individual trial may have both confirmatory and exploratory aspects.

Confirmatory Trial

A confirmatory trial is an adequately controlled trial in which the hypotheses are stated in advance and evaluated. As a rule, confirmatory trials are necessary to provide firm evidence of efficacy or safety. In such trials the key hypothesis of interest follows directly from the trial's primary objective, is always pre-defined, and is the hypothesis that is subsequently tested when the trial is complete. In a confirmatory trial it is equally important to estimate with due precision the size of the effects attributable to the treatment of interest and to relate these effects to their clinical significance.

Equivalence or Noninferiority Trial

In some cases, an investigational product is compared to a reference treatment without the objective of showing superiority. This type of trial is divided into two major categories according to its objective; one is an 'equivalence' trial and the other is a 'noninferiority' trial. Bioequivalence trials fall into the former category. In some situations, clinical equivalence trials are also undertaken for other regulatory reasons such as demonstrating the clinical equivalence of a generic product to the marketed product when the compound is not absorbed and therefore not present in the blood-stream. Many active control trials are designed to show that the efficacy of an investigational product is no worse than that of the active comparator, and hence falls into the latter category. Another possibility is a trial in which multiple doses of the investigational drug are compared with the recommended dose or multiple doses of the standard drug. The purpose of this design is simultaneously to show a dose-response relationship for the investigational product and to compare the investigational product with the active control.

Superiority Trial

Scientifically, efficacy is most convincingly established by demonstrating superiority to a placebo in a placebo-controlled trial, by showing superiority to an active control treatment, or by demonstrating a dose-response relationship. This type of trial is referred to as a 'superiority' trial. For serious illnesses, when a therapeutic treatment which has been shown to be efficacious by superiority trial(s) exists, a placebo-controlled trial may be considered unethical. In that case, the scientifically sound use of an active treatment as a control should be considered. The appropriateness of placebo control vs. active control should be considered on a trial by trial basis.

Dose-Response Trial

How a response is related to the dose of a new investigational product is a question to which answers may be obtained in all phases of development, and by a variety of approaches. Dose-response trials may serve a number of objectives, among which the following are of particular importance: the confirmation of efficacy; the investigation of the shape and location of the dose-response curve; the estimation of an appropriate starting dose; the identification of optimal strategies for individual dose adjustments; the determination of a maximal dose beyond which additional benefits would be unlikely to occur. These objectives should be addressed using the data collected at a number of doses under investigation, including a placebo (zero dose) wherever appropriate. There are various sample size calculation methods available for dose-response trials with different endpoints.

Parallel Design

A parallel design is a design in which each patient receives one and only one treatment, usually in a random fashion. A parallel design can be two or more treatment groups with one or more control groups. Parallel designs are commonly used in clinical trials because they are simple, universally accepted, and applicable to acute conditions.

Crossover Design

A common and generally satisfactory use of the 2×2 crossover design is to demonstrate the bioequivalence of two formulations of the same medication. In this particular application in healthy volunteers, carryover effects on the relevant pharmacokinetic variable are most unlikely to occur if the washout time between the two periods is sufficiently long. However, it is still important to check this assumption during analysis on the basis of the data obtained, for example, by demonstrating that no drug is detectable at the start of each period.

Factorial Design

In a factorial design two or more treatments are evaluated simultaneously through the use of varying combinations of the treatments. The simplest example is the 2×2 factorial design in which subjects are randomly allocated to one of the four possible combinations of two treatments, A and B say. These are: A alone; B alone; both A and B; neither A nor B. In many cases this design is used for the specific purpose of examining the interaction of A and B. The statistical test of interaction may lack power to detect an interaction if the sample size was calculated based on the test for main effects. This consideration is important when this design is used for examining the joint effects of A and B, in particular, if the treatments are likely to be used together. Another important use of factorial design is to establish the dose-response characteristics of the simultaneous use of treatments C and D, especially when the efficacy of each monotherapy has been established at some dose in prior trials. A number, m, of doses of C is selected, usually including a zero dose (placebo), and a similar number, n, of doses of D; the full design then consists of $m \times n$ treatment groups, each receiving a different combination of doses of C and D. The resulting estimate of the response surface may then be used to help identify an appropriate combination of doses of C and D for clinical use.vspace*-4pt

6.1.2 *Clinical Trial Endpoint*

Clinical trial endpoints can be classified as safety and efficacy endpoints for the purpose of evaluation. Efficacy endpoints can be further classified as primary or secondary endpoints. Primary endpoints measure outcomes that will answer the most important question being asked by a trial, such as whether a new treatment will reduce the incidence of heart attacks or mortality or prolong survival.

Secondary endpoints ask other important relevant questions in the same study so that they may potentially be put in the drug label. It is important to consider a reasonable number of secondary endpoints because if every endpoint is added that will imply some sort of statistical penalties such as multiplicity adjustment.

An endpoint may be a binary (e.g., death), continuous (e.g., hemoglobin level), or time-to-event clinical outcome (e.g., survival time).

In choosing an endpoint, it is important to ensure that it (Wang and Bakhai, 2006):

(1) Is clinically meaningful and related to the intent-to-treat disease
(2) Answers the important question to be answered by the trial
(3) Is practical so that it can be assessed in all subjects in the same way
(4) Is easily assessed with reasonable precision such that the study will have adequate statistical power or the size of the trial is feasible

6.1.3 *Superiority and Noninferiority Designs*

In designing a clinical trial, a sponsor must decide on the target number of patients who will participate. The sponsor's goal is often to have adequate statistical power to demonstrate, when the NME is in fact effective, the trial outcomes with statistical significance. The number of patients required depends on the question to be answered from the trial. For example, to show the effectiveness of a new drug in a noncurable disease such as metastatic kidney cancer requires many fewer patients than in a highly curable disease such as seminoma if the drug is compared to a placebo.

The larger the sample size is in the trial, the greater the statistical power will be. However, in designing a clinical trial, this consideration must be balanced with the fact that more patients make for a more expensive trial. The power of a trial will depend on the assumption about the treatment difference. For example, a trial of a lipid-lowering drug versus placebo with 100 patients in each group might have a power of 90% to detect a difference between patients receiving the study drug and patients receiving the placebo of 10 mg/dL or more, but it will only have a power of 0.70 to detect a difference of 5 mg/dL.

When testing a null hypothesis $H_o : \varepsilon \leq 0$ against an alternative hypothesis $H_a : \varepsilon > 0$, where ε is the treatment effect (difference in response), the type-I error rate function is defined as

$$\alpha(\varepsilon) = \Pr\{\text{reject } H_o \text{ when } H_o \text{ is true}\}.$$

Note: alternatively, the type-I error rate can be defined as $\sup_{\varepsilon \in H_o}\{\alpha(\varepsilon)\}$. Similarly, the type-II error rate function β is defined as

$$\beta(\varepsilon) = \Pr\{\text{fail to reject } H_o \text{ when } H_a \text{ is true}\}.$$

For hypothesis testing, knowledge of the distribution of the test statistic under H_o is required. For sample-size calculation, knowledge of the distribution of the test statistic under a particular H_a is also required. To control the overall type-I error rate at level α under any point of the H_o domain, the condition $\alpha(\varepsilon) \leq \alpha^*$ for all $\varepsilon \leq 0$ must be satisfied, where α^* is a threshold that is usually larger than 0.025 unless it is a Phase III trial. If $\alpha(\varepsilon)$ is a monotonic function of ε, then the maximum type-I error rate occurs when $\varepsilon = 0$, and the rejection region should be derived under this condition. For example, for the null hypothesis $H_o : \mu_2 - \mu_1 \leq 0$, where μ_1 and μ_2 are the means of the two treatment groups, the maximum type-I error rate occurs on the boundary of H_o when $\mu_2 - \mu_1 = 0$. Let $T = \frac{\hat{\mu}_2 - \hat{\mu}_1}{\hat{\sigma}}$, where $\hat{\mu}_i$ and $\hat{\sigma}$ are the sample mean and pooled sample standard deviation, respectively. Further, let $\Phi_o(T)$ denote the cumulative distribution function (c.d.f) of the test statistic on the boundary of the null hypothesis domain, and let $\Phi_a(T)$ denote the c.d.f. under H_a. Given this information, under the large sample assumption, $\Phi_o(T)$ is the c.d.f. of the standard normal distribution, $N(0,1)$, and $\Phi_a(T)$ is the c.d.f. of $N(\frac{\sqrt{n}\varepsilon}{2\sigma}, 1)$, where n is the total sample size and σ is the common standard deviation (Figure 6.1).

The power of the test statistic T under a particular H_a can be expressed

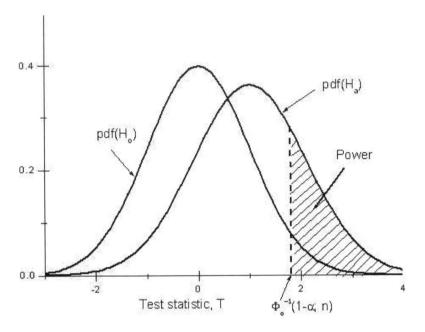

Figure 6.1:   Power as a Function of α and n

as follows:

$$\text{Power}\,(\varepsilon) = \Pr(T \geq \Phi_o^{-1}(1 - \alpha; n) | H_a) = 1 - \Phi_a(\Phi_o^{-1}(1 - \alpha; n); n), \quad (6.1)$$

which is equivalent to

$$\text{Power}\,(\varepsilon) = \Phi\left(\frac{\sqrt{n}\varepsilon}{2\sigma} - z_{1-\alpha}\right), \quad (6.2)$$

where Φ is the c.d.f. of the standard normal distribution, ε is treatment difference, and $z_{1-\beta}$ and $z_{1-\alpha}$ are the percentiles of the standard normal distribution. Figure 6.1 is an illustration of the power function of α and the sample size n. The total sample size is given by

$$n = \frac{4(z_{1-a} + z_{1-\beta})^2 \sigma^2}{\varepsilon^2}. \quad (6.3)$$

More generally, for an balanced design with sample size ratio $r = n_1/n_2$ and a margin δ ($\delta > 0$ for a superiority test and $\delta < 0$ for a non-inferiority test), the sample size is given by

$$n_2 = \frac{(z_{1-\alpha} + z_{1-\beta})^2 \sigma^2 (1 + 1/r)}{(\varepsilon - \delta)^2}. \quad (6.4)$$

Equation (6.4) is a general sample size formulation for two-group designs with a normal, binary, or survival endpoint. When using the formulation, the corresponding "standard deviation" σ should be used (see Chang, 2007b, Table 2.1).

We now derive the standard deviation for the time-to-event endpoint. Under an exponential survival model, the relationship between hazard (λ), median (T_{median}), and mean (T_{mean}) survival time is very simple:

$$T_{Median} = \frac{\ln 2}{\lambda} = (\ln 2)T_{mean}. \tag{6.5}$$

Let λ_i be the population hazard rate for group i. The corresponding variance σ_i^2 can be derived in several different ways.

Let T_0 and T_s be the accrual time period and the total trial duration, respectively. We then can prove that the variance for uniform patient entry is given by

$$\sigma^2(\lambda_i) = \lambda_i^2 \left[1 + \frac{e^{-\lambda_i T_s}(1 - e^{\lambda_i T_0})}{T_0 \lambda_i} \right]^{-1}. \tag{6.6}$$

See Chang (2007b) for the proof of (6.6).

In practice, to have the drug benefit patients, statistical significance is not enough; the drug must demonstrate its clinical significance and be commercially viable. Statistical and clinical significance are requirements for FDA approval for marketing the drug. Commercial viability ensures financial incentive to the sponsor such that it are willing to make the drug. Both clinical significance and commercial viability can be expressed in terms of the observed treatment effect over the control:

$$\hat{\delta} > \delta_{\min},$$

where $\delta_{\min}$ is usually an estimation.

For convenience, denote PE (probability of efficacy) for the probability of having both statistical significance and $\hat{\delta} > \delta_{\min}$, i.e.,

$$PE = \Pr\left(p < \alpha \text{ and } \hat{\delta} > \delta_{\min}\right).$$

This PE is a better probabilistic measure for trial success than power alone. For this reason, PE is implemented in the following algorithm (Algorithm 6.1) in addition to power. Figure 6.2 shows the differences between power and PE curves under different scenarios. It is interesting to know that when the parameter $\delta = \delta_{\min}$, power approaches 100% as sample size increases, but PE $\leq$ 50% regardless of sample size.

Algorithm 6.1: Probability of Efficacy (PE)

Objective: To calculate power and PE for a two-group design.

Input $\mu_1, \sigma_1, \mu_2, \sigma_2$ for the two groups, n, one-sided α, $\delta_{\min}$, and nRuns.

power:= 0; PE:= 0

For $iRun := 1$ **To** nRuns

$\qquad \bar{x}_1 := 0; \bar{x}_2 := 0; s_1 = 0; s_2 := 0;$

$\qquad$ **For** $i := 1$ **To** n

$\qquad\qquad$ Generate x_1 from $N\left(\mu_1, \sigma_1^2\right)$

$\qquad\qquad \bar{x}_1 := \bar{x}_1 + x_1/n$

$\qquad\qquad s_1 := s_1 + x_1^2/n$

$\qquad\qquad$ Generate x_2 from $N\left(\mu_2, \sigma_2^2\right)$

$\qquad\qquad \bar{x}_2 := \bar{x}_2 + x_2/n$

$\qquad\qquad s_2 := s_2 + x_2^2/n$

$\qquad$ **Endfor**

$\qquad s_e := \sqrt{(s_1 - \bar{x}_1^2)/n + (s_2 - \bar{x}_2^2)/n}$

$\qquad T := (\bar{x}_2 - \bar{x}_1)/s_e$

$\qquad$ **If** $T \geq t_{1-\alpha, n-1}$ **Then** power $:=$ power+1/nRuns

$\qquad$ **If** $T \geq t_{1-\alpha, n-1}$ and $\bar{x}_2 - \bar{x}_1 > \delta_{\min}$ **Then** PE $:=$ PE+1/nRuns

Endfor

Return {power, PE}

§

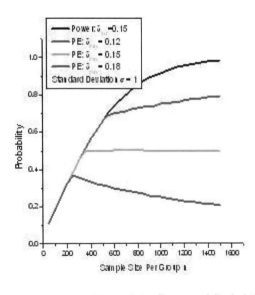

- Increasing sample size does not make a drug better, but it improves the precision of the estimate.

- Statistical significance only proves treatment effect $\delta > 0$

- Power $= \Pr(p < \alpha)$

- PE $= \Pr(p < \alpha \,\& \,\delta_{obs} > \delta_{min})$

$\qquad > \Pr(\text{Lower-CI-Limit} > \delta_{min})$

$\delta_{min} =$ the minimal treatment difference with both clinical and commercial values.

Figure 6.2:   Power and Probability of Efficacy (PE)

6.1.4 Two-Group Equivalence Trial

The equivalence test for the two parallel groups can be stated as

$$H_0 : |\mu_T - \mu_R| \geq \delta \text{ versus } H_a : |\mu_T - \mu_R| < \delta, \qquad (6.7)$$

where the subscripts T and R refer to the test and reference groups, respectively. If the null hypothesis is rejected, then we conclude that the test drug and the reference drug are equivalent. It is obvious that the test is equivalent to two one-sided tests:

$$\begin{cases} H_{01} : \mu_T - \mu_R \geq \delta \text{ versus } H_a : \mu_T - \mu_R < \delta \\ H_{02} : \mu_R - \mu_T \geq \delta \text{ versus } H_a : \mu_R - \mu_T < \delta \end{cases} \qquad (6.8)$$

To reject H_0, if and only if we reject H_{01} and H_{02} simultaneously. The null hypotheses H_{01} and H_{02} are rejected, respectively, if

$$T = \frac{\bar{x}_T - \bar{x}_R - \delta}{\sqrt{\frac{\hat{\sigma}_T^2}{n_T} + \frac{\hat{\sigma}_R^2}{n_R}}} < -t_{1-\alpha,n-1} \text{ and } T = \frac{\bar{x}_R - \bar{x}_T - \delta}{\sqrt{\frac{\hat{\sigma}_T^2}{n_T} + \frac{\hat{\sigma}_R^2}{n_R}}} < -t_{1-\alpha,n-1},$$
$$(6.9)$$

where $t_{\alpha,n}$ is 100α percentile from the student t-distribution with n degrees of freedom.

For the power calculation, we assume $\mu_T - \mu_R = \varepsilon$ and $\hat{\sigma}_x = \hat{\sigma}_y = \sigma$. The approximate power formulation is given by Chow et al. (Chow, Shao and Wang, 2003; Chang, 2008).

Since the power is larger than

$$\text{power} = 1 - 2\check{T}_v (t_{1-\alpha,v}; \tau_0), \quad \tau_0 = -\frac{\delta - |\varepsilon|}{\hat{\sigma}\sqrt{\frac{1}{n_T} + \frac{1}{n_R}}}. \qquad (6.10)$$

Replacing the t-distribution with the standard normal distribution under a large sample size assumption, the conservative sample size estimation is given by

$$n_R = \frac{\left(z_{1-\alpha} + z_{1-\beta/2}\right)^2 \sigma^2 \left(1 + 1/r\right)}{\left(|\varepsilon| - \delta\right)^2}, \qquad (6.11)$$

where $r = n_T/n_R$.

The exact solution should be based on the noncentral bivariate t-distribution (Owen, 1965)

$$\text{power} = 1 - \check{T}_v (t_{1-\alpha,v}; \tau_1) - \check{T}_v (t_{1-\alpha,v}; \tau_2), \qquad (6.12)$$

where $\check{T}_v$ is the noncentral t-distribution with the degrees of freedom $v = n_1 + n_2 - 2$ and the noncentral parameters $\tau_1 = \dfrac{\delta - \varepsilon}{\hat{\sigma}\sqrt{\frac{1}{n_T} + \frac{1}{n_R}}}$ and $\tau_2 = \dfrac{\delta + \varepsilon}{\hat{\sigma}\sqrt{\frac{1}{n_T} + \frac{1}{n_R}}}$.

Alternatively (and much simpler to implement than the noncentral bivariate t-distribution), we can use Monte Carlo to get a precise sample size estimation and evaluate the performance of (6.10) and (6.11). See Algorithm 6.2.

Algorithm 6.2: Power for Equivalence Trial
Objective: Return power for equivalence trial
Input $\mu_T, \sigma_T, \mu_R, \sigma_R$ for the two groups, n, δ, α, and nRuns.
power:= 0
For $iRun := 1$ **To** nRuns
    $\bar{x}_T := 0; \bar{x}_R := 0; s_T = 0; s_R := 0;$
    For $i := 1$ **To** n
        Generate x from $N\left(\mu_T, \sigma_T^2\right)$
        $\bar{x}_T := \bar{x}_T + x/n$
        $s_T := s_T + x^2/n$
        Generate y from $N\left(\mu_R, \sigma_R^2\right)$
        $\bar{x}_R := \bar{x}_R + y/n$
        $s_R := s_R + y^2/n$
    Endfor
    $s_e := \sqrt{(s_T - \bar{x}_T^2)/n + (s_R - \bar{x}_R^2)/n}$
    $T_1 := (\bar{x}_T - \bar{x}_R - \delta)/s_e$
    $T_2 := (\bar{x}_R - \bar{x}_T - \delta)/s_e$
    If $T_1 < -t_{1-\alpha, n-1}$ and $T_2 < -t_{1-\alpha, n-1}$ **Then**
        power:=power+1/nRuns
    Endif
Endfor
Return power
§

6.2 Adaptive Trial Simulation

6.2.1 *Adaptive Trial Design*

Compared to a classic trial design with static features, an adaptive design allows for changing or modifying the characteristics of a trial based on cumulative information. Adaptive design can increase the probability of success, reduce the cost, reduce the time to market, and deliver the right drug to the right patient. Two popular definitions of adaptive design are: (1) Chow-Chang's definition: an adaptive design is a clinical trial design that allows adaptations or modifications to aspects of the trial after its initiation without undermining the validity and integrity of the trial (Chow and Chang, 2005) and (2) The PhRMA Working Group's definition: adaptive design refers to an adaptive design as a clinical trial design that uses accumulating data to decide on how to modify aspects of the study as it continues, without undermining the validity and integrity of the trial (Gallo et al., 2006).

Commonly used types of adaptive trials include standard group sequential design, sample size re-estimation, drop-loser design, adaptive dose-finding study, and response-adaptive randomization.

There are many different methods for hypothesis-driven adaptive designs, for which we are going to present a unified approach using combinations of stage-wise p-values. There are four major components of adaptive designs in the frequentist paradigm: (1) type-I error rate or α - control: determination of stopping boundaries, (2) type-II error rate β: calculation of power or sample size, (3) trial monitoring: calculation of conditional power or futility index, and (4) analysis after the completion of a trial: calculations of adjusted p-values, unbiased point estimates, and confidence intervals. The mathematical formulation for these components will be discussed and simulation algorithms for calculating the operating characteristics of adaptive designs will be developed.

6.2.2 Hypothesis-Based Adaptive Design Method

Stopping Boundary

Consider a clinical trial with K stages and at each stage a hypothesis test is performed followed by some actions that are dependent on the analysis results. Such actions can be early futility or efficacy stopping, sample size re-estimation, modification of randomization, or other adaptations. The objective of the trial (e.g., testing the efficacy of the experimental drug) can be formulated using a hypothesis test:

$$H_o \text{ versus } \bar{H}_o. \tag{6.13}$$

Generally, the test statistics T_k at the kth stage can be a function $\eta(p_1, p_2, ..., p_k)$, where p_i is the one-sided p-value from the ith stage subsample and $\eta(p_1, p_2, ..., p_k)$ is a strictly increasing function of all p_i ($i = 1, 2, ...k$).

The stopping rules are given by

$$
\begin{cases}
\text{Stop for efficacy} & \text{if } T_k \le \alpha_k \,, \\
\text{Stop for futility} & \text{if } T_k > \beta_k, \\
\text{Continue with adaptations} & \text{if } \alpha_k < T_k \le \beta_k,
\end{cases}
\tag{6.14}
$$

where $\alpha_k < \beta_k$ $(k = 1, ..., K - 1)$, and $\alpha_K = \beta_K$. For convenience, α_k and β_k are called the efficacy and futility boundaries, respectively.

To reach the kth stage, a trial has to pass the 1 to $(k - 1)^{th}$ stages. Therefore, the c.d.f. of T_k is given by

$$
\psi_k(t) = \Pr(\alpha_1 < T_1 < \beta_1, ..., \alpha_{k-1} < T_{k-1} < \beta_{k-1}, T_k < t)
$$

$$
= \int_{\alpha_1}^{\beta_1} ... \int_{\alpha_{k-1}}^{\beta_{k-1}} \int_{-\infty}^{t} f_{T_1...T_k} \, dt_k \, dt_{k-1}...dt_1,
\tag{6.15}
$$

where $f_{T_1...T_k}$ is the joint p.d.f. of $T_1, ...,$ and T_k.

Type-I Error Control, p-value, and Power

When H_0 (or $\delta = 0$) is true, $\psi_k(t)$ is the stagewise p-value p_c if the trial stopped at the kth stage, i.e.,

$$
p_c(t; k) = \psi_k(t|H_0).
\tag{6.16}
$$

The stagewise error rate (α spent) π_k at the kth stage is given by

$$
\pi_k = \psi_k(\alpha_k|H_0).
\tag{6.17}
$$

The stagewise power of rejecting H_o at the kth stage is given by

$$
\varpi_k = \psi_k(\alpha_k|H_a).
\tag{6.18}
$$

When efficacy is claimed at a certain stage, the trial is stopped. Therefore, type-I errors at different stages are mutually exclusive. Hence the experiment-wise type-I error rate can be written as

$$
\alpha = \sum_{k=1}^{K} \pi_k.
\tag{6.19}
$$

Similarly, power can be written as

$$
power = \sum_{k=1}^{K} \varpi_k.
\tag{6.20}
$$

Equation (6.17) is the key to determining the stopping boundaries for adaptive designs, as illustrated in the next several chapters.

There are several possible definitions of (adjusted) p-values. Here we are most interested in the so-called stagewise-ordering p-values, defined as

$$p(t; k) = \sum_{i=1}^{k-1} \pi_i + p_c(t; k). \qquad (6.21)$$

The adjusted p-value is a measure of overall statistical strength against H_o. The later the H_o is rejected, the larger the adjusted p-value is, and the weaker the statistical evidence (against H_o) is. A late rejection leading to a larger p-value is reasonable because the alpha at earlier stages has been spent. An important characteristic of the adjusted p-value is that when the test statistic t is on a stopping boundary a_k, p_k must be equal to the alpha spent so far.

Selection of Test Statistics

To form the test statistic $\eta\,(p_1, p_2, ..., p_k)$, there are many possible combinations of p-values such as:

(1) linear combination

$$T_k = \Sigma_{i=1}^k w_{ki} p_i, \ \ k = 1, ..., K, \qquad (6.22)$$

where $w_{ki} > 0$ are constants.

(2) product of stagewise p-values (Fisher combination, Bauer and Kohne, 1994),

$$T_k = \prod_{i=1}^k p_i, \ \ k = 1, ..., K, \qquad (6.23)$$

and

(3) linear combination of inverse-normal stagewise p-values (Lehmacher and Wassmer, 1999; Cui, Hung, and Wang, 1999; Lan and DeMets, 1983)

$$T_k = \Sigma_{i=1}^k w_{ki} \Phi^{-1}\,(1 - p_i), \ \ k = 1, ..., K, \qquad (6.24)$$

where weight, $w_{ki} > 0$, $\sum_{i=1}^k w_{ki}^2 = 1$, can be constant or a function of data from previous stages, and K is the number of analyses planned in the trial.

Note that p_k is the naive p-value from the subsample at the kth stage, while $p_c(t; k)$ and $p(t; k)$ are stagewise and stagewise-ordering p-values, respectively.

Method for Stopping Boundary Determination

After selecting the type of test statistic, we can determine the stopping boundaries α_k and β_k by using (6.15), (6.20), and (6.22) under the null hypothesis (6.13). Once the stopping boundaries are determined, power and sample size under a particular H_a can be obtained using (6.18), (6.21), and (6.23) in conjunction with the Monte Carlo method.

After selecting the test statistic, we can choose one of the following approaches to fully determine the stopping boundaries:

(1) Classical Method: Choose certain types of functions for α_k and β_k. The advantage of using a stopping boundary function is that there are only limited parameters in the function to be determined. After the parameters are determined, the stopping boundaries are then fully determined using (6.18), (6.20), and (6.22), regardless of the number of stages. Commonly used boundaries are OB-F (O'Brien and Fleming, 1979), Pocock's (Pocock 1977), and Wang-Tsiatis' boundaries (Wang and Tsiatis, 1987).

(2) Error-Spending Method: Choose certain forms of functions for π_k such that $\Sigma_{k=1}^{K}\pi_k = \alpha$. Traditionally, the cumulative quantity $\pi_k^* = \Sigma_{i=1}^{k}\pi_i$ is called the error-spending function, which can be either a function of stage k or the so-called information time based on the sample size fraction. After determining the function π_k or equivalently π_k^*, the stopping boundaries α_k and β_k ($k = 1, ..., K$) can be determined using (6.18), (6.20), and (6.22).

(3) Nonparametric Method: Choose nonparametric stopping boundaries, i.e., no function is assumed; instead, use computer simulations to determine the stopping boundaries via a trial-error method. The non-parametric method does not allow for changes to the number and timing of the interim analyses.

(4) Conditional Error Function Method: One can rewrite the stagewise error rate for a two-stage design as

$$\pi_2 = \psi_2(\alpha_2|H_o) = \int_{\alpha_1}^{\beta_1} A(p_1)\, dp_1, \tag{6.25}$$

where $A(p_1)$ is called the conditional error function. For a given α_1 and β_1, by carefully selecting $A(p_1)$, the overall α control can be met (Proschan and Hunsberger, 1995). However, $A(p_1)$ cannot be an arbitrary monotonic function of p_1. In fact, when the test statistic (e.g., sum of p-values, Fisher's combination of p-values, or inverse-normal p-values) and constant stopping boundaries are determined, the conditional error function $A(p_1)$ is determined. For example, in the three commonly used adaptive methods, MSP, MPP, and MINP (see next sections), $A(p_1)$ are given by

$$A(p_1) = \alpha_2 - p_1 \text{ for MSP,}$$
$$A(p_1) = \alpha_2/p_1 \text{ for MPP,} \tag{6.26}$$
$$A(p_1) = (\alpha_2 - \sqrt{n_1}p_1)/\sqrt{n_2} \text{ for MINP,}$$

where n_i are subsample sizes for the ith stage.

On the other hand, if an arbitrary (monotonic) $A(p_1)$ is chosen for a test statistic (e.g., sum of p-values or inverse-normal p-values), the stopping boundaries α_2 and β_2 may not be constant any more. Instead, they are usually functions of p_1.

(5) Conditional Error Method: In this method, for a given α_1 and β_1, $A(p_1)$ is calculated on the fly or in real time, and only for the observed p_1 under H_o. Adaptations can be made under conditions that keep $A(p_1|H_o)$ unchanged.

Note that α_k and β_k are usually only functions of stage k or information time, but they can be functions of response data from previous stages, i.e., $\alpha_k = \alpha_k(t_1, ..., t_{k-1})$ and $\beta_k = \beta_k(t_1, ..., t_{k-1})$. In fact, using variable transformation of the test statistic to another test statistic, the stopping boundaries often change from response independent to response dependent. For example, in MSP (see next sections), we use stopping boundary $p_1 + p_2 \leq \alpha_2$, which implies that $p_1 p_2 \leq \alpha_2 p_2 - p_2^2$. In other words, the MSP stopping boundary at the second stage, $p_1 + p_2 \leq \alpha_2$, is equivalent to the MPP boundary at the second stage, $p_1 p_2 \leq \alpha_2 p_2 - p_2^2$ — a response-dependent stopping boundary.

(6) Recursive Design Method: Based on Müller-Shäfer's conditional error principle, this method recursively constructs two-stage designs at the time of interim analyses, making the method a simple but very flexible approach to a general K-stage design (Müller-Shäfer, 2004; Chang, 2007b).

6.2.3 *Method Based on the Sum of p-values*

Chang (2007a) proposed an adaptive design method in which the test statistic is defined as the sum of the stagewise p-values (MSP):

$$T_k = \Sigma_{i=1}^k p_i, \ k = 1, ..., K. \tag{6.27}$$

The type-I error rate at stage k can be expressed as (assume $\beta_i \leq \alpha_{i+1}, i = 1...$)

$$\pi_k = \int_{\alpha_1}^{\beta_1} \int_{\alpha_2-p_1}^{\beta_2} \cdots \int_{\alpha_{k-1}-\sum_{i=1}^{k-2} p_i}^{\beta_{k-1}} \int_0^{\alpha_k-\sum_{i=1}^{k-1} p_i} dp_k dp_{k-1} \cdots dp_2 dp_1 \tag{6.28}$$

where for the nonfutility binding rule let $\beta_i = \alpha_k$, $i = 1...$, i.e.,

$$\pi_k = \int_{\alpha_1}^{\alpha_k} \int_{\max(0,\alpha_2-p_1)}^{\alpha_k} \cdots \int_{\max(0,\alpha_{k-1}-\sum_{i=1}^{k-2} p_i)}^{\alpha_K} \\ \int_0^{\max(0,\alpha_k-\sum_{i=1}^{k-1} p_i)} dp_k dp_{k-1} \cdots dp_2 dp_1. \tag{6.29}$$

We set up $\alpha_k > \alpha_{k-1}$ and if $p_i > \alpha_k$, then no interim efficacy analysis is necessary for stage $i + 1$ to k because there is no chance to reject H_o at these stages.

To control type-I error, it is required that

$$\Sigma_{i=1}^{K} \pi_i = \alpha. \tag{6.30}$$

Theoretically, (6.29) can be carried out for any k. Here, we provide the analytical forms for $k = 1$ to 5, which should satisfy most practical needs.

$$\pi_1 = \alpha_1 \tag{6.31}$$

$$\pi_2 = \frac{1}{2}\left(\alpha_2 - \alpha_1\right)^2 \tag{6.32}$$

$$\pi_3 = \alpha_1\alpha_2\alpha_3 + \frac{1}{3}\alpha_2^3 + \frac{1}{6}\alpha_3^3 - \frac{1}{2}\alpha_1\alpha_2^2 - \frac{1}{2}\alpha_1\alpha_3^2 - \frac{1}{2}\alpha_2^2\alpha_3 \tag{6.33}$$

$$
\begin{aligned}
\pi_4 = {} & \frac{1}{8}\alpha_3^4 - \alpha_1\alpha_2\alpha_3\alpha_4 + \frac{1}{24}\alpha_4^4 - \frac{1}{3}\alpha_1\alpha_3^3 - \frac{1}{6}\alpha_1\alpha_4^3 - \frac{1}{6}\alpha_3^3\alpha_4 \\
& + \frac{1}{2}\alpha_1\alpha_2\alpha_3^2 + \frac{1}{2}\alpha_1\alpha_2\alpha_4^2 + \frac{1}{2}\alpha_1\alpha_3^2\alpha_4 + \frac{1}{2}\alpha_2^2\alpha_3\alpha_4 \\
& - \frac{1}{4}\alpha_2^2\alpha_3^2 - \frac{1}{4}\alpha_2^2\alpha_4^2
\end{aligned} \tag{6.34}
$$

$$
\begin{aligned}
\pi_5 = {} & \alpha_1\alpha_2\alpha_3\alpha_4\alpha_5 + \frac{1}{30}\alpha_4^5 + \frac{1}{120}\alpha_5^5 - \frac{1}{8}\alpha_1\alpha_4^4 - \frac{1}{24}\alpha_1\alpha_5^4 - \frac{1}{24}\alpha_4^4\alpha_5 \\
& + \frac{1}{3}\alpha_1\alpha_2\alpha_4^3 + \frac{1}{6}\alpha_1\alpha_2\alpha_5^3 + \frac{1}{6}\alpha_1\alpha_4^3\alpha_5 + \frac{1}{6}\alpha_3^3\alpha_4\alpha_5 - \frac{1}{2}\alpha_1\alpha_2\alpha_3\alpha_4^2 \\
& - \frac{1}{2}\alpha_1\alpha_2\alpha_3\alpha_5^2 - \frac{1}{2}\alpha_1\alpha_2\alpha_4^2\alpha_5 - \frac{1}{2}\alpha_1\alpha_3^2\alpha_4\alpha_5 - \frac{1}{2}\alpha_2^2\alpha_3\alpha_4\alpha_5 \\
& - \frac{1}{6}\alpha_2^2\alpha_4^3 - \frac{1}{12}\alpha_2^2\alpha_5^3 - \frac{1}{12}\alpha_3^3\alpha_4^2 - \frac{1}{12}\alpha_3^3\alpha_5^2 + \frac{1}{4}\alpha_1\alpha_3^2\alpha_4^2 \\
& + \frac{1}{4}\alpha_1\alpha_3^2\alpha_5^2 + \frac{1}{4}\alpha_2^2\alpha_3\alpha_4^2 + \frac{1}{4}\alpha_2^2\alpha_3\alpha_5^2 + \frac{1}{4}\alpha_2^2\alpha_4^2\alpha_5
\end{aligned} \tag{6.35}
$$

π_i is error spent at the ith stage, which can be predetermined or specified as error spending function $\pi_k = f(k)$. The stopping boundary can be solved through numerical iterations. Specifically, (1) determine π_i $(i = 1, 2, ..., K)$; (2) from $\pi_1 = \alpha_1$, solve for α_1; from $\pi_2 = \frac{1}{2}\left(\alpha_2 - \alpha_1\right)^2$, obtain $\alpha_2, ...$; from $\pi_K = \pi_K(\alpha_1, ..., \alpha_{K-1})$, obtain α_K. It is interesting to know that π_k includes the term $\Pr(T_k < \alpha_k | H_o) = \frac{\alpha_k^k}{k!}$, where T_k is given by (6.27) and $0 \leq \alpha_k \leq 1$ (Exercise 6.8).

For a larger value k, the Monte Carlo method for multiple integrations in Chapter 2 can be used because the numerical integration algorithm (6.36) is computationally inefficient when k is large:

$$\pi_k = \sum_{i_1=1}^{k} \sum_{i_2=1}^{k} \cdots \sum_{i_{k-1}=1}^{k} \max(0, \alpha_k - \sum_{i=1}^{k-1} p_i) \Delta_{i_1} \Delta_{i_2} \ldots \Delta_{i_{k-1}}, \qquad (6.36)$$

where

$$\Delta_{i_j} = \max(0, \alpha_{i_j} - \alpha_{i_{j-1}}).$$

For two-stage designs, using (6.31) and (6.32), we have the following formulation for determining the stopping boundaries:

$$\alpha = \alpha_1 + \frac{1}{2}(\alpha_2 - \alpha_1)^2. \qquad (6.37)$$

To calculate the stopping boundaries for a given α and α_1, solve (6.37) for α_2. Various stopping boundaries can be chosen based on (6.37). See Table 6.1 for numerical examples of stopping boundaries.

Table 6.1: Stopping Boundaries with MSP

α_1	0.000	0.0025	0.005	0.010	0.015	0.020
α_2	0.2236	0.2146	0.2050	0.1832	0.1564	0.1200

Note: One-sided $\alpha = 0.025$. $\alpha_2 = \beta_1 = \beta_2$.

The stagewise-ordering p-value can be obtained by replacing α_1 with t in (6.37) if the trial stops at stage 2. That is

$$p(t;k) = \begin{cases} t, & k = 1, \\ \alpha_1 + \frac{1}{2}(t - \alpha_1)^2, & k = 2, \end{cases} \qquad (6.38)$$

where $t = p_1$ if the trial stops at stage 1 and $t = p_1 + p_2$ if it stops at stage 2.

It is interesting to know that when $p_1 > \alpha_2$, there is no point in continuing the trial because $p_1 + p_2 > p_1 > \alpha_2$, and futility should be claimed. Therefore, statistically it is always a good idea to choose $\beta_1 \leq \alpha_2$. However, because the nonbinding futility rule is adopted currently by regulatory bodies, it is better to use stopping boundaries with $\beta_1 = \alpha_2$.

The condition power is given by (Chang, 2007b)

$$cP = 1 - \Phi\left(z_{1-\alpha_2+p_1} - \frac{\hat{\delta}}{\hat{\sigma}}\sqrt{\frac{n_2}{2}}\right), \quad \alpha_1 < p_1 \leq \beta_1, \qquad (6.39)$$

where $n_2 =$ sample size per group at stage 2; $\hat{\delta}$ and $\hat{\sigma}$ are observed treatment difference and standard deviation, respectively.

To obtain power for group sequential design using MSP, Monte Carlo simulation can be used. Algorithm 6.3 was developed for this purpose. To obtain efficacy stopping boundaries, one can let $\delta = 0$, then the power from the simulation output is numerically equal to α. Using the trial-and-error method, adjust $\{\alpha_i\}$ until the output power $= \alpha$. The final set of $\{\alpha_i\}$ is the efficacy stopping boundary.

Algorithm 6.3: K-Stage Group Sequential with MSP (large n)
Objective: return power for a two-group K-stage adaptive design.
Input treatment difference δ and common σ, one-sided α, $\delta_{\min}$, stopping boundaries $\{\alpha_i\}$ and $\{\beta_i\}$, stagewise sample size $\{n_i\}$, number of stages K, nRuns.
power:= 0
For $iRun := 1$ **To** nRuns
      $T := 0$
      For $i := 1$ **To** K
            Generate u from $N(0, 1)$
            $z_i = \delta\sqrt{n_i/2}/\sigma + u$
            $p_i = 1 - \Phi(z_i)$
            $T := T + p_i$
            If $T > \beta_i$ **Then Exitfor**
            If $T \leq \alpha_i$ **Then** power := power+1/nRuns
      Endfor
Endfor
Return power
§

6.2.4   *Method with Product of p-values*

This method is referred to as MPP. The test statistic in this method is based on the product (Fisher's combination) of the stagewise p-values from the subsamples (Bauer and Kohne, 1994; Bauer and Rohmel 1995), defined as

$$T_k = \Pi_{i=1}^k p_i, \ \ k = 1, ..., K. \tag{6.40}$$

$$\pi_k = \int_{\alpha_1}^{\beta_1} \int_{\alpha_2/p_1}^{\beta_2} \int_{\alpha_3/(p_1 p_2)}^{\beta_3} \cdots \int_{\alpha_{k-1}/(p_1 \cdots p_{k-2})}^{\beta_{k-1}} \int_0^{\alpha_k/(p_1 \cdots p_{k-1})} dp_k \cdots dp_1. \tag{6.41}$$

For the nonfutility boundary, choose $\beta_1 = 1$. It is interesting to know that when $p_1 < \alpha_2$, there is no point in continuing the trial because

$p_1 p_2 < p_1 < \alpha_2$ and efficacy should be claimed. Therefore, it is suggested that we choose $\beta_1 > \alpha_2$ and $\alpha_1 > \alpha_2$. In general, if $p_k \leq \max(a_k, \ldots a_n)$, stop the trial. In other words, α_k should monotonically decrease in k. The relationships between error-spent π_i and stopping boundary α_i at the ith stage are given up to three stages:

$$\pi_1 = \alpha_1, \tag{6.42}$$

$$\pi_2 = \alpha_2 \ln \frac{1}{\alpha_1}, \tag{6.43}$$

$$\pi_3 = \alpha_3 \left(\ln \alpha_2 - \frac{1}{2} \ln \alpha_1 \right) \ln \alpha_1, \tag{6.44}$$

$$\pi_4 = \alpha_4 \bigg((\ln \alpha_1 - \ln \alpha_3 - \ln \alpha_2) \ln \alpha_2 \\ + \frac{1}{2} (\ln \alpha_3 - \ln \alpha_1) \ln \alpha_1 \bigg) \ln \alpha_1, \tag{6.45}$$

$$\pi_5 = -\alpha_5 \bigg[\left(-\frac{1}{2} \ln^3 \alpha_2 - \frac{1}{2} \left(\ln^2 \alpha_2 \right) \zeta - (\ln \alpha_2) \eta \right) \ln \alpha_1 \\ + \frac{1}{2} \left(\eta + 3 \ln^2 \alpha_2 + 2 (\ln \alpha_2) \zeta \right) \ln^2 \alpha_1 \\ + \frac{1}{3} \left(-6 \ln \alpha_2 - \frac{3}{2} \zeta \right) \ln^3 \alpha_1 + \frac{7}{8} \ln^4 \alpha_1 \bigg], \tag{6.46}$$

where $\zeta = \ln \alpha_4 + 2 \ln \alpha_5$ and $\eta = \ln \alpha_4 \ln \alpha_5 + \frac{1}{2} \ln^2 \alpha_5$.

The closed form of π_k for any k-stage design with Fisher's combination is provided by Wassmer (1999).

Numerical examples of stopping boundaries for two-stage adaptive designs with MPP are presented in Table 6.2.

Table 6.2: Stopping Boundaries with MPP

α_1	0.001	0.0025	0.005	0.010	0.015	0.020
α_2	0.0035	0.0038	0.0038	0.0033	0.0024	0.0013

Note: One-sided $\alpha = 0.025$.

The stagewise-ordering p-value for a two-stage design can be obtained using

$$p(t; k) = \begin{cases} t, & k = 1, \\ \alpha_1 - t \ln \alpha_1, & k = 2, \end{cases} \tag{6.47}$$

where $t = p_1$ if the trial stops at stage 1 ($k = 1$) and $t = p_1 p_2$ if the trial stops at stage 2 ($k = 2$).

The condition power is given by (Chang, 2007b)

$$cP = 1 - \Phi\left(z_{1-\frac{\alpha_2}{p_1}} - \frac{\hat{\delta}}{\hat{\sigma}}\sqrt{\frac{n_2}{2}}\right), \alpha_1 < p_1 \le \beta_1. \tag{6.48}$$

Algorithm 6.4 is a Monte Carlo simulation algorithm for K-stage group sequential design. To obtain efficacy stopping boundaries, one can let $\delta = 0$, then the power from the simulation output is numerically equal to α. Using the trial-and-error method, adjust $\{\alpha_i\}$ until the output power $= \alpha$. Then the final set of $\{\alpha_i\}$ is the efficacy stopping boundary.

Algorithm 6.4: K-Stage Group Sequential with MPP (large sample)

Objective: return power for a two-group K-stage adaptive design.

Input treatment difference δ and common σ, one-sided α, $\delta_{\min}$, stopping boundaries $\{\alpha_i\}$ and $\{\beta_i\}$, stagewise sample size $\{n_i\}$, number of stages K, nRuns.

```
power:= 0
For iRun := 1 To nRuns
    T := 1
    For i := 1 To K
        Generate u from N(0,1)
        z_i = δ√(n_i/2)/σ + u
        p_i = 1 − Φ(z_i)
        T := T · p_i
        If T > β_i Then Exitfor
        If T ≤ α_i Then power := power+1/nRuns
    Endfor
Endfor
Return power
§
```

6.2.5 *Method with Inverse-Normal p-values*

This method is based on inverse-normal p-values (MINP), in which the test statistic at the kth stage T_k is a linear combination of the inverse-normal of stagewise p-values. The weights can be fixed constants. MINP (Lecherman and Wassmer, 1999) can be viewed as a general method, which includes standard group sequential design and the Cui-Hung-Wang method for sample size re-estimation (Cui, Hung, and Wang, 1999) as special cases.

Let z_k be the stagewise normal test statistic at the kth stage. In general, $z_i = \Phi^{-1}(1 - p_i)$, where p_i is the stagewise p-value from the ith stage subsample.

In a group sequential design, the test statistic can be expressed as

$$T_k^* = \sum_{i=1}^{k} w_{ki} z_i, \tag{6.49}$$

where the prefixed weights satisfy the equality $\sum_{i=1}^{k} w_{ki}^2 = 1$ and the stage-wise statistic z_i is based on the subsample for the ith stage.

Note that when w_{ki} is fixed, the standard multivariate normal distribution of $\{T_1^*, ..., T_k^*\}$ will not change regardless of adaptations as long as z_i $(i = 1, ..., k)$ has the standard normal distribution. To be consistent with the unified formations, in which the test statistic is on a p-scale, we use the transformation $T_k = 1 - \Phi(T_k^*)$ such that

$$T_k = 1 - \Phi\left(\sum_{i=1}^{k} w_{ki} z_i\right), \tag{6.50}$$

where $\Phi =$ the standard normal c.d.f.

The stopping boundary and power for MINP can be calculated using only numerical integration or computer simulation using Algorithm 6.5.

In Table 6.3 are numerical examples of stopping boundaries for two-stage adaptive designs, generated using ExpDesign Studio^{TM} 5.0.

Table 6.3: Stopping Boundaries with MINP

α_1	0.0010	0.0025	0.0050	0.0100	0.0150	0.0200
α_2	0.0247	0.0240	0.0226	0.0189	0.0143	0.0087

Note: One-sided $\alpha = .025$, $w_1 = w_2$.

The conditional power for a two-stage design with MINP is given by

$$cP = 1 - \Phi\left(\frac{z_{1-\alpha_2} - w_1 z_{1-p_1}}{w_2} - \frac{\hat{\delta}}{\hat{\sigma}}\sqrt{\frac{n_2}{2}}\right), \quad \alpha_1 < p_1 \leq \beta_1, \tag{6.51}$$

where weights satisfy $w_1^2 + w_2^2 = 1$.

The stopping boundary and power can be obtained using Algorithm 6.5.

Algorithm 6.5: K-Stage Group Sequential with MINP (large n)

Objective: Return power for K-stage adaptive design

Input treatment difference δ and common σ, one-sided α, $\delta_{\min}$, stopping boundaries $\{\alpha_i\}$ and $\{\beta_i\}$, stagewise sample size $\{n_i\}$, weights $\{w_{ki}\}$, number of stages K, nRuns.

power:= 0
For $iRun := 1$ **To** nRuns
    For $i := 1$ **To** K
        Generate u from $N(0,1)$
        $z_i = \delta\sqrt{n_i/2}/\sigma + u$
    Endfor
    For $k := 1$ **To** K
        $T_k^* := 0$
        For $i := 1$ **To** k
            $T_k^* := T_k^* + w_{ki}\, z_i$
        Endfor
        $T_k; = 1 - \Phi(T_k^*)$
        If $T_k > \beta_k$ **Then Exitfor**
        If $T_k \leq \alpha_k$ **Then** power := power+1/nRuns
    Endfor
Endfor
Return power
§

Chang (2007b) has implemented Algorithms 6.3–6.5 using SAS and R for normal, binary, and survival endpoints. The implementation of Algorithm 6.5 in JavaScript is presented in Appendix A.

6.2.6 *Method Based on Brownian Motion*

All three methods mentioned above, MSP, MPP, and MINP, have fixed weights w_{ki} regardless of the time changes for the interim analyses. For example, if the equal weights for all stages were initially decided, then whether the interim analysis was performed on 10% or 80% patients, the weights will not change. Theoretically you can change the weights without peeking at the data. In contrast, Lan and DeMets (1983) developed an adaptive design method with time-variable weights based on Brownian motion.

First-Time Hitting of Standard Brownian Motion

It can be proved, using the reflection principle (Taylor and Karlin, 1998, p. 491–493), that the probability of the first passing (boundary C) before time $t > 0$ can be expressed as:

$$\Pr\{M(t) \geq C\} = 2\left[1 - \Phi\left(\frac{C}{\sqrt{t}}\right)\right]. \tag{6.52}$$

Equation (6.51) can be used directly to control type-I error (see the next section).

Lan–DeMets Error-Spending Method

Brownian motion was first introduced by Lan and DeMets (1983) to adaptive design with a prefixed error spending function, which allows for changing the timing and the number of analyses.

When the maximum sample-size N is fixed, i.e., without sample size re-estimation, the Brownian motion can be constructed as follows:

$$B_k = \Sigma_{i=1}^k z_i \sqrt{I_i}, \qquad (6.53)$$

where the information time $I_i = \frac{N_i}{N}$, $N_i = \Sigma_{j=1}^k n_j$.

From (6.52), the following properties of Brownian motion can be obtained using simple calculations:

(1) $E[B_N(I)] = \theta\sqrt{N}$
(2) $var(B_N(I)) = I$
(3) $cov(B_N(I_1), B_N(I_2)) = \min(I_1, I_2)$

Note that B_k is a linear function of information time $I_k \in [0, 1]$.

The Lan–DeMets method is similar to but different from the MINP method because the weight $w_{ki} = \sqrt{I_i}$ is not a prefixed constant and $\sum_{i=1}^k w_{ki}^2 = \sum_{i=1}^k I_i \neq 1$ when $k \neq K$. Instead, it is a prefixed function of information time. Note that the Lan–DeMets method uses the same stopping boundaries as classical group sequential design (GSD), because for each fixed information time, the test statistic is equivalent to that in classical GSD. For two-stage design, the stopping boundaries and power can be obtained through simulations.

We now use Brownian motion to illustrate the error-spending method. If H_o is rejected whenever (within information time interval 0 and 1) the Brownian motion particle crosses the boundary $\alpha^*(I_k) = 2\left[1 - \Phi\left(\frac{C}{\sqrt{I_k}}\right)\right]$ for the first time, then we can control overall α by letting the maximum crossing probability $\Pr\{M(1) \geq C\} = \alpha$, and solving (6.52) for C. That is, from $2[1 - \Phi(C)] = \alpha$, we can immediately obtain $C = z_{1-\alpha/2} = \Phi^{-1}(1 - \alpha/2)$. We now designate the error-spending function to be the first passing probability (6.52), i.e.,

$$\alpha^*(I_k) = \begin{cases} 2\left[1 - \Phi\left(\frac{z_{1-\alpha/2}}{\sqrt{I_k}}\right)\right], & I_k > 0 \\ 0, & I_k = 0 \end{cases}. \qquad (6.54)$$

Note that $\alpha^*(t)$ is an increasing function in t or information time I_k and $\alpha^*(1) = \alpha$, the one-sided significance level.

Because Brownian motion is not observable between two interim analyses, we can assign an accumulated crossing probability between two interim analyses to the information time point I_k. However, these assignments or aggregations of crossing probabilities to different discrete time points will not inflate the overall cross probability if the choice of time points for the interim analyses is independent of the observed data z_i. Otherwise, the overall cross probability or the type-I error could be inflated.

The error-spending function can be any nondecreased error-spending function $\alpha^*(t)$ with a range of $[0,1]$. When $\alpha^*(I_k) = \alpha^*(I_{k-1})$, the kth stage interim analysis is used either for futility stopping or modifying the design (such as its randomization), but not for efficacy stopping. Note that (6.56) is the error-spending function very close to the O'Brien-Fleming stopping boundaries (called OF-like stopping boundary). Other commonly used error-spending functions include Pocock-like function $\alpha^*(t) = \alpha \log[1 + (e-1)t]$ (Kim and DeMets,1992) and power family $\alpha^*(t) = \alpha t^\theta, \theta > 0$.

When the error-spending function $\alpha^*(t)$ is prefixed and timing of the analyses is not dependent on the observed (unblind) data from the trial, then the overall type-I error rate is

$$\sum_{k=1}^{K} \pi_k = \sum_{k=1}^{K} [\alpha^*(I_k) - \alpha^*(I_{k-1})] = \alpha^*(1) - \alpha^*(0) = \alpha. \qquad (6.55)$$

This is true even when the number of analyses K and the timing of the analyses I_k are not predetermined. This is the most attractive feature of the error-spending method. We now can see that this error-spending function can be applied to MSP, MPP, and MINP directly without any difficulty (Exercise 6.7).

To be consistent with other methods (MSP, MPP, MINP), we use the test statistic on the p-scale:

$$T_k = 1 - \Phi(B_k). \qquad (6.56)$$

The corresponding stopping rules are given in (6.14). For the two-stage design with an O'Brien-Fleming-like error-spending function (6.54), the stopping boundaries are given by Table 6.4. You should keep in mind that O'Brien-Fleming-like and O'Brien-Fleming are two types of stopping boundaries that are very close but have different boundaries (Proschan, Lan, and Wittes, 2006; Chang, 2008).

Table 6.4: OF-like Error-Spending Stopping Boundaries

I_k	0.3	0.4	0.5	0.6	0.7	0.8
α_1	0.00004	0.00039	0.00153	0.00381	0.00738	0.01221
α_2	0.22347	0.02490	0.02454	0.02380	0.02271	0.02142

Note: One-sided $\alpha = .025$. Computed by ExpDesign Studio^{TM} 5.0

6.2.7 *Design Evaluation — Operating Characteristics*

Stopping Probabilities

The stopping probability at each stage is an important property of an adaptive design, because it provides the time-to-market and the associated probability of success. It also provides information on the cost (sample size) of the trial and the associated probability. In fact, stopping probabilities are used to calculate the expected samples that represent the average cost or efficiency of the trial design and the duration of the trial.

There are two types of stopping probabilities: unconditional probability of stopping to claim efficacy (reject H_o) and unconditional probability of futility (accept H_o). The former refers to the efficacy stopping probability (ESP), and the latter refers to the futility stopping probability (FSP). From (6.18), it is obvious that the ESP at the kth stage is given by

$$ESP_k = \psi_k(\alpha_k) \qquad (6.57)$$

and the FSP at the kth stage is given by

$$FSP_k = 1 - \psi_k(\beta_k). \qquad (6.58)$$

Expected Duration of an Adaptive Trial

Stopping probabilities can be used to calculate the expected trial duration, which is definitely an important feature of an adaptive design. The conditionally (on the efficacy claim) expected trial duration is given by

$$\bar{t}_e = \sum_{k=1}^{K} ESP_k \, t_k, \qquad (6.59)$$

where t_k is the time from the first-patient-in to the kth interim analysis.

The conditionally (on the futility claim) expected trial duration is given by

$$\bar{t}_f = \sum_{k=1}^{K} FSP_k \, t_k. \qquad (6.60)$$

The unconditionally expected trial duration is given by

$$\bar{t} = \sum_{k=1}^{K} (ESP_k + FSP_k) \, t_k. \qquad (6.61)$$

Expected Sample Sizes

Expected sample size is a commonly used measure of the efficiency (cost and timing of the trial) of the design. Expected sample size is a function of the treatment difference and its variability, which are unknowns. Therefore, expected sample size is really based on hypothetical values of the parameters. For this reason, it is beneficial and important to calculate the expected sample size under various critical or possible values of the parameters. The total expected sample size per group can be expressed as

$$N_{\text{exp}} = \sum_{k=1}^{K} n_k \left(ESP_k + FSP_k\right) = \sum_{k=1}^{K} n_k \left(1 + \psi_k(\alpha_k) - \psi_k(\beta_k)\right). \quad (6.62)$$

It can also be written as

$$N_{\text{exp}} = N_{\text{max}} - \sum_{k=1}^{K} n_k \left(\psi_k(\beta_k) - \psi_k(\alpha_k)\right), \quad (6.63)$$

where $N_{\text{max}} = \sum_{k=1}^{K} n_k$ is the maximum sample size per group.

Conditional Power and Futility Index

Conditional power is the conditional probability of rejecting the null hypothesis during the rest of the trial based on the observed interim data. Conditional power is commonly used for monitoring an ongoing trial. Similar to ESP and FSP, conditional power is dependent on the population parameters or treatment effect and its variability. The conditional power at the kth stage is the sum of the probability of rejecting the null hypothesis at stage $k+1$ to K (K does not have to be predetermined), given the observed data from stages 1 through k.

$$cP_k = \sum_{j=k+1}^{K} \Pr\left(\cap_{i=k+1}^{j-1} (a_i < T_i < \beta_i) \cap T_j \le \alpha_j \mid \cap_{i=1}^{k} T_i = t_i\right), \quad (6.64)$$

where t_i is the observed test statistic T_i at the ith stage. For a two-stage design, conditional power can be expressed as

$$cP_1 = \Pr\left(T_2 \le \alpha_2 | t_1\right). \quad (6.65)$$

Specific formulations of conditional power for two-stage designs with MSP, MPP, and MINP were provided in earlier sections.

The futility index is defined as the conditional probability of accepting the null hypothesis:

$$FI_k = 1 - cP_k. \quad (6.66)$$

Algorithm 6.6 can be used to obtain the operating characteristics of a group sequential design, which can be modified for other adaptive designs and other adaptive design methods (e.g., MPP, MINP).

Algorithm 6.6: Operating Characteristics of a Group Sequential Design

Objective: return power, average sample size per group (AveN), futility stopping probability (FSP_i), and efficacy stopping probability (ESP_i) for a two-group K-stage adaptive design with MSP.

Note: the mean difference has distribution $N\left(\delta, 2\sigma^2\right)$.

Input treatment difference δ and common σ, one-sided α, stopping boundaries $\{\alpha_i\}$ and $\{\beta_i\}$, stagewise sample size $\{n_i\}$, number of stages K, nRuns.

power:= 0
For $iRun := 1$ **To** nRuns
    $T := 0$
For $i := 1$ **To** K
    $FSP_i := 0$
    $ESP_i := 0$
Endfor
    For $i := 1$ **To** K
        Generate u from $N(0,1)$
        $z_i = \delta\sqrt{n_i/2}/\sigma + u$
        $p_i = 1 - \Phi\left(z_i\right)$
        $T := T + p_i$
        If $T > \beta_i$ **Then**
            $FSP_i := FSP_i + 1/$nRuns
            Exitfor
        Endif
        If $T \le \alpha_i$ **Then**
            $ESP_i := ESP_i + 1/$nRuns
            power := power+1/nRuns
            Exitfor
        Endif
    Endfor
Endfor
$aveN := 0$
For $i := 1$ **To** K
    $aveN := aveN + (FSP_i + ESP_i)n_i$
Endfor
Return $\{$power, $aveN, \{FSP_i\}, \{ESP_i\}\}$
§

6.2.8 *Sample Size Re-Estimation*

Sample size determination is critical in clinical trial designs. It is estimated there are about 5000 patients per NDA on average (PAREXEL source book, 2008). The average cost per patient ranges from \$20,000 USD to \$50,000 USD. A small but adequate sample size will allow sponsors to use their resources efficiently, shorten the trial duration, and deliver the drug to patients earlier.

From an efficacy point of view, sample size is often determined by the power for the hypothesis test of the primary endpoint. However, the challenge is the difficulty in getting precise estimates of the treatment effect and its variability at the time of protocol design. If the effect size of the NME is overestimated or its variability is underestimated, the sample size will be underestimated and consequently the power will be too low to have a reasonable probability of detecting the clinical meaningful difference. On the other hand, if the effect size of the NME is underestimated or its variability is overestimated, the sample size will be overestimated and consequently the power will be higher than necessary, which could lead to unnecessary exposure of many patients to a potentially harmful compound when the drug, in fact, is not effective. A commonly used adaptive design, called sample size re-estimation (SSR), emerged for this purpose.

A sample size re-estimation (SSR) design refers to an adaptive design that allows for sample size adjustment or re-estimation based on review of interim analysis results. There are two types of sample size re-estimation procedures, namely, sample size re-estimation based on blinded and unblinded data. In the first scenario, the sample adjustment is based on the (observed) pooled variance at the interim analysis to recalculate the required sample size, which does not require unblinding the data. In this scenario, the type-I error adjustment is practically negligible. In the second scenario, the effect size and its variability are re-assessed, and sample size is adjusted based on the unblinded information. The statistical method for the adjustment can be based on observed effect size or the conditional power.

For a two-stage SSR, the sample size for the second stage can be calculated based on the target conditional power:

$$
\begin{cases}
n_2 = \frac{2\hat{\sigma}^2}{\hat{\delta}^2} \left(z_{1-\alpha_2+p_1} - z_{1-cP} \right)^2, & \text{for MSP}, \\
n_2 = \frac{2\hat{\sigma}^2}{\hat{\delta}^2} \left(z_{1-\alpha_2/p_1} - z_{1-cP} \right)^2, & \text{for MPP}, \\
n_2 = \frac{2\hat{\sigma}^2}{\hat{\delta}^2} \left(\frac{z_{1-\alpha_2}}{w_2} - \frac{w_1}{w_2} z_{1-p_1} - z_{1-cP} \right)^2, & \text{for MINP}
\end{cases}
\tag{6.67}
$$

where, for the purpose of calculation, $\hat{\delta}$ and $\hat{\sigma}$ are taken to be the observed treatment effect and standard deviation at stage 1; cP is the target conditional power.

For a general K-stage design, the sample size rule at the kth stage can be based on the observed treatment effect in comparison with the initial assessment:

$$n_j = \min\left(n_{j,\max}, \left(\frac{\delta}{\bar{\bar{\delta}}}\right)^2 n_j^0\right), j = k, k+1, ..., K, \qquad (6.68)$$

where n_j^0 is the original sample size for the jth stage, δ is the initial assessment for the treatment effect, $\bar{\delta}$ is the updated assessment after interim analyses, given by

$$\bar{\delta} = \frac{\sum_{i=1}^k n_i \hat{\delta}_i}{\sum_{i=1}^k n_i} \text{ for MSP and MPP}, \qquad (6.69)$$

$$\bar{\delta} = \sum_{i=1}^k w_{ki}^2 \hat{\delta}_i \text{ for MINP}. \qquad (6.70)$$

We now can develop algorithms for sample size re-estimation using MSP, MPP, and MINP. As samples, Algorithm 6.7 is devised for two-stage SSR based on conditional power using MSP and Algorithm 6.8 is provided for K-stage SSR using MINP. Both algorithms return power and PE as simulation outputs.

Algorithm 6.7: Two-Stage Sample Size Re-Estimation with MSP

Objective: Return power and PE for two-stage adaptive design

Input treatment difference δ and common σ, stopping boundaries $\alpha_1, \alpha_2, \beta_1, n_1, n_2$, target conditional power for SSR, sample size limits $n_{\max}$, clinical meaningful and commercial viable $\delta_{\min}$, and nRuns.

power := 0
PE := 0
For $iRun$:= 1 **To** nRuns
    $T := 0$
    Generate u from $N(0,1)$
    $z_1 = \delta\sqrt{n_1/2}/\sigma + u$
    $p_1 = 1 - \Phi(z_1)$
    If $p_1 > \beta_1$ **Then Exitfor**
    If $p_1 \leq \alpha_1$ **Then** power := power+1/nRuns
    If $p_1 \leq \alpha_1$ **And** $\hat{\delta}_1 \geq \delta_{\min}$ **Then** PE := PE+1/nRuns
    If $\alpha_1 < p_1 \leq \beta_1$ **Then**

$$n_2 := \frac{2\sigma^2}{\hat{\delta}_1^2}\left(z_{1-\alpha_2+p_1} - z_{1-cP}\right)^2$$

Generate u from $N(0,1)$

$z_2 = \delta\sqrt{n_2/2}/\sigma + u$

$p_2 = 1 - \Phi(z_2)$

$T := p_1 + p_2$

If $T \leq \alpha_2$ **Then** power := power+1/nRuns

$\hat{\delta} = (\hat{\delta}_1 n_1 + \hat{\delta}_1 n_2)/(n_1 + n_2)$

If $T \leq \alpha_2$ **And** $\hat{\delta} \geq \delta_{\min}$ **Then** PE := PE+1/nRuns

    Endif

Endfor

Return {power, PE}

§

Algorithm 6.7 can be easily modified using MPP.

Algorithm 6.8: K-Stage Sample Size Re-estimation with MINP (large sample size)

Objective: Return power and PE for K-stage adaptive design

Note: sample size re-estimation will potentially increase the overall sample size only by the subsample size for the last stage n_K.

Input treatment difference δ and common σ, one-sided α, $\delta_{\min}$, stopping boundaries $\{\alpha_i\}$ and $\{\beta_i\}$, stagewise sample size $\{n_i\}$, sample size limits $\{n_{i,\max}\}$number of stages K, weights $\{w_{ki}\}$, nRuns.

power:= 0

PE := 0

For $iRun := 1$ **To** nRuns

    For $i := 1$ **To** K

        Generate u from $N(0,1)$

        $z_i = \delta\sqrt{n_i/2}/\sigma + u$

    Endfor

    For $k := 1$ **To** K

        $T_k^* := 0$

        For $i := 1$ **To** k

            $T_k^* := T_k^* + w_{ki} z_i$

            $\bar{\delta} = \bar{\delta} + w_{ki}^2\hat{\delta}_i$

        Endfor

        $T_k; = 1 - \Phi(T_k^*)$

        If $T_k > \beta_k$ **Then Exitfor**

        If $T_k \leq \alpha_k$ **Then** power := power+1/nRuns

        If $T_k \leq \alpha_k$ **And** $\bar{\delta} \geq \delta_{\min}$ **Then** PE := PE+1/nRuns

        If $\alpha_k < T_k \leq \beta_k$ **Then**

> **For** $j := k$ **To** K
> $$n_j := \min\left(n_{j,\max}, \left(\tfrac{\delta}{\delta}\right)^2 n_j^0\right)$$
> **Endfor**
> **Endif**
> **Endfor**
Endfor
Return {power, PE}
§

The stagewise adjusted p-value can be calculated using the Monte Carlo method. Specifically, if the trial is stopped at the $\tilde{k}^{th}$ stage with $T_{\tilde{k}} = t_{\tilde{k}}$, we replace $\alpha_{\tilde{k}}$ with $t_{\tilde{k}}$, the conditional probability $P\left(T_{\tilde{k}} > t_{\tilde{k}}\right)$ is the stagewise p-value, and the stagewise ordering p-value is given by

$$p = \sum_{i=1}^{\tilde{k}-1} \pi_i + P\left(T_{\tilde{k}} > t_{\tilde{k}}\right). \tag{6.71}$$

As an example, Algorithm 6.9 was developed for an obtained stagewise ordering p-value using Monte Carlo simulation.

Algorithm 6.9: Stagewise p-value of Adaptive Design SSR

Objective: Return stagewise ordering p-value

Note: sample size re-estimation will potentially increase the overall sample size only by the subsample size for the last stage n_K.

Input treatment difference δ and common σ, one-sided α, $\delta_{\min}$, stopping boundaries $\{\alpha_i\}$ and $\{\beta_i\}$, where $\alpha_{\tilde{k}}$ is replaced with $t_{\tilde{k}}$, stagewise sample size $\{n_i\}$, sample size limits $\{n_{i,\max}\}$, number of stages K, weights $\{w_{ki}\}$, nRuns.

> power:= 0
> **For** $iRun := 1$ **To** nRuns
> > **For** $i := 1$ **To** $\tilde{k}$
> > > Generate u from $N(0,1)$
> > > $z_i = \delta\sqrt{n_i/2}/\sigma + u$
> > **Endfor**
> > **For** $k := 1$ **To** $\tilde{k}$
> > > $T_k^* := 0$
> > > **For** $i := 1$ **To** k
> > > > $T_k^* := T_k^* + w_{ki} z_i$
> > > > $\bar{\delta} = \bar{\delta} + w_{ki}^2 \hat{\delta}_i$
> > > **Endfor**
> > > $T_k; = 1 - \Phi\left(T_k^*\right)$

If $T_k > \beta_k$ **Then Exitfor**
If $T_k \leq \alpha_k$ **And** $k = \tilde{k}$ **Then** power := power+1/nRuns
If $\alpha_k < T_k \leq \beta_k$ **Then**
    For $j := k$ **To** $\tilde{k}$
$$n_j := \min\left(n_{j,\max}, \left(\tfrac{\delta}{\delta}\right)^2 n_j^0\right)$$
    Endfor
  Endif
Endfor
Endfor
Return power
§

6.2.9 *Pick-Winner Design*

A drop-loser design (DLD) is an adaptive design consisting of multiple stages. At each stage, an interim analysis is performed and the losers (i.e., inferior treatment groups) are dropped based on prespecified criteria (Figure 6.1). With appropriate criteria, there is a good chance that the best arm(s) are retained. In addition, if there is a control arm, it is usually also retained for the purpose of comparison. This type of design can be used in Phase II/III combined trials. A Phase II clinical trial is often a dose-response study, where the goal is to assess whether there is a treatment effect. If there is a treatment effect, the goal becomes finding the appropriate dose level (or treatment groups) for the Phase III trials. This type of traditional design is not efficient with respect to time and resources because the Phase II efficacy data are not pooled with data from Phase III trials, which are the pivotal trials for confirming efficacy. Therefore, it is desirable to combine Phases II and III so that the data can be used efficiently. Such a combined study is called adaptive seamless Phase II/III design, which is one of the most attractive adaptive designs. In a seamless design, there is usually a so-called learning phase that serves the same purpose as a traditional Phase II trial, followed by a confirmatory phase that serves the same objectives as a traditional Phase III trial (Figure 6.3). Compared to traditional designs, a seamless design can reduce sample size and time-to-market for a positive drug candidate. The main feature of a seamless design is the drop-loser mechanism. Sometimes it also allows for adding new treatment arms. A seamless design usually starts with several arms or treatment groups. At the end of the learning phase, inferior arms (losers) are identified and dropped from the confirmatory phase so that the required sample size can be reduced.

Bauer and Kieser (1999) provided a two-stage method for this purpose, where investigators can terminate the trial entirely or drop a subset of treatment groups for lack of efficacy after the first stage. As pointed out by Sampson and Sill (2005), the procedure of dropping the losers is highly flexible, and distributional assumptions are kept to a minimum. However, because of the generality of the method, it is difficult to construct confidence intervals.

Here we discuss a very simple but somewhat conservative approach for two-stage seamless design (seamless trial with more stages can be designed similarly). Assume there are m_1 comparisons among M treatment groups at the first stage. These comparisons can be expressed as m_1 null hypotheses:

$$H_{oi}, \ i = 1, ..., m_1. \tag{6.72}$$

The corresponding p-values are $p_{1i}, \ i = 1, ...m_1$. With a Bonferroni adjustment (if there is a common control group for all the comparisons, the Dunnett method is better), the Bonferroni adjusted p-value is $\tilde{p}_{1i} = m_1 p_{1i}$.

Decision rules are described as follows:

At stage 1: (1) If $m_1 p_{1i} \leq \alpha_1$, then reject H_{oi} ($i = 1, ..., m_1$); (2) If $m_1 p_{1i} > \beta_1$, then accept H_{oi} ($i = 1, ..., m_1$); (3) If $\beta_1 \geq m_1 p_{1\min} > \alpha_1$, then continue to the second stage and make adaptations (e.g., adjust sample size and add new arms) if necessary, where $p_{1\min} = \min\{p_{11}, ..., p_{1m_1}\}$.

At stage 2: (1) Choose a set of comparisons based on the corresponding p-values $\tilde{p}_{1i}$ or other criteria such as safety, for the second stage. Assume there are m_2 comparisons at the second stage. (2) Based on the second stage data, the naive stagewise p-values are calculated as p_i and the Bonferroni adjusted p-value is $\tilde{p}_{2i} = m_2 p_{2i}$.

Decision rules at stage 2 if MSP is used: If $\tilde{p}_{1i} + \tilde{p}_{2i} = m_1 p_{1i} + m_2 p_{2i} \leq \alpha_2$, then reject H_{oi} ($i = 1, ..., m_2$), otherwise don't reject the null. The global null can be rejected as long as $m_1 p_{1\min} + m_2 p_{2\min} \leq \alpha_2$, where $p_{2\min} = \{p_{21}, ..., p_{2m_2}\}$.

The algorithm for this approach is presented in Algorithm 6.10, where only the best winner and the control are picked for the second stage. If a method other than MSP is used, the decision rule can be changed accordingly without any difficulty.

Algorithm 6.10: Two-Stage Pick-Winner Design With MSP

Objective: Return power of drop-loser design with normal endpoint.

Input: number of arms m, number of simulation runs nRuns, $\{\mu_i\}$, σ, n_1, n_2, α

    For iRun :=1 **To** nRuns;

        $Z_{\max} := 0; i_{\max} := 1$

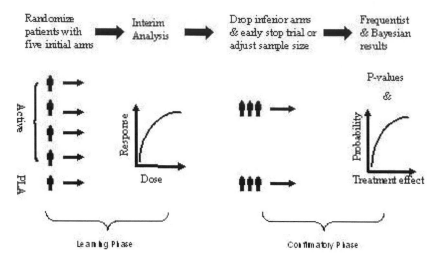

Figure 6.3:   Pick-Winner Adaptive Design

Generate $\hat{\mu}_0$ from $N\left(\mu_0, \sigma^2/n_1\right)$
For $i := 1$ **To** m;
     Generate $\hat{\mu}_i$ from $N\left(\mu_i, \sigma^2/n_1\right)$
     $z_i := \frac{(\hat{\mu}_i - \hat{\mu}_0)}{\sigma}\sqrt{n_1/2}$
     If $z_i > z_{\max}$ **Then**
         $z_{\max} = z_i$
         $i_{\max} = i$
     Endif
Endfor
     Generate $\hat{\mu}_{i_{\max}}$ from $N\left(\mu_{i_{\max}}, \sigma^2/n_2\right)$
     $z := \frac{(\hat{\mu}_{i_{\max}} - \hat{\mu}_0)}{\sigma}\sqrt{n_2/2}$
     $T = m \cdot \Phi\left(-z_{\max}\right) + \Phi\left(-z\right)$
     If $T \leq \alpha$ **Then** power:=power $+1/\text{nRuns}$
Endfor
Return power
§

6.2.10   *Adaptive Design Case Studies*

Case Study 6.1: Acute Coronary Syndrome

     The trial, known as EARLY ACS (early glycoprotein IIb-IIIa inhibition in non-st-segment elevation acute coronary syndrome: a randomized, placebo-controlled trial evaluating the clinical benefits of early front-loaded eptifibatide in the treatment of patients with non-st-segment elevation acute coronary syndrome), evaluates the benefit of an approved drug ABC compared to placebo in reducing death and other major adverse cardiac events, including heart attack, within 96 hours and up to 30 days following randomization. The initial sample size is designed to be 10,000 patients at 500 sites worldwide featuring sample size re-estimation at interim analysis.

Motivation of Simulation: The pivotal trial for NDA approval of drug ABC was conducted 6–8 years ago. Since then, standard care has changed. The patent drug company and its potential strategic alliance on work in the final stage of the partnership: risk assessment. Questions of interest included: (1) What would be the chance of success for ABC against placebo with such a trial? (2) What would be the optimal design to maximize success? What sample size would be needed for such a trial?

To perform the simulation, we need to build the model and collect historical data. ACS data from the two pivotal studies for the original approval and two oral GP IIb-IIIa inhibitor studies at DCRI were used for this modeling and simulation project. There were a total of 13,057 patients in the database.

Logistic regression was used in modeling with 30 initial risk factors selected including race, gender, age ($\leq$ 65 years and > 65 years), smoking status, heart rate, SBP/DBP, prior hypertension, prior MI, stroke, chronic renal insufficiency, enzymatic MI at enrollment, ST depression, etc. Final risk factors: 12 risk factors, both clinically and statistically significant, were considered in the simulations using the random walk method (RWM) based on partition of the patients' data under various patient and site selection criteria for the clinical trial protocol. Figure 6.4 presents some of the key simulation results.

Case Study 6.2: Adaptive Design for NHL Trial

A Phase III two parallel group non-Hodgkin's lymphoma trial was designed with three analyses. The primary endpoint is progression-free survival (PFS); the secondary endpoints are (1) overall response rate (ORR) including complete and partial response and (2) complete response rate (CRR). The estimated median PFS is 7.8 months and 10 months for the control and test groups, respectively. Assume a uniform enrollment with an accrual period of 9 months and a total study duration of 23 months. The estimated ORR is 16% for the control group and 45% for the test group. A classic design with a fixed sample size of 375 subjects per group will allow for detecting a 3-month difference in median PFS with 82% power at a one-sided significance level of $\alpha = 0.025$. The first interim analysis (IA) will

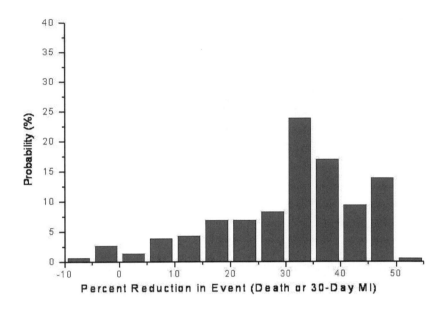

Figure 6.4:   Early ACS Trial

be conducted on the first 125 patients/group (or total $N_1 = 250$) based on
ORR. The objective of the first IA is to modify the randomization. Specifically, if the difference in ORR (test control) is $\Delta_{ORR} > 0$, enrollment will
continue. If $\Delta_{ORR} \leq 0$, then enrollment will stop. If enrollment is terminated prematurely, there will be one final analysis for efficacy based on PFS
and possible efficacy claimed on the secondary endpoints. If enrollment continues, there will be an interim analysis based on PFS and the final analysis
of PFS. When the primary endpoint (PFS) is significant, the analyses for
the secondary endpoints will be performed for the potential claim on the
secondary endpoints. During the interim analyses, patient enrollment will
not stop. The number of patients at each stage is approximately as shown
in Figure 6.5.

The OB-F stopping boundaries on the p-scale are $\alpha_1 = 0.0002$, $\alpha_2 =
0.0068$, $\alpha_3 = 0.022$ for stage 1, 2, and 3, respectively. For simplicity, the
same stopping boundaries are used for PFS, ORR, and CR. The actual trial
was successful and the drug was approved for the indication.

**Case Study 6.3: Adaptive Dose-Finding for Prostate Cancer
Trial**

In this case study, the traditional 3+3 escalation rule (TER) and continual reassessment method (CRM, see Chang, 2007b) were used in the

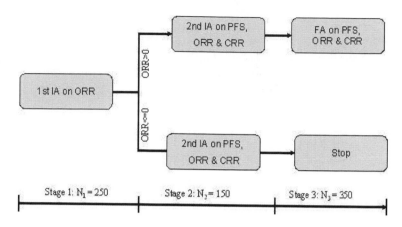

Figure 6.5: Multiple-Endpoint Adaptive Design

simulation. The trial is designed to establish the dose-toxicity relationship and identify the MTD for a compound in patients with metastatic androgen independent prostate cancer. Based on preclinical data, the estimated MTD is 230 mg/m². The modified Fibonacci sequence is chosen for dose levels (Table 6.5). There are eight dose levels anticipated, but more dose levels can be added if necessary. The initial dose level is 30 mg/m², which is 1/10 of the minimal effective dose level (mg/m²) for 10% deaths (MELD10) in mice after verification that no lethal and no life-threatening effects were seen in another species. The toxicity rate (DLT rate) at the MTD is defined for this indication as 17%.

Table 6.5: Dose Levels and DLT Rates

Dose level i	1	2	3	4	5	6	7	8
Dose x	30	45	68	101	152	228	342	513
DLT rate	0.01	0.02	0.03	0.05	0.12	0.17	0.22	0.4

Table 6.6: Adaptive Dose-Response Simulation Results

Method	Mean N	Mean DLTs	Mean MTD	SdMTD
TER	24.5	2.71	5.97	1.43
STER	26.0	3.03	5.87	1.44
CRM	8.0	1.63	6.03	1.05
CRM	16.0	3.11	5.95	0.92

In the CRM, the following logistic model is used

$$p = \frac{1}{1 + 150 \exp(-a\,i)}, \tag{6.73}$$

where i = dose level (we can also use actual dose) and the prior distribution for parameter a is flat over $[0, 3]$.

Note the true MTD is dose level 6 ($228\ mg/m^2$). The simulation results are summarized in Table 6.6. The average predicted MTD (dose level) is 5.33 with TER and 5.27 with STER, which are underestimated. In contrast, the average MTD for the two CRMs with sample size 8 and 16 patients accurately predicts the true MTD. From a precision point of view, even with a smaller sample size, the standard deviation of MTD (SdMTD) is much smaller for CRM than both TER and STER. It can be seen that increasing sample size in CRM may not materially increase precision, but could increase the DLTs or responses, which is not desirable. In the current scenario, the CRM design with eight patients is the best among the four designs. However, we should be aware that the performance of CRM is dependent on the goodness of the model specification.

6.3 Summary

Clinical trial simulation (CTS) is a powerful tool for supporting strategic decision making in clinical trials. CTS is very intuitive and easy to implement with minimal cost and can be done in a short time. The utilities of CTS include (1) sensitivity analysis and risk assessment, (2) estimation of probability of success (power), (3) design evaluation and optimization, (4) cost, time, and risk reduction, (5) clinical development program evaluation and prioritization, (6) prediction of long-term benefit using short-term outcomes, (7) validation of trial design and statistical methods, and (8) streamlining communication among different parties. Within regulatory bodies, CTS has been frequently used for assessing the robustness of results, validating statistical methodology, and predicting long-term benefits in accelerated approvals.

In classical design, CTS not only can be used to simulate the power of a hypothesis test for a complex trial, but also allows us to calculate the probability of efficacy, which is often a better measure for the probability of success of a prospective trial.

CTS plays an important role in adaptive design for the following reasons: First, statistical theory for adaptive designs is often complicated under some relatively strong assumptions, and CTS is useful in modeling very complicated situations with minimum assumptions not only to control type-I error, but also to calculate power, and to generate many other important operating characteristics such as the expected sample size, conditional power, and unbiased estimates. Second, CTS can be used to evaluate the robustness of the adaptive design against protocol deviations. Moreover, CTS can be used as a tool to monitor trials, predict outcomes, identify potential problems, and provide early remedies.

Compared to a classical trial design with static features, an adaptive design allows for changing or modifying the characteristics of a trial based on cumulative information. Adaptive design can increase the probability of success, reduce the cost, reduce the time-to-market, and deliver the right drug to the right patient. Commonly used types of adaptive trials include standard group sequential design and designs that allow for sample size re-estimation, dropping losers, adaptive dose finding, and response-adaptive randomization.

There are four major components of adaptive designs in the frequentist paradigm: (1) type-I error rate or α-control: determination of stopping boundaries, (2) calculation of power or sample size and PE, (3) trial monitoring: calculation of conditional power or futility index, and (4) analysis after the completion of the trial: calculations of adjusted p-values, unbiased point estimates, and confidence intervals.

We have provided a uniform formulation for hypothesis-based adaptive designs based on combinations of stage-wise p-values and derived closed forms for stopping boundaries for MSP and MPP up to five-stage adaptive trials. We have also devised simulation algorithms for determining stopping boundaries and power for any K-stage adaptive trials using MSP, MPP, and MINP. We have discussed how to expend the error-spending approach by the Lan–DeMets method to MSP, MPP, and MINP. This error-spending method is valid (controls the overall type-I error) as long as the choice of timing for interim analyses is not dependent on the observed data in the trial.

Evaluation of trial designs beyond the power of hypothesis testing is obviously important. We have extensively reviewed the operating characteristics of adaptive designs, including power, efficacy, and futility stopping probabilities, the maximum and expected sample size, conditional power and futility index, adjusted p-value, and confidence intervals. The mathematical formulations provided allow us to implement these operating characteristics in Monte Carlo.

Monte Carlo simulations play an important role in deciding adaptations in adaptive trials such as sample size re-estimation, dropping losers, and trial optimization as well. By combining the techniques in this and previous chapters, we can confidently accomplish clinical development planning and portfolio optimization.

6.4   Exercises

Exercise 6.1: Explain the terms exploratory and confirmatory trials; noninferiority, superiority, equivalence, and dose-response trials; parallel, crossover, and factorial designs; classical and adaptive trials.

Exercise 6.2: Explain the differences between power and PE. Why is PE a better measure than power for measuring the potential success of a trial?

Exercise 6.3: Develop algorithms of PE for binary and survival endpoints, respectively.

Exercise 6.4: What is an adaptive design and why is it important? What are the common types of adaptive designs?

Exercise 6.5: Explain the terms: SSR, drop-loser design, efficacy and futility stopping probabilities, maximum and expected sample size, conditional power and futility index, adjusted p-value.

Exercise 6.6: Discuss the applications of CTS.

Exercise 6.7: Derive the stopping boundaries for K-stage adaptive designs ($K = 2, 3, 4,$ and 5) with the test statistic $T_k = \frac{1}{k}\sum_{i=1}^{k} p_i$, ($k = 1, 2, 3, 4, 5$) for the kth stages.

Exercise 6.8: Let $T_k = \sum_{i=1}^{k} p_i$, where p_k are independent variables with uniform distributions on $[0,1]$. Prove:

(1)

$$\Pr(T_k < \alpha_k) = \frac{\alpha_k^k}{k!},$$

where $0 \leq \alpha_k \leq 1$;

(2) The p.d.f of T_k is given by

$$\mathbf{f}_k(x) = \begin{cases} \frac{1}{(k-1)!} \sum_{i=0}^{k}(-1)^i \binom{k}{i}(x-i)^{k-1} \delta(x-i) & \text{for } 0 \leq x \leq n \\ 0, \text{ otherwise} \end{cases},$$

where the indication function $\delta(x-i)$ is defined as 1 if $x - i > 0$ and 0, otherwise.

(3) As $k \to \infty$, T_k tends to the normal distribution $N(k/2, k/12)$.

Exercise 6.9: Prove that the error-spending function can be used for MSP or MPP directly without changing the overall type-I error as long as the information time for the interim analyses does not depend on observed data in the trial. (Hint: prove any random combination of adaptive designs (different number of stages and timing) has the expected overall type-I error rate $= \alpha$.)

Exercise 6.10: Use MC to study the overall type-I error rate for the error-spending approach, assuming that the BF-like spending function

(6.54) is used but the information time I is determined by the observed data, particularly, $I_k = p_{k-1}^c$, where p_{k-1} is the stagewise p-value at stage $k-1$ and constant $c \in [-2, 2]$. Study the effect of c on the overall type-I error rate for a three-stage, two-arm adaptive design without sample size adjustment.

Exercise 6.11: Can you develop an algorithm using Brownian motion with a shift to simulate the power?

Exercise 6.12: Devise an algorithm and implement it for a two-stage SSR design using MSP and output both the average sample size and rejecting probability at each stage.

Exercise 6.13: Devise an algorithm for a two-stage adaptive design with SSR based on conditional power and MPP.

Exercise 6.14: Devise an algorithm for a two-stage SSR design with the outputs of power and PE using MPP, MSP, and MINP.

Exercise 6.15: Develop an MC algorithm and implement it for K-stage SSR (MSP, MPP, MINP) design with outputs of as many operating characteristics of adaptive design as you can.

Exercise 6.16: Discuss how to use MPP and MINP for the drop-loser design with normal, binary, and survival endpoints.

Exercise 6.17: Implement the algorithms provided in this chapter.

Exercise 6.18: Case Study — Cancer Trial

After a cancer drug was approved for marketing, there were off-label uses, in which physicians combined the drug with other cancer drugs for treating patients. The experiences in these off-label uses from the physicians were very different. Therefore, there is a need to have a valid study as to which drug combination(s) is the best among these off-label therapeutic combinations: (1) ABC + thalomid + dexamethasone (VTD), (2) ABC + dexamethasone (VD), and (3) ABC + melphalan +prednisone (VMP). The primary objective of the study is to assess progression-free survival for each of the treatment arms. However, the sponsor company didn't want to make a huge investment on this study; they limited the sample size to about 300 patients.

Discuss in a group the adaptive options including types of adaptive designs, sample size, etc.

Exercise 6.19: Discuss the adaptive design options for an NME with dose selection and possible multiple indications or target populations.

Chapter 7

Clinical Trial Management and Execution

This chapter will cover the following topics:

- Clinical Trial Management
- Patient Recruitment and Projection
- Randomization
- Dynamic and Adaptive Drug Supply
- Statistical Trial Monitoring

7.1   Introduction

The overall aim of project management, according to PRINCE (Projects in Controlled Environments, International Standard Organization, ISO 9001) method, is to deliver required products with specified quality on time within budget. To carry a project needs a project plan and a team or organization. A plan is a document specifying technical, resourcing, quality, and exception issues. A project team or organization is a project board consisting of people with a set of responsibilities. Successful execution of a project plan demands controls. There are two types: Managerial controls assess progress throughout the project with various defined assessments and checkpoint (actual versus planned achievements) meetings. The other type of control concerns the product or deliverable.

It is important to have a technique or tool to facilitate planning, executing, and monitoring, and to document clinical trial activities. In what follows, we will discuss different techniques combined with the Monte Carlo method to carry out various tasks in clinical trial management and execution, including project management using critical path analysis (CPA) and dynamic programming, global patient recruitment projection and improvement, adaptive randomization algorithm, trial monitoring with conditional power, and dynamic drug supply.

7.2   Clinical Trial Management

7.2.1   *Critical Path Analysis*

Clinical trials require the use of human test subjects and thus could potentially impact the well-being of the subjects. Successful management of a clinical trial is essential to data quality, patients' safety, and time-to-market for the drug.

Pharmaceutical companies can spend 12 to 15 years and up to $900 million to bring a drug to market. About 45 percent of this cost is accrued during the clinical trial phase. Additionally, studies indicate that 75 percent of all trials conducted in the United States are behind schedule by one to six months (Microsoft, 2005).

Because improving time-to-market for new drugs is critical for pharmaceutical companies, managing the clinical trial process is one of the most significant places for improvement. However, there are many challenges: (1) Lengthy and complex trial design and planning process often involve hundreds to thousands of patients and support staff, (2) extraordinary efforts and time required for getting valid data and cleaning up, (3) great efforts required to remain compliant with regulatory requirements good clinical practice (GCP), (4) each trial involves many intervening tasks, and (5) multiple trials run simultaneously, competing for resources (finance, staff, and patients). Software such as CTMS (Clinical Trial Management System) and MicroSoft Project can be helpful in managing these challenges.

The critical path method (CPM), or critical path analysis (CPA), is a mathematically based algorithm for finding a shortest path or longest path (scheduling a set of project activities). It is an important tool for effective project management.

The essential elements in the CPM include: (1) a list of events, e.g., start of patient enrollment, end of patient treatment, database lock, statistical analysis, etc., (2) the dependencies and duration between the events. The process between two adjacent events is usually called activity. Collectively these activities with constraints are graphically presented as networks (e.g., Figure 7.1). Each box in Figure 7.1 can represent a set of sub-tasks. The network is the graphical representation of the project.

In the scenario of finding the shortest path, there are multiple ways to accomplish the project and the goal is to find the fastest (or cheapest) way to achieve the goal. For example, there are several alternative ways to drive from office to home, and you want to find the shortest or fastest one; or you may be asked to manage a clinical trial within a challenging time and/or budget, but are provided the options of insourcing and outsourcing.

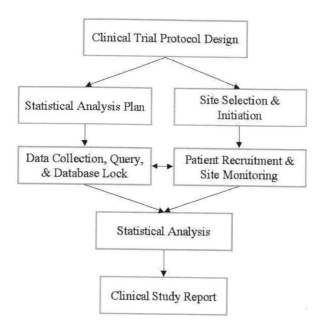

Figure 7.1: Clinical Trial Execution Flowchart

In the scenario of critical path scheduling, the CPM calculates the longest path of planned activities to the end of the project, and the earliest and latest that each activity can start and finish without making the project longer. This process determines which activities are "critical" (i.e., on the longest path) and which have "total float" (i.e., can be delayed without making the project longer). These results allow managers to prioritize activities for effective management of project completion, and to shorten the planned critical path of a project by pruning critical path activities and shortening the duration of the critical path (e.g., add resources). In practice, there are often mixed scenarios of shortest and longest paths. However, the term critical path analysis should not be confused with other critical path analysis, e.g., FDA Critical Path Initiatives (2004). Regarding software tools available for project management, please see, e.g., the list at http://en.wikipedia.org/wiki/List_of_project_management_software.

7.2.2 Logic-Operations Research (OR) Networks—Shortest Path

Let's discuss the scenario that we need to find a shortest path among several alternatives in the networks — the logic-OR networks.

Suppose that we have a network with vertices $1, 2, ..., n$, where each of the vertices represents an event (e.g., arriving at a bus stop). Certain pairs of vertices (i, j) are directly linked by an arc (Figure 7.2). Such an arc represents an activity with an associated positive value (length) d_{ij}. A path is a sequence of arcs and its length is the sum of the corresponding d_{ij}. The task is to find the shortest path from vertex 1 to vertex n, i.e., min $\{d_{1n}\}$.

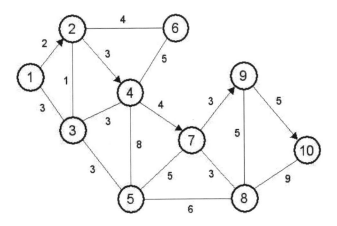

Figure 7.2:   Network and Critical Path Analysis

In our discussion, assume there is no isolated event, i.e., there is at least one path between any two vertices. For any vertex i, there are finite numbers of alternative paths from i to n. Let f_i be the length of the shortest of these paths. It is obvious that $f_n = 0$ and for each $i < n$,

$$f_i = \min_j \{d_{ij} + f_j\},$$

where vertex j is directly linked to vertex i by an arc.

The following proposition ensures a unique solution for the shortest distance f_1.

Theorem 7.1   *The following equation (7.1) has a unique solution for f_i, $i < n$, subject to the condition that $f_n = 0$, and f_i is the length of a shortest path from vertex i to vertex n:*

$$f_i = \min_j \{d_{ij} + f_j\} \tag{7.1}$$

where the minimization includes every vertex j which is directly linked to i by an arc.

For the proof of the theorem, see (Bather, 2000, p. 28–29).

Backwards Induction

It is easy to develop a backwards induction algorithm for finding the shortest path based on (7.1). Specifically, f_i are determined from n to 1 in terms of their direct links (arcs). We illustrate by the network example in Figure 7.2.

The solution, giving the length of the shortest path to vertex 10 for each i, is found by working from right to left on the network:

$$
\begin{array}{lcccccccccc}
i = & 10 & 9 & 7 & 8 & 4 & 5 & 3 & 2 & 1 & 6 \\
f_i = & 0 & 5 & 8 & 9 & 12 & 13 & 15 & 15 & 17 & 17
\end{array}
$$

The f_i satisfy equation (7.1) and, for each vertex i, the solution indicates a direction as shown by the arrows. Thus, the shortest path from 1 to 10 is: $1 \rightarrow 2 \rightarrow 4 \rightarrow 7 \rightarrow 9 \rightarrow 10$, and its length is given by

$$f_1 = 2 + 3 + 4 + 3 + 5 = 17.$$

In reality, the length d_{ij} is often a random variable; we need to assess the average f_1 and its variability.

Directed Networks

So far, we have been concerned with networks in which the links between vertices can be traversed in either direction. Clinical trial management more often relies on one-way links called directed arcs. The use of directed networks has little effect on the problem of finding shortest paths. Consider a network with vertices $i, j = 1, 2, ..., n$ and a subset of the possible ordered pairs $< i, j >$ which specifies the directed arcs. We write $i \rightarrow j$, if (i, j) is a directed arc. A path consists of a sequence:

$$i_1 \rightarrow i_2 \rightarrow \cdots \rightarrow i_n.$$

It will be assumed that the network is acyclic. In other words, there are no paths with $i_1 = i_k$. Then we can always rearrange the order of the vertices so that every directed arc $i \rightarrow j$ has $i < j$.

Theorem 7.2 *If a directed network is acyclic, then the vertices can be renumbered in such a way that $i < j$ for each directed arc $i \rightarrow j$.*

Proof. (Bather, 2000) There must be at least one vertex in the network which is not the endpoint of an arc. Otherwise, we can construct a cycle in the following way. Start at any vertex j and replace it by the initial point i of an arc $i.....j$. Then i is the endpoint of another arc, so we can replace it by the initial point and so on. This process generates a path by reversing the direction of each arc and it must eventually determine a cycle when one of the vertices is repeated. Having identified a vertex which is not an endpoint, we assign the number 1 to it and then consider the reduced network obtained by removing this vertex and every arc of the form $1.....j$. The reduced network is acyclic, so it must contain a vertex which is not an endpoint and this is renumbered as vertex 2. By successively reducing the number of vertices to $n - 1, n - 2, ..., 2, 1$ in this way we can rearrange the original network to obtain the required property. □

7.2.3 *Logic-AND Networks—Longest Path*

Let's now discuss the scenario that we need to find a longest path among the networks, in which all the events (denoted by the vertices) have to be accomplished — the logic-AND networks.

Methodologically, the difference in finding the shortest and longest path is trivial: we just need to switch min to max in the previous section. Particularly, (7.1) becomes

$$f_i = \max_j \{d_{ij} + f_j\} \tag{7.2}$$

where f_i now denotes the longest path from vertex i to vertex n.

The events on the critical path are often called milestones. They are critical to the success of the entire project. After the critical path and the starting time of the first event is determined, schedules for the milestones can be calculated. The CPM also computes the earliest and latest possible starting times for each activity. This calculation is of particular interest for activities which are not on the critical path (or paths), since these activities might be slightly delayed or re-scheduled as a manager desires without delaying the entire project.

Relation to Linear Programming

Critical path analysis is treated as an application of linear programming in operations research, rather than a sequential approach or backwards induction approach discussed above.

Suppose that our project network has n vertices or nodes, labeled 1 for the first event and n for the last event. Let the event times be $x_1, x_2, ..., x_n,$

respectively. The start of the project at x_1 is defined as time 0. The time to complete the activity between event i and event j is denoted by value $d_{ij} > 0$. The critical path scheduling problem is to minimize the time of project completion (x_n) subject to the constraints that each event cannot occur until each of the predecessor activities has been completed. Mathematically,

$$
\begin{aligned}
&\text{Minimize}\ :\ z = x_n, \\
&\text{subject to}\ :\ x_1 = 0 \text{ and} \\
&x_j - x_i - d_{ij} > 0 \text{ for each activity}(i, j).
\end{aligned}
\tag{7.3}
$$

This is a typical linear programming problem since the objective value to be minimized and each of the constraints are linear equations. Therefore, it can be solved with a linear programming algorithm. However, backwards induction is more efficient because it takes advantage of the network structure of the problem.

7.2.4 Algorithms for Critical Path Analysis

We present three commonly used algorithms for critical path analysis.

Algorithm 7.1: Activity-on-Branch Representation
(Event Numbering Algorithm)
Step 1: Give the starting event number 0.
Step 2: Give the next number to any unnumbered event whose predecessor events are each already numbered.
Repeat Step 2 until all events are numbered.
§

Algorithm 7.2: Earliest Event Time Algorithm
(Fundamental Scheduling Procedures)
Step 1: Let $E_0 = 0$.
Step 2: For $j = 1, 2, 3, ..., n$ (where n is the last event), let
$$E_j := \max\{E_i + D_{ij}\},$$
where the maximum is computed over all activities (i, j) that have j as the ending event.
§

Algorithm 7.3: Latest Event Time Algorithm
Step 1: Let L_n equal the required completion time of the project.

Note: L_n must equal or exceed E_n.

Step 2: For $i = n - 1, n - 2, ..., 0$, let
$$L_i := \min\{L_j - D_{ij}\}$$
where the minimum is computed over all activities (i, j) that have i as the starting event.

§

In a clinical trial, because of the great impact of a possible trial delay and because it is often easy to obtain casual labor at low rates in this situation, it is recommended to take the approach with the least time with the greatest resources available.

To summarize, the steps in critical path analysis are:

(1) Defining activities and events in the project, e.g., protocol design starting, protocol finish, first-patient-in, last-patient-out, database look, statistical analysis, clinical study report, NDA, and marketing
(2) Determining the order dependence
(3) Determining the time (can be a random variable) required for the completion of each task
(4) Finding the path using critical path analysis (backwards induction) and/or Monte Carlo simulations

7.3 Patient Recruitment and Projection

7.3.1 *Clinical Trial Globalization*

In recent years, clinical trial globalization and outsourcing have increased dramatically (Figure 7.3). A research study conducted in 2008 shows that there were 188,428 study sites for 8,143 clinical trials based on the data posted on www.clinicalTrials.org by 12 April 2007. As pointed out by Woodcock (Woodcock, 2008), industries regulated by the FDA have changed from primarily domestic to largely global over the past 20 years: (1) food imported from all over the globe, (2) source materials originated in developing countries, (3) clinical trials conducted worldwide, (4) drug API (active pharmaceutical ingredients) manufactured in third world countries. In this paradigm shift from a local to a global approach, there are increasing signs that drug sponsors, regulatory agencies, and human subject protection programs are joining forces to increase training and oversight of investigators based abroad to enhance GxP compliance and homogenization. The fast increase in clinical trial demands for contract research organization (CRO) services is higher than ever globally, especially in countries such as China, India, and Russia. The low trial densities (0.4 in China, 0.7 in India, and 7.7 in Russia), defined as the number of recruiting sites divided by the country population in millions, in those countries indicate the potential for conducting more clinical trials and the high growth rates (47% in China, 19.6% in India, and 33% in Russia) in clinical trials indicate a strong globalization trend.

The driving forces behind globalization include rising development costs and cycle times, growing volume and scope of clinical trials, and domestic patient source competitions for clinical trials.

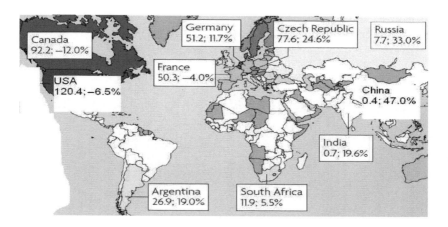

Figure 7.3:   Density of Active Clinical Sites of Clinical Trials
(Source: Thiers 2008)

However, there are challenges coming from different sources in the globalization transition (Thoelke, 2008) including (1) clinical trial agreements — a US contract is rarely directly transferable to a developing or ex-US region; instead, there are multiple-way contracts involving a sponsor, a sponsor representative, an institution, and an investigator; (2) the cost — everything associated with the trial may need to be covered by the sponsor; a comparator drug must be supplied and reimbursed; equipment costs have to be considered; all other protocol medications must be reimbursed; the tax implications on the import of the comparator drug can be significant; cash transfers may also be taxed; investigator travel, global infrastructure, and GMC requirements should also be considered; (3) common and important questions — Is the practice of medicine the same? Do they have the same medications available? Supportive Care? Diagnostics? Is the quality of data as good as the US? Can they do EDC? What about quality of life? Endpoints? Will the FDA accept the data? How many patients can come from outside the US? All these important questions will impact business decisions; (4) governance and regulatory issues — scope of harmonization, globalization versus localization, large parties of engagement, differences in culture, economic status, medical practice, treatment options available; (5) data and statistical analysis issues — data format (CDISC), collection, storage and sharing, statistical analysis criteria/methods, heterogeneity, subgroup analysis, multiple endpoints, and drug labeling.

Despite the complexity of the issues, the globalization process of clinical trials can be modeled and simulated using a very general method, i.e., the diffusion model. The diffusion equation can be viewed as a macroconsequence caused by the micro-behavior of random movement of many small particles or individual behaviors.

$$\frac{dx_i}{dt} = k_{ij}\left(x_j - x_i\right), \tag{7.4}$$

where $0 \leq x_k \leq 1$ is the trial density in the kth country and k_{ij} is the diffusion coefficient. This model can also be used for other globalization processes.

7.3.2   *Target Population and Site Selection*

Clinical trial recruitment (CTR) initiatives, if implemented correctly, can be highly successful, time can be dramatically reduced, and recruitment targets can be met ahead of schedule. Every day saved in the progression to marketing authorization can equate to patient health improvements and millions of dollars made in sales revenue.

Statistics show most clinical trial delays happen during enrollment (Thompson Medstat, 2004): overall, 34% of sites fail to attract a single subject; 27% of screened subjects fail to randomize; 76% of all Phase II and 3 studies are more than 90 days late.

The following key factors often contribute to clinical trial delays (Decisionview, 2009): (1) isolated, global teams have difficulty collaborating, (2) study teams lack a standardized approach to clinical enrollment, (3) study managers are unable to adjust plans when enrollment veers off course, and (4) global, disparate data are difficult to gather.

Every year, several million people participate in clinical trials. This level of participation represents less than 10% of the more than 60 million people who have severe, chronic, and life-threatening illnesses in the United States, according to data from PhRMA. Globally, the densities (per million populations) of actively recruiting clinical trial sites are 120.3 (US), 92.2

(Canada), 50.3 (France), 51.2 (Germany), 26.9 (Argentina), 11.9 (South Africa), and 77.6 (Czech Republic). Globalization is a way to improve the recruitment of clinical trials, but it is not without challenges.

Patient recruitment accounts for a quarter to one half of the time spent conducting a typical clinical trial. A survey indicates that the most frequent barriers to clinical trial participation cited by patients are inability to find a trial, study center being too far away, insufficient information, fear of reduction in quality of life, fear of receiving a placebo, concern about potential side effects, fear of being treated like a "guinea pig," physician reluctance to refer patients to clinical trials, lack of information about clinical trial benefits, and concern that insurance will not cover treatment (Avitabile, 2006).

Lynette Chiapperino and Gail Radcliffe (Stark, 2009) summarized the top twelve mistakes causing a trial delay or failure:

- Trial designer writes impossible protocols.
- Time, cost, quality — pick any two.
- Last site visit not reviewed.
- No action item list.
- Site isolation.
- Data points and endpoints don't match.
- Those boring repetitive entries.
- Unhappy trends, clues, issues.
- Undocumented trends, clues, issues.
- Unkept promises.
- Test results come late from the lab.
- Out-of-date ranges and test methods not identified.

There are common strategies to improve CTR, including clinical trial branding, advertising, patient-advocacy relations, site-specific support, and Web education programs (Figure 7.4).

Clinical trial branding is building trial awareness among patients by developing a recognizable acronym for the clinical study that will resonate with patients and investigators. Advertising clinical trial recruitment in newspapers, radio, television, and other media is a commonly used approach. Working with patient-advocacy organizations and discussing the requirements for inclusion of information about clinical trials in their communications materials are effective ways to have key messages reach a motivated target audience. Site-specific support programs involve tactics designed to encourage local public affairs contacts and the physicians at each clinical study site to enroll more patients faster in the trial. A clinical trial website can help patients to learn more about the trial.

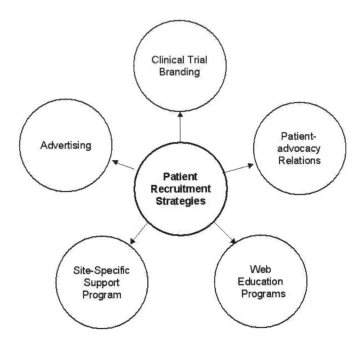

Figure 7.4:   Clinical Trial Recruitment Strategies

Patient retention is just as important as patient recruitment on average; nearly 25% of volunteers drop out before completing the study. Patients welcome good customer service; hence, the best way to keep patients enrolled in a clinical trial is to treat them as indispensable customers (Avitabile, 2006).

7.3.3   Time-to-Event Projection

In practice, it is not unusual that recruitment is slower than expected despite the strategic efforts mentioned above. In such a case, we can either increase the number of study sites or modify the inclusion/exclusion criteria. Before we make modifications, we need to assess the impact of the delay, which can be illustrated with the following survival analysis in terms of Monte Carlo simulation.

When the enrollment delays for a time-to-event (survival) trial or the number of events is fewer than what was initially anticipated at interim observations (note that the reason for fewer events can also be a consequence of a better drug effect), the solution can be one of the following or a combination to meet the power required for the hypothesis test: (1) not prolonging the recruitment period, but prolonging the trial follow-up so we have enough events to obtain power for the hypothesis test, (2) prolonging enrollment time to get the number of patients as initially projected, (3) increasing the number of clinical sites for the study to meet the recruitment timeline. Options (1) and (2) will delay the timeline, but (3) may not. The question is which option or combination is the best? To answer the question, we can launch a Monte Carlo simulation and provide the cost-time-power trade-off curve under various scenarios. Then, we check the results against the company's position to make a decision. In what follows, we will discuss such a simulation model.

Patient survival presumably follows the exponential distribution starting at the randomization. The hazard rate is constantly updated based on the information available. The relationship between number of deaths and number of patients enrolled over time can be derived as follows.

Let $S(t)$ be the survival function, i.e., the probability of a patient surviving at least at age t, $F(t) = 1 - S(t)$ be the probability of dying before age t, $f(t) = dF(t)/dt$ the probability density function, $R(t)$ enrollment rate, D the number of deaths or events, and T_I the enrollment duration.

Assuming no censoring before time T, i.e., no early dropouts, the number of deaths D can be written as

$$D = \int_0^T \int_0^t R(\tau)\,d\tau\, f(t - \tau)\,dt. \tag{7.5}$$

Given $S(t) = exp(-\lambda t)$, $f(t) = \lambda exp(-\lambda t)$, and $R(t) = \hat{R}$ (constant) if $t \le T_I$ and $R(t) = 0$ otherwise, the number of deaths can be calculated as follows:

$$D = R\lambda \int_0^T \int_0^{\min(T_I, t)} \exp(-\lambda(t - \tau))\,d\tau dt \tag{7.6}$$

or

$$D = \begin{cases} R\left(T - \frac{1}{\lambda} + \frac{1}{\lambda}e^{-\lambda T}\right) & \text{if } T \le T_I, \\ R\left(T_I - \frac{1}{\lambda}\left(e^{-\lambda T_I} - 1\right)e^{-\lambda T}\right) & \text{if } T > T_I. \end{cases} \tag{7.7}$$

From (7.7), we can obtain the time when there is the desired number of events D:

$$T = \begin{cases} -\frac{1}{\lambda}\ln\left(\frac{\lambda D}{\hat{R}} - T\lambda + 1\right) & \text{if } T \le T_I, \\ -\frac{1}{\lambda}\ln\left(\lambda\left(T_I - \frac{D}{\hat{R}}\right)\frac{1}{\exp(\lambda T_I - 1)}\right) & \text{if } T > T_I. \end{cases} \tag{7.8}$$

Example 7.1:

Suppose a trial required N = 300 patients to be enrolled in 9 months, the median survival time t_m = 7.91 months, and the total study duration = 23 months. Therefore, T_I = 9 months, R = $300/9$ = 33.333, $\lambda = ln2/t_m$ = 0.0876. Keep in mind that the power for the logrank test is actually determined by the number of deaths, not the number of patients.

Algorithm 7.4 can be used to project the number of events using the following input parameters: current accrual rate $\hat{R}$, hazard rate $\hat{\lambda}$ (estimated from the interim data using (7.7)), hazard rate for exponential dropouts ω, time T_A of interim projection, patient enrollment time left T_I, study ending time T_E. In the algorithm, k represents the number of deaths observed by time T_A, D_n is the additional number of patients to be enrolled in drugs T_A and T_I, t_{0i} enrollment time and t_i survival time, τ_i censoring time for the ith patient, respectively, and $\breve{E}(\cdot)$ the exponential distribution.

Algorithm 7.4: Projection of Number of Events
Objective: return the projected number of events at T_E.
Input $\hat{R}$, $\hat{\lambda}$, ω, T_I, T_A, k, D_n, and nRuns.
AveD := 0; VarD := 0; avePower := 0
For iRun:=1 **To** nRuns
    D := k
    For i := 1 **To** D_n
        Generate enrollment time t_{0i} from $U(T_A, T_I)$
        Generate survival time t_i from $\breve{E}\left(\hat{\lambda}\right)$
        Generate censoring time τ_i from $\breve{E}(\omega)$
        If $\tau_i \geq t_i$ and $t_{0i} + t_i \leq T_E$ **Then** $D := D + 1$
    Endfor
    aveD := aveD+D/nRuns
    varD := varD+D^2/nRuns
    power := f(D)
    avePower := avePower + power
Endfor
varD := varD-aveD·aveD
Return {aveD, varD}
§

Algorithm 7.5 can be used to project the trail duration using the following input parameters: $\hat{R}$, $\hat{\lambda}$ (estimated from the interim data), ω, T_I, T_A, k, and the total deaths observed D_E.

Algorithm 7.5: Projection of Trial Duration
Objective: return the projected trial duration.
Input $\hat{R}$, $\hat{\lambda}$, ω, T_I, T_A, D_E, and nRuns.
$T_E := 0$; $\text{ave}T_E := 0$, $\text{var}T_E := 0$
For iRun:=1 **To** nRuns
D := k
    For $i := 1$ **To** D_n
        Generate enrollment time t_{0i} from $U\left(T_A, T_I + T_A\right)$
        Generate survival time t_i from $\breve{E}\left(\hat{\lambda}\right)$
        Generate censoring time τ_i from $\breve{E}\left(\omega\right)$
        If $\tau_i \geq t_i$ **Then** $A[D++] := t_{0i} + t_i$
    Endfor
Sort the array $A[\cdot]$ in ascending order
$T_E := $ the $(D_E)^{th}$ element.
$\text{ave}T_E := \text{ave}T_E + T_E/\text{nRuns}$
$\text{var}T_E := \text{var}T_E + T_E^2/\text{nRuns}$
Endfor
$\text{var}T_E := \text{var}T_E - \text{ave}T_E \cdot \text{ave}T_E$
Return $\{\text{ave}T_E, \text{var}T_E\}$
§

7.4 Randomization

Randomization is a crucial part of randomized clinical trials. The purpose of randomization is to minimize the imbalance between the treatment groups regarding the potential confounding variables and consequently maximize (usually) the power to detect the treatment difference. However, when there are a large number of potential confounders related to sample size, it is difficult to keep a balance between the two groups for all the variables. Therefore, analysis of covariance (ANCOVA) rather than analysis of variance (ANOVA) is often used during the analysis.

In a blind, randomized trial, a patient is informed of the chance of receiving a treatment, but cannot predict or know exactly the treatment he/she received. Randomization is not the same as random sampling. Randomization is used to reduce selection bias. The intention to treat prevents biased outcomes.

7.4.1 *Simple Randomization*

Randomization may have no restriction, i.e., a single sequence of random assignment. This type of randomization is known as simple randomization.

Simple randomization is the simplest randomization method, in which each patient will receive treatment based on a randomization schedule generated based on a single fixed probability associated with a randomization ratio. Algorithm 7.6 was devised for simple randomization for a two-group trial.

Algorithm 7.6: Simple Randomization
Objective: return randomization schedule with simple randomization
Input randomization ratio r and number of patient nPatient
For $i :=$ **To** nPatients
    Generate x from $U(0,1)$
    If $x \leq r/(1+r)$ **Then** TrtCode$_i := 0$
    If $x > r/(1+r)$ **Then** TrtCode$_i := 1$
Endfor
Return {TrtCode$_i$}
§

Given a balanced design with randomization $r = 1 : 1$ and $n_1 + n_2 = n$, the probability of imbalance is given by (Rosenberger, 2002)

$$\Pr\left(|n_1 - n_2| > r\right) = 2\left[1 - \Phi\left(\frac{r}{\sqrt{n}}\right)\right]. \tag{7.9}$$

Under homogeneous variance between groups, balanced design is the most powerful design; the required sample size ratio of imbalanced versus balanced design is given by

$$R = \frac{2 + n_2/n_1 + n_1/n_2}{4}. \tag{7.10}$$

When the sample size is relatively large, simple randomization is expected to produce equal sized treatment groups, but it is not always the case. Blocking is used to ensure a close balance between groups during randomization. Within each block the number of participants in each group will be exactly equal. However, such a blocking technique tends to increase the predictability of randomization.

7.4.2 *Stratified Randomization*

Stratification ensures that the numbers of participants receiving each intervention are closely balanced within each stratum. Stratified randomization is achieved by performing a separate randomization procedure within each of two or more subsets of participants. Algorithm 7.7 can be used for such a randomization, where nS = number of strata, nP = number of patients, and nG = number of treatment groups.

Algorithm 7.7: Stratified Randomization
Objective: Return a stratified randomization schedule with
Input nS, nP, nG
    For k:= **To** nS
        For m:=1 **To** nP
            For j:=1 **To** nG
                Generate x from U_c (nG)
                For i:=1 **To** nG
                    If $i/\text{nG} < x \le i/\text{nG}$ **Then** Return i
                Endfor
            Endfor
        Endfor
Endfor
§

Another randomization algorithm used in practice is the so-called minimization procedure. Minimization is not really randomization per se. Indeed, it is the only nonrandom method which is acceptable as an alternative to randomization. Minimization ensures balance between intervention groups for several patient factors. Randomization lists are not set up in advance. The first patient is truly randomly allocated; for each subsequent patient, the treatment allocation is identified based on the minimization of the imbalance between groups at that time.

7.4.3 *Adaptive Randomization*

Response-adaptive randomization is a randomization technique in which the allocation of patients to treatment groups is based on the response (outcome) of the previous patients. The purpose of such a randomization is to provide a better chance of randomizing patients to a superior treatment group based on knowledge about the treatment effect at the time of randomization. As a result, response-adaptive randomization takes ethical concerns into consideration. The well-known response-adaptive models are the randomized play-the-winner (RPW) model and optimal RPW.

Randomized Play-the-Winner Model
The randomized play-the-winner (RPW) model is a simple probabilistic model used to sequentially randomize subjects in a clinical trial (Wei and

Durham, 1978; Coad and Rosenberger, 1999). The RPW model can be used for clinical trials comparing several treatments with binary outcomes. In the RPW model, it is assumed that the previous subject's outcome will be available before the next patient is randomized. Taking a trial with two parallel groups as an example, at the start of the clinical trial, an urn contains a_0 balls representing treatment A and b_0 balls representing treatment B, where a_0 and b_0 are positive integers. Denote these balls as either type A or type B balls. When a subject is recruited, a ball is drawn and replaced. If it is a type A ball, the subject will receive treatment A; if it is a type B ball, the subject will receive treatment B. When a subject's outcome is available, the urn is updated as follows: A success on treatment A (B) or a failure on treatment B (A) will generate an additional a_1 (b_1) type-A (type-B) ball in the urn. In this way, the urn builds up more balls representing the more successful treatment (Figure 7.5).

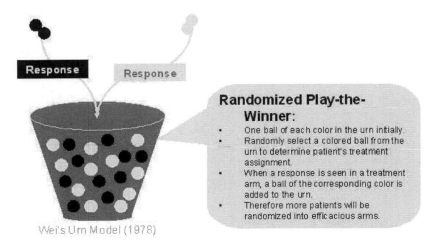

Figure 7.5:   Randomized Play-the-Winner

There are some interesting asymptotic properties with RPW. Let n_a/n (or n_b/n) be the proportion of subjects assigned to treatment A (or B) out of n subjects. Also, let $q_a = 1 - p_a$ and $q_b = 1 - p_b$ be the failure probabilities. Further, let F be the total number of failures. Then, we have (Wei and Durham, 1978)

$$\begin{cases} \lim\limits_{n\to\infty} \frac{n_a}{n_b} = \frac{q_b}{q_a}, \\ \lim\limits_{n\to\infty} \frac{n_a}{n} = \frac{q_b}{q_a+q_b}, \\ \lim\limits_{n\to\infty} \frac{F}{n} = \frac{2q_a q_b}{q_a+q_b}. \end{cases} \tag{7.11}$$

Since treatment assignment is based on the response of the previous patient in RPW model, it is not optimized with respect to any clinical endpoint. It is desirable to randomize the treatment assignment based on some optimal criteria such as minimizing the expected number of treatment failures. This leads to the so-called optimal RPW model.

Optimal RPW Model

The optimal randomized play-the-winner model (ORPW) is intended to minimize the number of failures in the trial. There are three commonly used efficacy endpoints in clinical trials, namely, the simple proportion difference $(p_a - p_b)$, the relative risk (p_a/p_b), and the odds ratio $(p_a q_b/p_b q_a)$, where $q_a = 1 - p_a$ and $q_b = 1 - p_b$ are failure rates. These can be estimated consistently by replacing p_a by $\hat{p}_a$ and p_b by $\hat{p}_b$, where $\hat{p}_a$ and $\hat{p}_b$ are the proportions of observed successes in treatment groups A and B, respectively. Suppose that we wish to find the optimal allocation $r = n_a/n_b$ such that it minimizes the expected number of treatment failures $n_a q_a + n_b q_b$ which is given by (Rosenberger and Lachin, 2002):

$$r^* = \arg \min_r \{n_a q_a + n_b q_b\} \tag{7.12}$$

$$= \arg \min_r \{\frac{r}{1+r} n\, q_a + \frac{1}{1+r} n\, q_b\}.$$

For a simple proportion difference, the asymptotic variance is given by

$$\frac{p_a q_a}{n_a} + \frac{p_b q_b}{n_b} = \frac{(1+r)(p_a\, q_a + r\, p_b\, q_b)}{nr} = K, \tag{7.13}$$

where K is some constant. Solving (7.13) for n yields

$$n = \frac{(1+r)(p_a\, q_a + r\, p_b\, q_b)}{rK}. \tag{7.14}$$

Substituting (7.14) into (7.12), we obtain

$$r^* = \arg \min_r \left\{ \frac{(r\, p_a + q_b)(p_a q_a + r\, p_b q_b)}{r\, K} \right\}. \tag{7.15}$$

Taking the derivative of (7.15) with respect to r and equating to zero, we have

$$r^* = \left(\frac{p_a}{p_b}\right)^{\frac{1}{2}}. \tag{7.16}$$

This r^* in (7.16) does not depend on K. For the other two measures (relative risk and odds ratio), the optimal allocations can be derived similarly. The results are summarized in Table 7.1.

Table 7.1: Asymptotic Variance with RPW

Measure	Optimal r^*	Asymptotic variance
Proportion difference	$\left(\dfrac{p_a}{p_b}\right)^{\frac{1}{2}}$	$\dfrac{p_a\,q_a}{n_a} + \dfrac{p_b\,q_b}{n_b}$
Relative risk	$\left(\dfrac{p_a}{p_b}\right)^{\frac{1}{2}}\left(\dfrac{q_b}{q_a}\right)$	$\dfrac{p_a\,q_b^2}{n_a q_a^3} + \dfrac{p_b\,q_b}{n_b q_a^2}$
Odds ratio	$\left(\dfrac{p_b}{p_a}\right)^{\frac{1}{2}}\left(\dfrac{q_b}{q_a}\right)$	$\dfrac{p_a\,q_b^2}{n_a q_a^3 p_b^2} + \dfrac{p_b q_b}{n_b q_a^2 p_b^2}$

(Source: Chow and Chang, 2006, p. 61)

Because the optimal allocation depends on the unknown binomial parameters, the unknown success probabilities in the optimal allocation rule can be replaced by the current estimate of the proportion of successes (i.e., $\hat{p}_{a,n}$ and $\hat{p}_{b,n}$) observed in each treatment group thus far. Algorithm 7.8 was developed for the randomized play-the-winner model, where n_{0i} and m_i ($i = a$ or b) are the initial and incremental number of balls; n is the total sample size.

Algorithm 7.8: Randomized Play-the-Winner
Objective: Generate treatment code based on RPW.
Input initial and incremental number of balls n_{0i} and m_i, and n
Initialize $\{n_i\} := \{n_{0i}\}$
For $i := 1$ **To** n
    Generate x from $U(0,1)$
    trtCode $:= 0$
    If $x \le n_a/(n_a + n_b)$ **Then** trtCode $:= 1$
    If response is observed in group i **Then**
        $n_i := n_i + m_i$
    Endif
Return trtCode
Endfor

7.5 Dynamic and Adaptive Drug Supply

7.5.1 *Conventional Drug Supply*

The conventional way for drug supply in a clinical trial separates the supply chains for each stratum or treatment group. In this approach, an initial drug shipment would be made for each stratum. Resupply shipments would then follow, based on fixed trigger levels for each stratum. However, keeping the supply chains separate requires a high initial outlay and can result in a lot of waste if a site does not enroll as anticipated. This conventional drug supply can be particularly problematic for adaptive trials.

As Hamilton and Ho (2004) described, to randomize a patient, a site would call the interactive voice response system (IVRS) and enter some basic patient identifiers such as ID number and date of birth, along with the stratum to which the patient belonged. The system would then access the randomization and treatment kit lists and read back to site personnel the blinded kit number assigned to that patient. A fax confirming patient information and assigned kit number would then be automatically generated by the system and sent to the site.

7.5.2 *Dynamic and Adaptive Drug Supply*

Stratified and adaptive randomization place a challenge on drug supply because the randomization list can't be predetermined. A conventional supply algorithm based on the site is often overly conservative and potentially wastes drugs.

To reduce waste in the drug supply process, efforts are devoted to the use of IVRS combined with allocation algorithms, as well as package design options. McEntegart (2003) proposed a scheme to force subject randomization into treatments for which stocks of medication are available. Dowlman (2001) describes savings that can be achieved if medications are not linked to subject numbers until the point of dispensation. Hamilton and Ho (2004) proposed a dynamic drug supply algorithm based on the patient-coverage concept and demonstrated through simulation a significant savings on drug supply.

Case Study 7.1: Dynamic Drug Supply

Hamilton and Ho (2004) dealt with a clinical study requiring stratification. In the initial planning stages for this study, it was determined that there would not be enough drug supply for clinic sites according to conventional seeding. They developed a more efficient algorithm for drug supply in terms of patient coverage, as opposed to the amount of medication remaining at each site. They focused on two key questions: (1) how much drug is required in order to randomize the next y patients, regardless of strata? and (2) given the current level of drug on hand, how many more patients can be randomized?

Their logistic steps for dynamic supply are:

(1) At site initiation, ship enough drugs to cover the first y patients enrolling the study, regardless of strata.
(2) After each patient is randomized, recalculate the patient coverage based on the randomization list and current levels of drug supply at the site.
(3) If the patient coverage falls below a lower resupply threshold x, ship enough drugs to replenish supply to an upper resupply threshold y. That is, ship enough drugs so that the next y patients can be enrolled the study, regardless of strata.

The implementation aspect of dynamic supply can be further elaborated as follows: In the original study, the dynamic drug supply scheme was implemented utilizing a telephone-based interactive voice response system (Figure 7.6). The system was designed in such a way that when a site completed regulatory and contractual requirements, sponsor personnel could go to a secure administrative web page and activate that site. Upon activation, the system would examine the randomization list for that site and calculate the amount of drug needed to cover the first y patients, regardless of strata. Notifications via email and fax would then be sent to the central drug repository indicating which drug kits to ship and the shipment number to appear on the waybill. When the site received the drug shipment, they were instructed to register the shipment number with the IVRS, making those drug kits available to be used to randomize patients at the site.

The steps to randomize a patient via IVRS are similar to the conversional approach. After each patient was successfully randomized, the IVRS would recalculate patient coverage at the site. If patient coverage dropped below x patients, another calculation was made by the IVRS to determine which kit types were necessary to bring the coverage back up to cover the next y patients. An automatic notification would then be sent to the central drug repository, indicating which drug kits were to be shipped to the site.

7.5.3 *Adaptive Drug Supply*

In an adaptive randomization trial, because the number of subjects on each treatment arm is not known at the start of the trial, overage in drug supply can be very substantial unless the adaptive procedure is explicitly accounted for in planning the drug supply (Patel, 2009). Adaptive drug supply can utilize data from the on-going trial to improve the efficiency of drug supply via Monte Carlo. Drug supply simulations can be used not only at the planning stage, but also during the trial for making adjustments to deviations from planning assumptions.

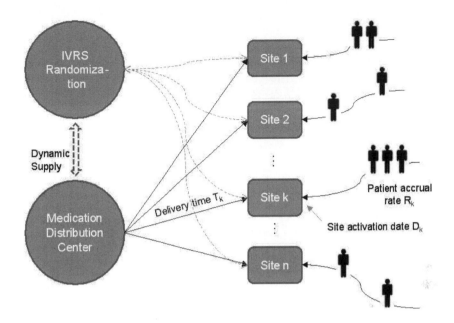

Figure 7.6: Sketch of Dynamic Medication Supply System

To utilize simulation, the initial step is to collectively gather the potential factors that impact (positive or negative) drug coverage for the trial. As Patel (2009) pointed out, the drug coverage may be, on one hand, exacerbated by the following factors: (1) number of sites increase, (2) unpredictably of dosing, (3) imbalanced allocation, (4) variable titration, (5) adaptive treatment allocation, (6) fast or uneven enrollment, (7) local country depots, (8) long shipping lead times; and, on the other hand, the coverage can be mitigated by: (1) short shipping lead times, (2) predictability of dosing, (3) long visit schedule, (4) slow, even enrollment (capped or controlled), (5) flexible packaging, (6) other tactics (e.g., site-to-site shipments).

Recommendations are to use pre-randomization based on all possible scenarios and associated probabilities for the next n patients at each site. The size of n can typically be 2 to 10 but is dependent on the time and cost required for the drug shipment, and available medication packaging (e.g., placebo, 1, 2, 3, ..., units). With all these random variables, we can do a dynamic shipment to ensure $x\%$ probability to cover the drug supply. The 'trigger/resupply' or 'floor/ceiling' system of inventory control with joint replenishment can be used with IVRS at centers and depots.

Algorithm 7.9 combined with Algorithm 7.10 provides a way to simulate adaptive drug supply, where m_i is the number of patients recruited during the time interval of drug shipment from warehouse to the ith clinic site, which is equal to the time required for drug shipment to the ith site multiplied by the patient accrual rate at the ith site. nSites is the number of clinic sites; p is the target probability of having sufficient drug at the site; the drug amount D_c will provide a p probability of covering the drug supply needed for the site; D_c is also used as the trigger level for resupply in the algorithm.

Algorithm 7.9: Adaptive Drug Supply
Objective: return the amount of drug required for a trial.
Input p and $\{m_i\}$ for sites.
mDrug $:= \sum_i n_{i0}$
$\{d_i\} := \{n_{i0}\}$
When each patient enrolled at site i
$\qquad D_c :=$ DrugCoverage(p)
$\qquad$ Calculate the drug inventory d_i at the site
$\qquad$ **If** $d_i < D_c$ **Then** mDrug$:=$ mDrug $+ D_c$
$\qquad$ **Return** mDrug
Endwhen

Algorithm 7.10: Function DrugCoverage (p)
Objective: Function used in Algorithm 7.7.
For $i := 1$ **To** 10000
$\qquad D_i := 0$
$\qquad$ **For** $j := 1$ **To** m_i
$\qquad\qquad$ Randomize patient j based on randomization rule.
$\qquad\qquad$ Determine the drug package x required for patient j.
$\qquad\qquad D_i := D_i + x$
$\qquad$ **Endfor**
Endfor
Sort D_i in ascending order
Return $D_{10000 \cdot pro}$

7.6 Statistical Trial Monitoring

7.6.1 *Necessities of Trial Monitoring*

To protect the integrity of a clinical trial, data monitoring is necessary. The monitoring, often carried out by an independent data monitor committee (DMC), includes safety and/or efficacy aspects.

As pointed out in FDA guidance (FDA, 2006), all clinical trials require safety monitoring, but not all trials require monitoring by a formal committee that may be external to the trial organizers, sponsors, and investigators. Data monitor committees (DMCs) have generally been established for large, randomized multi-site studies that evaluate treatments intended to prolong life or reduce the risk of a major adverse health outcome such as a cardiovascular event or recurrence of cancer. DMCs are generally recommended for any controlled trial of any size that will compare rates of mortality or major morbidity, but a DMC is not required or recommended for most clinical studies. DMCs are generally not needed, for example, for trials at early stages of product development. They are also generally not needed for trials addressing lesser outcomes, such as relief of symptoms, unless the trial population is at elevated risk of more severe outcomes.

To have a DMC will add administrative complexity to a trial and require additional resources, so we recommend that sponsors limit the use of a DMC to certain circumstances. The FDA guidance describes, mainly from a safety perspective, several factors to consider when determining whether to establish a DMC (a more commonly used name is DSMB — Data Safety Monitoring Board) for a particular trial. Particularly, the FDA suggests using a DMC when:

(1) The study endpoint is such that a highly favorable or unfavorable result, or even a finding of futility, at an interim analysis might ethically require termination of the study before its planned completion;
(2) There are prior reasons for a particular safety concern, as, for example, if the procedure for administering the treatment is particularly invasive;
(3) There is prior information suggesting the possibility of serious toxicity with the study treatment;
(4) The study is being performed in a potentially fragile population such as children, pregnant women, or the very elderly, or other vulnerable populations, such as those who are terminally ill or of diminished mental capacity;
(5) The study is being performed in a population at elevated risk of death or other serious outcomes, even when the study objective addresses a lesser endpoint;
(6) The study is large, of long duration, and multi-center.

Keep in mind that clinical trial investigators or physicians monitor patients on an individual basis, whereas the DMC review focuses on the aggregated data and safety trend with respect to the treatment(s).

So far, there is no official guidance from the FDA regarding interim analysis monitoring for an adaptive design, which will take both efficacy and safety into consideration. In adaptive design, "benefit-risk ratio" is

the key factor for interim decision making. When considering both efficacy and safety, there are common issues that affect a DMC's decision,
such as short-term versus long-term treatment effects, early termination
philosophies, response to early beneficial trends, response to early unfavorable trends, and response where there are no apparent trends (Ellenberg,
Fleming, and DeMets, 2002; Pocock, 2005). It is recommended that a DMC
be established to monitor the trial when an adaptive design is employed in
clinical trials, especially when many adaptations are considered for allowing
greater flexibility.

The stopping rule chosen in the design phase serves as a guideline to
a DMC (Ellenberg, Fleming, and DeMets, 2002) as it makes a decision
to recommend continuing or stopping a clinical trial. If all aspects of the
conduct of the clinical trial adhered exactly to the conditions stipulated
during the design phase, the stopping rule obtained during the design phase
could be used directly. However, there are usually complicating factors that
must be dealt with during the conduct of the trial.

DMC meetings are typically based on the availability of its members,
which may be different from the schedules set at the design stage. Enrollment may be different from the assumption made at the design phase. Deviation in the analysis schedule may affect the stopping boundaries; therefore,
the boundaries may need to be recalculated based on the actual schedules.

The true variability of the response variable is never known, but the
actual data collected at interim analysis may show that the initial estimates
in the design phase were inaccurate. Deviation in the variability estimation
could affect the stopping boundaries. In this case, we may want to know
the likelihood of success of the trial based on current data available, known
as conditional power. Similarly, the treatment effect may be different from
the initial estimation. This can lead to an adaptive design or sample size
re-estimation (Chapter 6).

7.6.2   Data Monitor Committee Charter

The monitoring of a clinical trial for scientific integrity is a dual respon-
sibility of the DMC and the sponsor. The DMC charter, developed and
approved by the sponsor and the DMC, is a central document for the monitoring. The DMC charter explicitly defines the roles and responsibilities
of the DMC and describes the procedures to be used in carrying out its
functions, such as meeting frequency and format, and voting procedures as
well. The DMC charter serves to delineate and make explicit the various
responsibilities of the sponsor, the DMC, and other parties (e.g., CROs)
involved.

There are different versions of DMC charters. However, the key contents are more or less the same. The following structure of the DMC charter is adapted from Fisher et al., 2001.

- Overview of IDMC Responsibilities:

  - Ethical responsibilities to study participants to monitor safety and efficacy
  - Scientific responsibilities to investigators and sponsor to monitor scientific integrity of the trial
  - Economic responsibilities to the sponsor to monitor the trial for futility

- Organization:

  - Composition
  - Selection of members

- Specific Functions:

  - Review the study protocol and any protocol amendments
  - Review data collection methods and safety monitoring procedures
  - Review and approve the DMC charter
  - Review and approve an interim analysis plan
  - Review interim monitoring reports and make recommendations to the steering committee

- Responsibilities of the Sponsor:

  - Make resources and information, including study documents, available to the DMC as necessary to carry out its designated functions
  - Monitor the study conduct and the collection and quality control of study data
  - Contract with the CRO for the preparation of interim monitoring reports
  - Inform the IDMC of any potential safety concern that is idiosyncratic or previously unreported
  - Provide analysis sets to the SAC containing data necessary for preparing DMC reports
  - Handle, financially and logistically, meeting arrangements of the DMC
  - Communicate regulatory information to relevant authorities

- Responsibilities of the CRO:

  - Prepare and distribute a draft DMC charter
  - Prepare and distribute a draft interim analysis plan
  - Prepare and distribute study reports based on data received from the sponsor

     – Prepare summary notes of each DMC meeting or conference call

- Conduct of DMC Meetings:

     – Meeting frequency and format (e.g., open, closed, executive sessions)
     – Definition of quorum and voting procedures
     – Procedures for recommendations to the steering committee
     – Summary notes
     – Confidentiality requirements
     – Conflict of interest guidelines

- Appendix I—Statistical Interim Monitoring Guidelines
- Appendix II—General Considerations for Early Termination

7.6.3   *Statistical Monitoring Tool*

Trial monitoring includes safety and efficacy aspects. For safety, there are no standard statistical procedures industry-wise accepted. For efficacy, commonly used monitoring tools for adaptive design include efficacy and futility stopping boundaries, conditional power, futility index, and the sample size re-estimation rule. The statistical formulations for the monitoring tools are discussed in the previous chapter. For a two-stage adaptive trial, the conditional power is given by

$$cP = \begin{cases} 1 - \Phi\left(B\left(\alpha_2, z_1\right) - \frac{\hat{\delta}}{\hat{\sigma}}\sqrt{\frac{n_2}{2}}\right) & \text{if } \alpha_1 < p_1 < \beta_2 \\ 0, \text{ otherwise}, \end{cases} \tag{7.17}$$

where

$$B\left(\alpha_2, z_1\right) = \begin{cases} z_{1-\alpha_2+p_1} & \text{for MSP} \\ z_{1-\frac{\alpha_2}{p_1}} & \text{for MPP} \\ \frac{z_{1-\alpha_2} - w_1 z_{1-p_1}}{w_2} & \text{for MINP}. \end{cases} \tag{7.18}$$

If the trial continues, i.e., $\alpha_1 < p_1 \le \beta_1$, for a target conditional power cP, we can solve (7.17) for the adjusted sample size for the second stage if this is featured by design:

$$n_2 = \frac{2\sigma^2}{\delta^2}\left(B\left(\alpha_2, z_1\right) - \Phi^{-1}\left(1 - cP\right)\right)^2. \tag{7.19}$$

For a K-stage design $(K > 2)$, the conditional power has to be calculated using simulation. See Algorithm 7.11.

Algorithm 7.11: Conditional Power for K-Stage Adaptive Design

Objective: return conditional power for a K-stage trial with normal endpoint using MSP

Input $K, n_1, ..., n_n, p_1, ..., p_k, \hat{\mu}, \hat{\sigma}, \alpha_{k+1}, ..., \alpha_n, \beta_{k+1}, ..., \beta_n$

cPower:=0

For iRun:=1 **To** nRuns

$\quad T := p_1 + ... + p_k$

$\quad$ **For** $i := k + 1$ **To** n

$\quad\quad$ Generate $\bar{x}_i$ from $N\left(\hat{\mu}, \frac{\hat{\sigma}^2}{n_i}\right)$

$\quad\quad p_i = \Phi\left(1 - \bar{x}_i \frac{\sqrt{n_i}}{\hat{\sigma}}\right)$

$\quad\quad T := T + p_i$

$\quad\quad$ **If** $p_i \leq \alpha_i$ **Then**

$\quad\quad\quad$ cPower:= cPower+1/nRuns

$\quad\quad\quad$ **Exitfor**

$\quad\quad$ **Endif**

$\quad\quad$ **If** $p_i > \beta_i$ **Then Exitfor**

$\quad$ **Endfor**

Endfor

Return cPower

Using the trial and error method, Algorithm 7.11 can be used to find the sample sizes required for a targeted conditional power.

There are several good books on trial monitoring, e.g., *Data Monitoring Committees in Clinical Trials* by Ellenberg, Fleming, and DeMets, 2002, and *Statistical Monitoring of Clinical Trials* by Proschan, Lan, and Wittes 2006, among others.

Case Study 7.2: Beta-Blocker Heart Attack Trial

"In the 1970s, it was thought that blockade of the beta-adrenergic receptors might be of benefit for patients with myocardial infarction. This led to the conduct of several clinical trials. Some of these trials treated patients with intravenous beta-blockers at the time of the acute MI; others began treatment intravenously at the time of the acute event and continued with oral beta-blockers after hospital discharge; still others began long-term oral treatment of patients after the acute recovery phase. Relevant to the development of the Beta-Blocker Heart Attack Trial (BHAT) were concerns that the long-term trials that had been conducted were inconclusive. In particular, some were underpowered, one used a beta-blocker that had unexpected serious toxicity, and some may have used inadequate doses of medication. Therefore, a workshop conducted by the National Heart, Lung, and Blood

Institute (NHLBI) recommended that another long-term trial with a sufficiently large sample size and using appropriate doses of a beta-blocker with
which there was considerable experience and a known toxicity profit, such
as propranolol, be conducted" (DeMets, 2006).

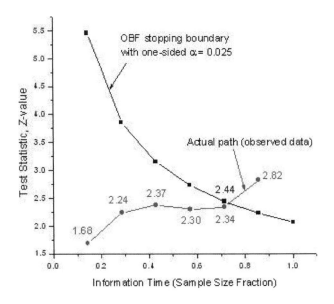

Figure 7.7:   BHAT Stopping Boundary and Actual Path

Patients aged 30 to 69 years who had a myocardial infarction 5 to 21
days prior to randomization were to be enrolled. The primary objective
of the study was to determine if long-term administration of propranolol
would result in a difference in all-cause mortality. The group sequential
design with six interim analyses (O'Brien-Fleming-like boundary with equal
information intervals) was used for the BHAT. The actual trial path (the
sequence of z-values from stage 1 to stage k) is presented in Figure 7.7.

A maximum of 4040 patients were to enroll. Participant enrollment began in 1978; a total of 3837 participants were actually enrolled. This trial
of 1884 survivors of an acute myocardial infarction showed a statistically
significant reduction in all-cause mortality, from 16.2% to 10.4%, during
a mean follow-up of 17 months. At this point, the BHAT was no longer
enrolling patients, but follow-up was continuing.

We are now ready to reproduce the group sequential design and then
change to a more flexible or adaptive design. For the latter we discuss how to
monitor and make adaptations according to the data observed. For a group

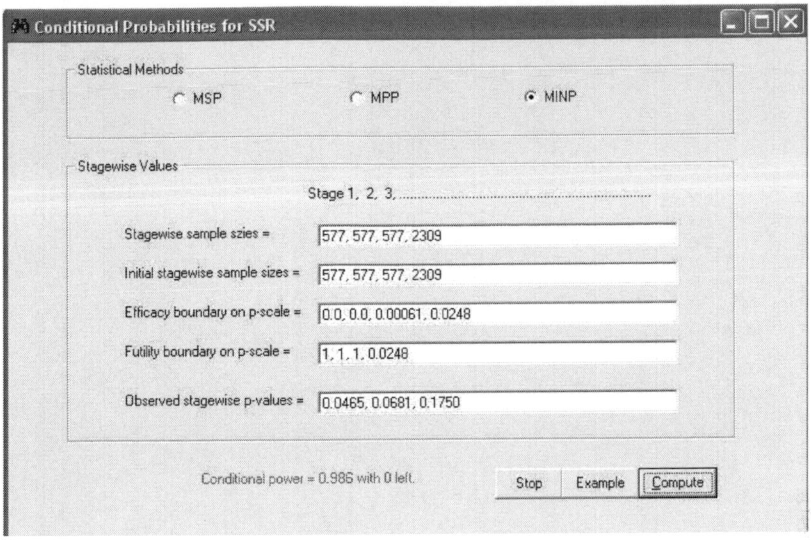

Figure 7.8: Conditional Power at Stage 4

sequential design with seven analyses with equal intervals and O'Brien-Fleming boundaries, 4040 patients will have 89.3% power (using either ExpDesign 5.0 or East 4.1) to detect a 28% relative change in mortality, from a three-year rate of 17.46% in the control (placebo) group to 13.75% in the intervention group, which was estimated from previous studies.

Suppose that we originally use an error-spending approach with an O'Brien-Fleming-like spending function featuring seven analyses at equal information intervals. After the third analysis, the efficacy results were somewhat promising, and the trend (Figure 7.7) showed that the trial was likely to be successful at the fifth interim analysis. Therefore, we want to do one more analysis (final analysis) for the study and eliminate the rest of the interim analyses. The final analysis is scheduled at the time for the original fifth interim analysis. Therefore, we calculate the stopping boundary using the same OF error-spending function but with four analyses at information time: $1/7$, $2/7$, $3/7$, and 1 (Figure 7.7). The new final stopping boundary is a naive p-value ≤ 0.0248 ($z = 1.9634$) using the distribution calculator in ExpDesign Studio 5.0 (Figure 7.8). The observed p-values at the first three IAs are 0.0465 ($z = 1.68$), 0.0125 ($z = 2.24$), and 0.0089 ($z = 2.37$), respectively. We want to check if the new design has sufficient power. If not, a sample size re-estimation may be required. We can accomplish this with ExpDesign Studio 5.0 as specified in the following steps: Note that the timing of the analyses is assumed to be independent of interim data. However, practically, we want to change the timing based on the data observed.

Fortunately, the potential type-I error rate inflation due to data-dependent timing is small ($< 10\%$) (Proschan et al., 2006). The results are summarized in Table 7.2.

Table 7.2: Table of Monitoring for Aldactone Study

AI time	Death placebo/test	Hazard ratio	Stage-wise P-value	Stopping boundary on p-scale	Condit. power
8/96	70/52	0.76	0.1100	0.0000	
3/97	136/109	0.83	0.2571	0.0000	
8/97	224/175	0.80	0.2868	0.0002	
3/98	304/241	0.81	0.0059	0.0009	
8/99	351/269	0.78	0.0048	0.0026	0.484
				0.0054	0.335
				0.0092	0.119
				0.0137	0.039
				0.0188	0.014

7.7   Summary

Clinical trials require the use of human test subjects and thus could potentially impact the well-being of the subjects. Successful management is essential to data quality, patients' safety, and time-to-market for the drug. Clinical trial management and execution includes many tasks such as trial project management, patient recruitment and projection, randomization, dynamic and adaptive drug supply, and statistical trial monitoring.

Managing the clinical trial process is one of the most significant places for improvement. However, there are many challenges: (1) lengthy and complex trial design and planning process often involving hundreds to thousands of patients and support staff, (2) extraordinary efforts and time required for getting valid data and cleaning up, (3) great efforts required to remain compliant with regulatory requirements (GCP), (4) each trial involves many intervening tasks, and (5) multiple trials run simultaneously, competing resources.

Critical path analysis (CPA) is a powerful tool for project management. Clinical trial tasks can be represented by directed or undirected networks. The goal can be to find the shortest path or longest path within the least time. These tasks can be represented by either a logic-OR or a logic-AND network. CPA, backwards induction, and linear programming can be used to solve the CTM task effectively.

Clinical trial recruitment (CTR) initiatives, if implemented correctly, can be highly successful, time can be dramatically reduced, and recruitment targets can be met ahead of schedule. The recent trend in clinical trial globalization has added new opportunities and challenges to CTR. Understanding those opportunities and challenges is significant to the success of CTR.

Projection of patient enrollment, time of interim analysis, and time of study ending are critical to clinical operation and management. In practice, it is not unusual that CTR is slower than expected despite the above mentioned strategic efforts. In such a case, we can increase the number of study sites, modify the inclusion/exclusion criteria, or prolong the trial if it is a survival study. To assess which method is preferable, Monte Carlo simulations can be conducted.

Randomization is an essential part of randomized clinical trials. The purpose of randomization is to minimize the imbalance between the treatment groups regarding potential confounding variables and improve trial efficiency by maximizing the power for detecting treatment differences.

From simple randomization, to blocking, stratified, and adaptive randomization, complexity gradually increases. Response-adaptive randomization is a randomization technique in which the allocation probability of patients to a treatment group is based on the outcomes of the previous patients. The purpose of such a randomization is to provide a better chance of randomizing patients to a superior treatment group based on knowledge about the treatment effect at the time of randomization. It can also be used to identify the optimal dose efficiently among several candidate doses.

Stratified and adaptive randomizations place a challenge on drug supply because the randomization list can't be predetermined. The conventional supply algorithm based on site is often overconservative and potentially wastes drugs. Adaptive drug supply can utilize data from the on-going trial to improve the efficiency of drug supply via Monte Carlo. Drug supply simulations can be used not only at the planning stage, but also during the trial for making adjustments to deviations from planning assumptions. To utilize simulation, the initial step is to collectively gather the potential factors that impact on drug coverage for the trial.

To protect the integrity of a clinical trial and the patients' well-being, trial monitoring is necessary. Monitoring can be carried out by an external independent data monitor committee or an internal DMC as guided by the relevant FDA guidance.

A commonly used statistical tool is conditional power in adaptive trials. Algorithm 7.11 can be used to simulate the conditional power for a K-stage design using MSP. We can also use commercial software (e.g., ExpDesign Studio and EAST) to calculate the conditional power for trial monitoring.

7.8   Exercises

Exercise 7.1: The time to complete a task is usually a random variable; thus the project with sequence of events (tasks) can be represented by random networks, in which the lengths of the arc d_{ij} are random variables. Develop a Monte Carlo algorithm (backwards induction or others) to assess the average f_1 and its variability.

Exercise 7.2: What new opportunities and challenges has clinical trial globalization brought to us?

Exercise 7.3: What are the common factors that lead to prolonging or failure of CTR? What are the common strategies to improve CTR?

Exercise 7.4: Modify Algorithms 7.2 and 7.3 using other distributions.

Exercise 7.5: Develop an algorithm for simple randomization for n parallel groups.

Exercise 7.6: Develop an algorithm for block randomization for two balanced groups.

Exercise 7.7: Develop an algorithm for block randomization for n parallel groups.

Exercise 7.8: Prove the results in Table 7.1.

Exercise 7.9: To utilize simulation for adaptive drug supply, the initial step is to gather a list of the potential factors that will impact (positively or negatively) on drug coverage for the trial. What are the factors?

Exercise 7.10: Review FDA guidance on DMC and answer the following questions: What are the purposes of a DMC? When is an external DMC needed?

Exercise 7.11: Develop algorithms for (1) conditional power for K-stage with binary endpoint using MSP, (2) conditional power for K-stage with normal endpoint using MPP and MINP.

Chapter 8

Prescription Drug Commercialization

This chapter will cover the following topics:

- Dynamics of Prescription Drug Marketing
- Stock-Flow Dynamic Model for Brand Planning
- Competitive Drug Marketing Strategy
- Compulsory Licensing and Parallel Importation

8.1 Dynamics of Prescription Drug Marketing

8.1.1 *Challenges in Innovative Drug Marketing*

There is critical public and political attention to high drug prices and large promotional budgets. Table 8.1 is a summary of big Pharma's profitability in 2004. Research (Schondelmeyer and Wrobel, 2004) indicates that US drug expenditures increased from approximately 7 billion USD (before rebates) in 1992 to 22 billion USD in 2002, a triple increase. Meanwhile, Hu and colleagues (Hu et al., 2007) reported that PhRM Research and Development spending increased from 12 billion to 36 billion in the same period, also a triple increase, whereas the number of FDA approvals remained flat from 1994 to 2004 (Figure 1.13 in Chapter 1). Since investment in Research and Development is expected to have a delayed reward, the comparison has different periods for Research and Development (1992–2002) and for FDA approvals (1994–2004). For this reason, the increase in prescription drug prices, more or less reflects an increase in Research and Development and commercial costs.

As to determination of drug prices, in the US, for instance, organizations such as HMOs determine the approved list of drugs to be prescribed by affiliated doctors ("formularies") based on drug prices. In Europe, governments maintain "positive" and "negative" lists, to reflect drugs that will and will not be reimbursed. Some countries have a tiered system, in which some drugs will be reimbursed at higher rates than others. In addition, both developing and developed nations have large uninsured population segments that are fully liable for the cost of drugs (Schondelmeyer and Wrobel, 2004).

Table 8.1: Big Pharma's Profitability, 2004

Company	Sales (in $M)	R & D as % Sales	Promotion % Sales	Net Profit Margin
Bristol-Myers Squibb	19,380	13%	30%	15%
Eli Lilly	13,858	19%	24%	22%
Johnson & Johnson	47,348	11%	30%	18%
Merck	22,939	18%	29%	27%
Pfizer	52,516	15%	30%	19%
Schering-Plough	8,272	19%	41%	10%
Wyeth	17,358	14%	25%	12%
Total	181,671	16%	30%	18%

(Data source: Pearlman, 2007)

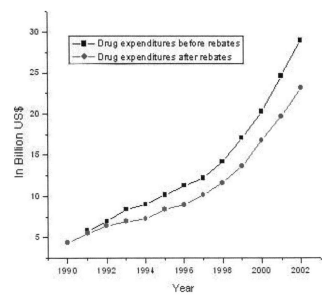

Figure 8.1:   US Medical Drug Expenditures, 2002
(Data source: Schondelmeyer and Wrobel, 2004)

In addition to price pressures, marketing for innovative therapies is also challenged by (1) evolving Medicare Part D drug benefits; an influx of generic therapies in costly therapeutic areas, (2) increasing involvement of consumers in healthcare decisions, (3) increased scrutiny of drug safety and off-label use, (4) the emergence of biosimilars, (5) declining marginal ROI for direct physician marketing, and (6) growing complexity in drug prescription and purchasing behaviors, due to trends such as formularies, internet pharmacies, and DTC-driven demand.

8.1.2 *Structure of the Pharmaceutical Market*

Structure of Pharmaceutical Prices

To understand the structure of pharmaceutical prices, let's start with pricing terms. There are many different price terms. List prices are published by manufacturers. The actual acquisition cost (AAC) is a transaction price used to describe the price paid by a pharmacy or provider when purchasing a drug product from either a drug manufacturer or wholesaler. This price is the appropriate conceptual basis for the payment policy. The wholesale acquisition cost (WAC) is a list price used for invoices between drug manufacturers and wholesalers. The average wholesale price (AWP) is a list price used for invoices between drug wholesalers. The direct price (DP) is a list price used for invoices between drug manufacturers and pharmacies or providers. The parties mainly involved in transactions include the manufacturer, wholesaler, and provider (e.g., pharmacy, physician, hospital, etc.); The class of trade eligible for prices is usually invited into independent pharmacies, chain pharmacies, mail order pharmacies, long term care pharmacies, hospitals, physicians, etc. (Figure 8.2).

Distribution Channels of Prescription Drugs

Distribution channels for prescription drugs include three primary levels: (1) manufacturers, (2) wholesalers, and (3) providers. Manufacturers and marketers reported $215.7 billion in revenue from prescription drugs in 2002 (Schondelmeyer and Wrobel, 2004), which were coming from various distribution channels (Figure 8.2). Manufacturers or marketers of prescription drugs most often sell their drug products to a middleman before the drug product reaches the pharmacy or physician. National wholesalers are the primary middleman, accounting for 45.7 percent of prescription drugs ($98.5 billion) in 2002, chain warehouses with 32.3 percent ($69.8 billion), and all others accounting for 22%.

Sources of Payment for Pharmaceuticals

Payments for prescription drug products may come from more than one source, including the patient as an individual, private insurance, public insurance, or government delivered and financed healthcare. Prescription drug programs are managed by pharmacy benefit managers and engage networks of pharmacies and providers to deliver prescription drugs. The disposition of various payment sources is depicted in Figure 8.3.

8.1.3   *Common Marketing Strategies*

Physicians are perhaps the most important players in pharmaceutical sales. Sales representatives from pharmaceutical companies call upon physicians regularly, providing information and free drug samples. Pharmaceutical companies are also developing processes to influence the people who influence the physicians. There are several channels by which a physician may be influenced, including self-influence through research, peer influence such as key opinion leaders, direct interaction with pharmaceutical companies, patients, and public or private insurance companies. There are also Web-based instruments that can be used to determine the influences and buying motives of physicians (www.wikipedia.com, 2009).

Big Pharma spends approximately $27B on its well-equipped army of 100,000 sales reps who visit the country's 600,000 physicians to detail and dispense free samples. This translates into more than one PCR (pharmaceutical company representative) for every five office-based physicians. With an annual budget of $160,000, it has been estimated that reps spend $500 per doctor per visit or $10,000 annually per physician. On average PCR visits occur weekly and last less than 2 minutes (Pearlman, 2007).

There are approximately 100,000 pharmaceutical sales representatives in the United States (Ebisch, 2005) pursuing some 830,000 pharmaceutical prescribers. Representatives often have a call list of about 200 physicians with 120 targets that should be visited in 1–2 week cycles.

Direct-to-patient marketing of prescription drugs has become important since the late 1970s. Many patients will inquire about, or even demand to receive, a medication they have seen advertised on television. Expenditures on direct-to-consumer (DTC) pharmaceutical advertising have more than quintupled in the last years since the FDA changed the guidelines, from $700 million in 1997 to more than $4.2 billion in 2005, according to the United States GAO (Government Accountability Office, 2006). Direct-to-consumer campaigns generally begin within a year after the approval of a product by the FDA.

In the United States, marketing and distribution of pharmaceuticals is regulated by the federal Prescription Drug Marketing Act of 1987. In general, pharmaceutical companies adhere to FDA regulatory guidelines which call for all DTC advertising and information to be accurate, to provide substantial evidence for any claims that are made, to provide a balance between the risks and benefits of the promoted drug, and to maintain consistency with labeling approved by the FDA. In the context of regulatory changes requiring legal review before issuing letters, the number of letters sent by the FDA to pharmaceutical manufacturers regarding violations of drug-

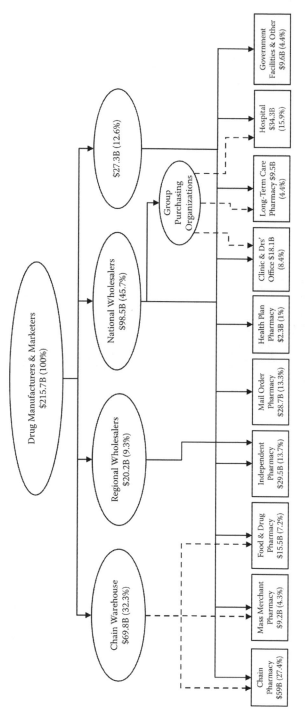

Figure 8.2: Channels of distribution for Prescription Drugs (2002).
(Sources: Adapted from Schondelmeyer and Wrobel, 2004)

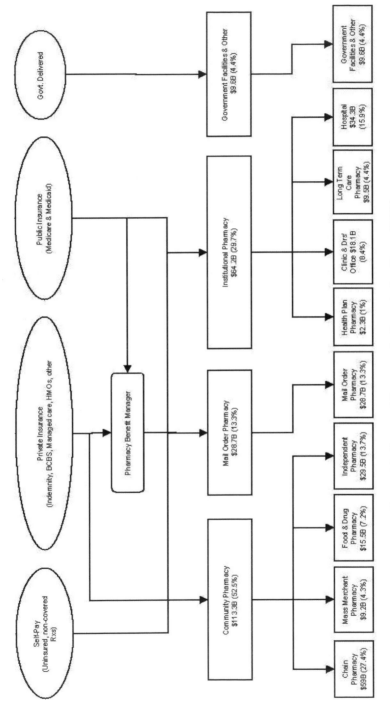

Figure 8.3: Source of Payment for Prescription Drugs (2002).
(Source: Adapted from Schondelmeyer and Wrobel, 2004)

advertising regulations fell from 142 in 1997 to only 21 in 2006 (Donohue et al. 2007).

The mass marketing to consumers of pharmaceuticals is controversial. Some feel it is better to leave the decision wholly in the hands of medical professionals; others feel that consumer education and participation in health is useful, but consumers need independent, comparative information about drugs. Mass marketing is banned in over 30 industrialized nations, but not in the US and New Zealand. Canada's limitations on pharmaceutical advertising ensure that commercials that mention the name of a product cannot in any way describe what it does (wikipedia.com, June 10, 2009).

8.2   Stock-Flow Dynamic Model for Brand Planning

8.2.1   *Traditional Approach*

Prescription drug marketing starts with a *brand plan*. A brand plan usually has both short (1–3 years) and longer term (over 10 years) objectives. The long term objective has to adopt the practice of cross-functional coordination in order to leverage various types of knowledge within the organization, assessing NCE market potential. The key outcome of the brand planning process is the concept of brand positioning, i.e., how the compound will be positioned with respect to its target audience, its expected benefits, its key reasons for trial/usage, etc. Brand positioning helps establish a series of product strategies created to leverage the collective knowledge of the disease market and effectively use resources to increase the uptake of the NCE.· Strategy areas include target influence, effect on pricing/reimbursement, publication strategy, impact on the regulatory environment, etc. Strategies resulting from the brand planning process are then rolled out to the operations personnel in various markets in order to determine the tactical approach to support them (Paich et al., 2009).

A financial projection for the NCE is usually derived from volume analysis, extrapolated from market financial projections. Analogs of other drugs in an indication marketplace, statistical and econometric models, and Monte Carlo simulation are often utilized.

However, traditionally this type of forecasting analysis boils down to two sets of aggregate assumptions about an indication marketplace and the position of the NCE within it (Figure 8.4). In the traditional approach, the expected indication sales are calculated from an extrapolation of historical data, modified by epidemiologic trends or expectations of advances in the efficacy of various treatment options. The sales projection is usually derived from analysis of product analogs, comparison of the NCE to existing treatment offerings in the marketplace, and team judgment regarding the level and type of marketing support for the compound. The projection includes three key concepts: (1) maximum or peak sales, (2) the average slope of revenue increase over time, and (3) the rate of the falloff from peak sales.

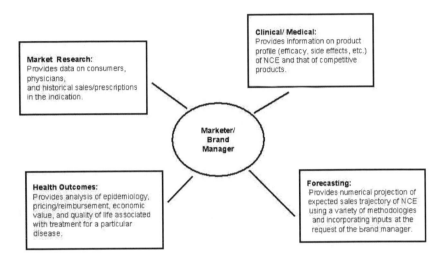

Figure 8.4:   (Source: Paich et al., 2009)

8.2.2   *Concept of the Stock-Flow Model*

Paich and colleagues (Paich et al., 2009) proposed a patient flow and portfolio simulation approach using techniques from operations research and system dynamics. Their approach can add value in at least two distinct ways.

(1) The dynamic modeling approach creates a means to test the linkages between cause and effect in various pharmaceutical settings. Such simulation-based models can be used to operationally define the expected outcomes of a set of strategic decisions, resulting in better strategic plans and a more complete understanding of the sets of key relationships governing them.

(2) Dynamic models provide a useful operational input to the forecasting process by establishing a framework to integrate the knowledge bases that exist within a pharmaceutical firm's functional divisions. The approach establishes practical boundaries in the realm of possible out-

comes from a commercial assessment, providing a solid foundation for reasonability checks of the commercial potential for an NCE. As such, dynamic models provide another lens through which the future behavior of a disease marketplace, and the position of a particular compound within it, can be seen.

Dynamic models represent an operational way to translate mental models from the implicit to the explicit, allowing for a set of specific business questions to be addressed and analyzed. Paich further elaborates these strategic questions as the following topics:

(1) How can we develop a more effective strategic brand plan?
(2) How can we better leverage the wealth of data and institutional knowledge about the disease indication, patient behavior, and physician preferences?
(3) How can we sanely check existing commercial assessment methodologies?
(4) How can we have an integrated tool to link the results of proposed strategies to the impact on the compound commercial assessment?

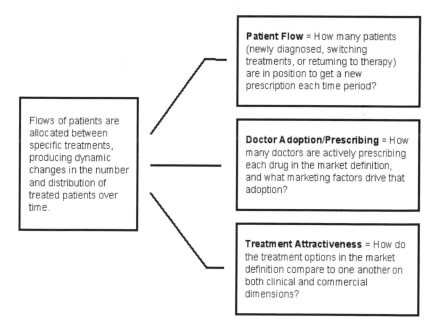

Figure 8.5: Three Sectors of the Standard Template Dynamic Model

The dynamic model includes three components: (1) patient flow, (2) doctor adoption, and (3) treatment attractiveness (Figure 8.5). These components are populated with data from epidemiology and a variety of physician and patient databases to ensure the entire model reflects actual market dynamics.

8.2.3   *Patient Flow*

Data on the number of prescriptions are often used by pharmaceutical companies for estimation of revenue for an NCE. However, rarely does the effort ask the fundamental question of the driving forces behind prescription generation (Figure 8.5). In the patient-flow component, the key is to formulate a patient segmentation, which conforms to data available. An example of a patient stock-flow diagram is depicted in Figure 8.6.

The concept of a mutually exclusive and collectively exhaustive (MECE) competitive set is useful here (Rasiel, 1999). MECE means that the treatment option set completely covers the spectrum of possible therapy choices, but does not double count patients who may be on more than one medication at a time. MECE provides a framework to facilitate consistent data collection, allows therapy changes to be categorized and quantified, and supports the projection of dynamic marketing behaviors using epidemiology data.

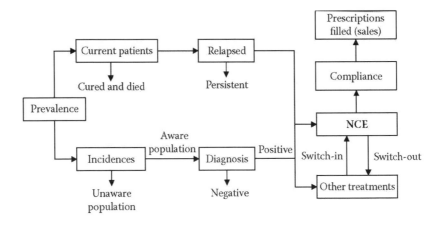

Figure 8.6:   Patient Flow Model

Compliance and persistence are often combined in traditional analysis of pharmaceutical markets into one metric to account for patients who do not take all of their prescribed medications. However, it is better to differentiate them for the purpose of marketing simulation and projection.

Compliance is a measure of agreement between the amount of prescribed medication and the amount taken. However, for revenue calculation, we define compliance as the agreement between the amount of prescribed medication and the amount of the prescription filled, because patients who continue to fill their prescriptions but do not take 100% of their prescribed dosage will be a source of revenue, although at a reduced rate due to the corresponding extension of time between prescription refills. Persistence relates to how long patients stay on any form of treatment before discontinuing prescription medication entirely.

8.2.4 *Doctor Adoption—Prescription*

In many pharmaceutical drug markets, historical data can be analyzed to determine how quickly drugs for a particular indication were adopted by prescribing physicians. Prospectively, market researchers often collect data on awareness of drugs that have yet to be launched and conduct surveys on doctors' expectations regarding their future prescribing patterns. Paich and colleagues (Paich et al., 2009) argue that this information, while useful, does not explicitly capture the mechanisms at play in both past and future adoption of pharmacological treatments by doctors, nor does it indicate how such dynamics interact with other parts of the marketplace to affect overall market performance. They believe the following aspects are important for model improvement: (1) understanding the operational physics driving adoption of pharmaceutical products, (2) determining the importance of certain marketing levers in driving that adoption, (3) relating the aspects of physician adoption to components of patient dynamics and various treatments in a competitive landscape, and (4) developing strategic forecasts based on an integrated view of marketplace dynamics.

To construct a physician adoption model, assume doctors meet with each other randomly with an equal probability. Therefore, the adoption rate at time t is proportional to the number of doctors who have adopted (N) the drug and the number of doctors who have the potential to adopt ($N_{max} - N$). Mathematically,

$$\frac{dN}{dt} = kN\left(N_{max} - N\right),\qquad(8.1)$$

where N_{max} is the maximum number of doctors who will ultimately adopt and k is the diffusion coefficient dependent on various factors in dynamic marketing (but usually considered as time independent).

Equation (8.1) can be rewritten as

$$\left(\frac{1}{N} + \frac{1}{N_{max} - N}\right) dN = kN_{max}dt. \tag{8.2}$$

After integration, (8.2) becomes

$$\ln \frac{N}{N_{max} - N} = kN_{max}\, t + c, \tag{8.3}$$

where constant c will be determined later using the initial condition. To do that we rewrite (8.3) as

$$\frac{N}{N_{max} - N} = \exp(c) \cdot \exp\left(kN_{max}\, t\right). \tag{8.4}$$

Applying the initial condition $N\,(t=0) = N_0$ (i.e., the number of doctors who adopted at time 0) in (8.4), we obtain

$$\exp\left(c\right) = \frac{N_0}{N_m - N_0}.$$

Therefore, the logistic model (8.4) can be written as:

$$p = \frac{p_0 \exp\left(kN_{max}t\right)}{1 + p_0 \exp\left(kN_{max}t\right)}, \tag{8.5}$$

where

$$p = \frac{N}{N_{max}} \text{ and } p_0 = \frac{N_0}{N_m - N_0} \approx \frac{N_0}{N_{max}}. \tag{8.6}$$

The key is to determine the diffusion coefficient k, which can be a function of market factors. To compose a list of these factors, the following questions might be helpful: What stages do physicians progress through in their acceptance of a new compound? What are the currently available treatment options for the indication? How do these therapies compare to one another and the NCE? If data are available logit regression can be used to determine k. If data are not or only partially available, Monte Carlo simulations are helpful, in which random numbers can be generated with various probability distributions. An example of a simulated prescription status is presented in Table 8.2.

Table 8.2: Example of Prescription Status

Year	2012	2013	2014	2015	2016
Prescription status	5%	40%	85%	92%	96%

8.2.5 Treatment Attractions

When physicians make prescribing decisions for patients with a particular disease, a set of product criteria is used to determine which drug is most appropriate to prescribe in a given situation. The key attributes in the decision making process vary by indication, but often include safety, tolerability, efficacy, convenience, and onset of action. The essential difference between safety and tolerability is that safety pertains to the actual risk to the health of a subject (e.g., death or disability), whereas tolerability is related to signs and symptoms that are temporary in nature, even though they may be severe (e.g., headache, constipation, vomiting).

Two simple models used by Paich and colleagues (Paich et al., 2009) are arithmetic logit choice and exponential logit choice formulations.

The arithmetic logit choice (ALC) formulation is given by

$$S_k\left(t\right) = \frac{U_k}{\sum_i U_i} + e_k,$$

where S_k = the share for treatment k; U_k = the utility or treatment attractiveness score for treatment k; $\sum U_i$ = the total of all utility scores in the MECE set; e_k = the error term for the calculation, indicated by the difference between the share calculation and the actual data to which it is being calibrated.

The exponential logit choice (ELC) formulation is given by

$$S_k\left(t\right) = \frac{e^{aU_k}}{\sum_i e^{aU_i}} + e_k,$$

where constant a can be determined using regression analysis. Certain dynamic modeling software platforms, such as VenSim® or AnyLogic®, have this capability as well.

Alternatively, factors contributing to treatment attractiveness can be assigned by the expert team. The importance and rating of each of these treatment attributes can be determined by team judgment for each of the MECE treatment sets, and can be designed to change over time.

8.2.6 Diffusion Model for Drug Adoption

A study (Domino et al., 2003) found that the diffusion of new behavioral health technologies, or the rate at which these products have spread through the market, has been very uneven. Differences in adoption and diffusion rates of psychotropic medications across insurance settings, geographic regions, or subpopulations characterized by age, gender, or ethnic groups have important implications for the quality of care received by persons with mental illnesses.

Case Study 8.1: Diffusion of New Pharmaceutical Drugs Worldwide

Desiraju and colleagues (Desiraju et al., 2004) used a diffusion model to study market characteristics for a new category of prescription drugs in both developing and developed countries. Using data from fifteen countries and a logistic specification in the Hierarchical Bayesian framework, they detected statistically the differences in diffusion speed and maximum penetration potential between developing and developed countries. Specifically, (1) compared to developed countries, developing nations tend to have lower diffusion speeds and maximum penetration levels; (2) developed countries have higher speeds. However, developing countries do not have higher diffusion speeds; (3) per capita expenditures on healthcare have a positive effect on diffusion speed (particularly for developed countries), while higher prices tend to decrease diffusion speed.

They also examined the diffusion speed, maximum penetration potential, and the effects of prices and per capita healthcare expenditures in fifteen countries: Belgium, South Africa, the United States, Spain, Italy, Mexico, Canada, The UK, France, The Netherlands, Brazil, Colombia, Venezuela, Australia, and Portugal.

The product growth model follows the logistic specification in Van den Bulte (2000). The model specifies the growth rate of sales for a new product in country i at time t as a function of cumulative sales at the beginning of period t, $X_i(t)$, and population $M_i(t)$:

$$\frac{dX_i(t)}{dt} = \frac{\theta_i}{a_i M_i(t)} X_i(t)(a_i M_i(t) - X_i(t)), \tag{8.7}$$

where parameters θ_i and a_i are to be estimated.

To work on discrete time points, we can rewritte (8.7) in a finite difference form:

$$X_{it} = \frac{\theta_i}{a_i M_{it}} X_{i,t-1}(a_i M_{it} - X_{i,t-1})\Delta t. \tag{8.8}$$

The amount of time required to move from one level of market penetration (say, $p_1\%$) to another (say, $p_2\%$) is $\frac{1}{\theta_i} \ln \frac{p_2(1-p_1)}{p_1(1-p_2)}$, which is inversely proportional to θ_i (Van den Bulte, 2000). Therefore, the parameter θ_i is a measure of the aggregate diffusion speed for the category in country i, and a comparison of diffusion speeds across countries can be made on the basis of their estimated θ_is.

They also adopted a hierarchical Bayes (HB) approach to obtain a posterior estimate of the diffusion rates and maximum penetrations by synchronizing the information strength across heterogeneous countries (Table 8.3). The HB approach allows for obtaining posterior estimates of diffusion parameters specific to each country in a statistically consistent manner that takes into account the uncertainty associated with the model and the available data.

Gibbs sampling (see Chapter 2) with WinBUGS was used to obtain the posterior distribution of the parameters. The first 20,000 draws are used for the burn-in period and the last 10,000 draws are used to generate all posterior parameter estimates and standard deviations.

Table 8.3: Posterior Diffusion Rate and Maximum Penetration

Country	Mean diffusion speed $\hat{\theta}_i$	Maximum penetration level $\hat{\alpha}_i$(Kg·s/million people)
Belgium	0.4259	1616
South Africa	0.4424	1113
US	0.2133	34,341
Spain	0.6823	1028
Italy	0.3635	1327
Canada	0.3361	19,320
UK	0.4415	1608
Mexico	1.5580	793
France	0.8946	1280
Netherlands	0.6194	1108
Brazil	0.2464	271
Colombia	0.3564	1277
Venezuela	0.3246	1361
Australia	0.2889	2101
Portugal	0.2608	1489
Average	0.4971	4669

(Source: Adapted from Desiraju et al., 2004)

Other ROI studies include those by the Association of Medical Publications (AMP) (2001), Wittink (2002), and Narayanan et al. (2002). Recent studies on pharmaceuticals using individual-physician-level data to understand the prescription behavior of physicians include those by Kamakura and Kossar (1998), who examined the adoption/timing of physician's drug prescription decisions, and Manchanda et al. (2003), who modeled physician prescription behavior within a framework that allows response parameters to be affected by the process by which detailing is set across physicians.

Berndt and colleagues (2003) used a similar approach to conduct a simulation study for H2-antagonist antiulcer drugs. They examined the role of consumption externalities in the demand for pharmaceuticals at both the brand level and over a therapeutic class of drugs. Externalities emerge when the use of a drug by others affects its value, and/or conveys information about efficacy and safety to patients and physicians. They found that consumption externalities influence both valuations and rates of diffusion.

After having parameter estimation in (8.7), it can be used as basis for Monte Carlo simulation, in which θ_i are treated as random variables.

8.2.7 *Strategy Framework for NCE Introductions*

Porter's Five Forces and the ubiquitous strengths, weaknesses, opportunities, and threats (SWOT) analysis are widely accepted approaches as common organizing principles by the pharmaceutical world for framing strategic issues. Paich and colleagues (Paich et al., 2009) developed an operating framework that provides a useful way to think about marketing strategy when entering/analyzing an indication marketplace, as shown in Figure 8.7.

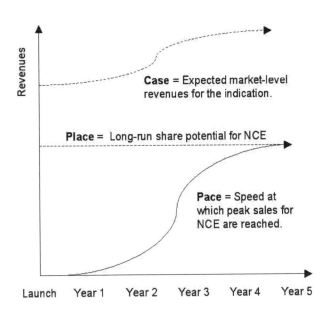

Figure 8.7:   Case, Place, and Pace Framework in NCEl
(Source: Paich et al., 2009)

The **Case** for a new compound is the set of aggregate, macro-economic market conditions of the indication being evaluated. Information on epidemiology, changing demographics, treatment paradigms, historical market revenue trends, and existing competitors all define the Case for an NCE considering entry into a new marketplace. Case issues are often summarized as revenue forecasts for an indication.

The **Place** for a new compound defines how it compares to the existing and future competition in terms of efficacy, safety, side effects, etc. In markets exhibiting specific treatment algorithms, Place may also include where the compound is expected to fall within a defined Lines of Therapy progression. In economic lingo, the Place of a compound in an indication determines its long-run market share potential—often referred to as peak sales in the pharmaceutical world.

The **Pace** for the new compound relates to the speed at which it can reach peak share potential—the shape of the expected sales trajectory. While Case and Place are generally functions of product attributes, disease epidemiology, and other aggregate conditions, the Pace for an NCE is more commonly under the influence of various strategic marketing decisions on the part of individual pharmaceutical firms. Effective Brand Planning leverages the observed dynamics of Patient Flow and Doctor Adoption to effectively increase the Pace at which an NCE is accepted in the marketplace. The resulting expected sales trajectory, commonly referred to as product uptake, is an important factor in the commercial assessment of the compound using financial metrics such as Net Present Value (NPV).

The sensitivity of dynamic modeling results based on various levels of calculated utility for that therapy option can be analyzed to determine the Place for a given NCE; these results can then be assessed in aggregate using the overall treatment attractiveness for the new compound or by the individual components of computed utility. The Pace is where marketing strategies can have the most influences.

8.2.8 *Data Source for Simulation*

In-house epidemiologists often can help inform the working team of data availability, possible segmentations, and configuring disease metrics that potentially impact the success of indication marketing.

For patient stock data, the U.S. Census Bureau (www.census.gov) and the Centers for Disease Control and Prevention (www.cdc.gov) post both historical and projected demographic data cut in a variety of different dimensions and update them periodically. Online resources such as PubMed provide a searchable repository of published research for various disease-specific data, drawing on peer-reviewed research studies and often forecast over some time interval. Advocacy groups or foundations focusing on specific indications also provide information on disease epidemiology at their respective web sites. The National Center for Health Statistics (NCHS) is a CDC division that collects and publishes cross-sectional survey data in the form of the National Health and Nutrition Examination Survey (NHANES) report. Currently treated nonpersistent-syndicated reports often estimate the treatment rate for diagnosed patients. Pharmacy claims databases can often be used as excellent sources for determining patient distribution across various treatment options, including patients designated as nonpersistent. Vendors such as MediPlus® from IMS Health, MarketScan® from MedStat, Caremark Rx, PharMetrics, Verispan from Scott-Levin, Surveillance Data, Synovate, and GE HealthCare specialize in these types of databases.

Integrated medical and pharmaceutical claims provide pharmaceutical executives with a picture of patient treatment patterns across a wide range of healthcare issues, and the PharMetrics database containing de-identified pharmaceutical and medical records is the largest and most complete of its kind. This health insurance claims database is contributed to by more than 70 geographically diverse payor organizations and captures the entire continuum of care for more than 57 million covered lives. The database is representative of the commercially insured population in the United States and contains information on all types of interactions a patient has with the healthcare system, including office visits, diagnoses, hospital stays, prescription treatments, and diagnostic procedures and tests (Steven Bloom, PharMetrics). This type of data can be used in a variety of analyses such as (1) developing and refining market segmentations, (2) informing brand positioning, (3) illustrating patterns and pathways of treatment, (4) identifying and valuing market opportunities, and (4) assessing the cost impact of treatment interventions.

Operationally, it is the flows of patients that are a primary driving factor in how pharmaceutical markets change over time. From an epidemiology standpoint, the movements of patients into a disease category through incidence or out of it through death or recovery dictate how the prevalence of an indication is likely to evolve. From a product standpoint, the flows associated with patients and their pharmaceutical treatments are what drive prescriptions and ultimately revenues in an indication marketplace (Paich et al., 2009).

8.3 Competitive Drug Marketing Strategy

In the patient-flow and portfolio dynamic model, competitors are basically treated as static opponents, but that does not reflect the marketing reality. In this section, we study models that treat a competitor as an opponent in the game.

The key to the marketing success of an NCE is to develop adaptive (rather than static) and thus robust *marketing mixes* or spend rates across available marketing and sales channels. This is because if your firm adopts a new and effective marketing mix, your competitors will detect that success quickly, thanks to market data subscription services such as IMS Health. Once alerted, your competitors will likely respond with counter-strategies to reverse your gains and retake market share. To prevent this, you need to anticipate likely competitor responses and design adaptive strategies to defeat these counter-measures (DecisionPath, www.decpath.com).

Dynamics in drug market shift continually involve competition, losing patent protection, new market entrants, new safety and/or efficacy studies, and changing FDA regulations and healthcare payer policies. Therefore, it is critical to develop marketing mix strategies that can promptly adapt to both environmental changes and anticipated responses by competitors. Key performance metrics include drug market share, net sales, profit, and overall value (NPV).

The following are important factors to be considered in marketing simulation: characteristics of the target market and current economic conditions, the drug companies competing in a particular market, the competing drugs, candidate marketing mix strategies, available business intelligence on the competitors' marketing practices and strategies, and other factors such as changes in regulations or reimbursement policies.

The CompeteRx simulation engine leverages a model published by researchers at MIT's Sloan School of Management that predicts market size and market share allocations. DecisionPath extended the Sloan model to address the problem of competitive behaviors through technologies including complex adaptive systems, game theory, system dynamics, and event-based programming. CompeteRx is unique in its ability to model and project adaptive behaviors, based on decision rules that capture anticipated competitor responses (www.decpath.com, March 2009).

8.3.1   *Pricing and Payer Strategies*

Pricing and payer strategies have never been more important to manufacturers and marketers of innovative drug therapies. In an era of rising health care costs, drug companies face mounting pressure to limit further increases, while managed care plans seek to control utilization of therapies through formularies and benefit designs (Analysis Group, www.analysisgroup.com, April 2009). The pricing and payer strategies included strategic pricing and finance (list pricing determination, scenario modeling), managed markets (price differentiation through segmentation, profitable contracting, rebates/discount programs), and health economics and outcomes research (cost effectiveness, budget impact, cost of illness).

Determining Product Value Proposition

Various experts, physicians, marketers, KOL, and pharmacists can perform evaluations for drug attractions from their own perspectives. However, their scores may be weighted differently for difference areas depending on their specialized area.

The value proposition can be determined by the attraction score. The attraction score can be calculated as follows:

$$AS_a = \frac{S_A}{S_A + S_B + S_C}. \tag{8.9}$$

Numerical examples of attraction scores are presented in Table 8.4.

Table 8.4: Determination of Product Value Proposition

Criterion	Product			Product A
	A	B	C	Attraction Score
	S_A	S_B	S_C	AS_a
Efficacy	8	3	6	0.42
Safety	7	6	5	0.39
Tolerability	5	7	2	0.36
Cost effectiveness	6	7	6	0.32
Convenience	9	5	8	0.43
Total	35	28	27	0.39

Note: Scores range from 1 to 10. AS ranges from 0 to 1.

Segmentation and Sensitivity Analysis

The price of a product will have an impact on its access and utilization. Therefore, the determination of optimal pricing strategy should be based on the characteristics (advantages and disadvantages) of the product in relation to the competitors and various patient or market segmentations (e.g., out-of-pocket costs). We can study the impact of price and other product attributes on access under relevant market scenarios, and investigate with clinicians, key opinion leaders, and patients concerning therapy decisions in the context of access levels (% formulary access and % shares of prescription).

Identify segments of customers with different underlying demand profiles and design contracting approaches tailored to each segment's specific circumstances. A segmentation approach, together with analysis of contract value, can make the difference in profitability.

It is important to identify the relative importance of each market channel (e.g., commercial, Medicare, Medicaid, LTC, hospital, federal) and of priority segments within each channel. Not all accounts represent equal opportunities in terms of market potential and ability to influence share through their formulary controls, nor do they respond similarly to pricing and contracting offerings (Analysis Group, Pricing and Strategy, www.analysisgroup.com, April 2009). The most effective, appropriate strategy for each account segment should be based on its unique characteristics and importance to the brand. An illustrative example is presented in Table 8.5.

Table 8.5: Segmenting Key Account

Top PBM	Top Insurer	Others
Express Scripts*	Aetna*	MedImpact
Prime Therapeutics	Regence*	HMSA
Walgreens*	BlueShield of CA	NMHCS
PacifiCare*	Kaiser Permanente	Coventry
Medco	Humana	Harvard Pilgrim
Wellpoint	United Healthcare	HIP (NY)
Caremark**	CIGNA*	Horizon (NJ)
Memberhealth**		Health Net
% Total lives:		
MCO: 65%	20%	15%
MMA: 55%	25%	20%

* — Tier 2, ** — Tier 3, others — not on formulary
(Source: Adapted from Analysis Group, 2009)

Payer contracting and rebate/discount programs are often helpful. However, successful contracting requires a comprehensive, fact-based analysis to determine the value of each plan, and to prioritize plans by their ability to affect product share through relative formulary position.

Customer segmentation may also be important. Each segmentation scheme can be evaluated based on its alignment with the brand's strategic objectives, ability to differentiate effectively among customers with different underlying response profiles and affinity for contracting offers, and simplicity in implementation and tracking over time.

8.3.2   *Marketing Strategies after Patent Expiration*

Chandon (2004) summarized five different strategies against generic pharmaceutical products: divest, innovate, provide more value for money, invest in generics, and reduce price (Figure 8.8).

Divest

This strategy involves cutting all promotional and research expenses once the brand faces direct competition from generics and redirecting the savings toward other brands or new compound development. This strategy leads to the lowest brand building (i.e., without brand support) and price competition (without challenging the price advantage of generics). This strategy makes the most sense when financial incentives of the generic are low and brand quality is highly differentiable from the generics. This strategy usually works over the short term. One of the major drawbacks of this strategy is that it could encourage generic makers to challenge drug patents more aggressively, knowing that the market will be theirs soon.

Innovate

In this approach, the innovative pharmaceutical company can launch new forms and dosages or demonstrate effectiveness for "new indications." They can also innovate by offering better services for doctors (e.g., hotline), and better communication on the illness. This strategy entails low price competition, but can improve the equity of the off-patent brand by offering additional patent protection. The trade-off is that innovations require investment in time and money, but success is not guaranteed.

Provide More Value for the Money

Introducing new and improved flavors, packaging, or delivery systems can lead to additional emotional or functional consumer benefits (e.g., higher compliance). The resulting differentiation enhances the awareness and image of the brand and hence increases its equity. However, these improvements can be easily copied by generics and thus often have only a short term effect and profit margins are limited.

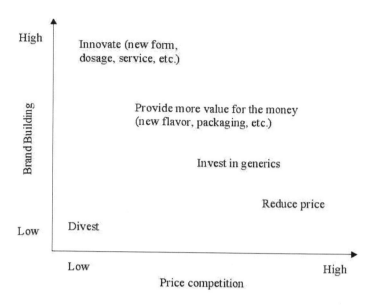

Figure 8.8: Marketing Strategies After Patent Expiration
(Source: Chandon, 2004)

Invest in Generics

Pharmaceutical companies can introduce their own generic and reduce the profitability of generic makers to deter them from entering the category. They can also license the drug before the expiration of the patent in exchange for royalties. The new copy will typically be priced higher than a true generic, but will benefit from first-mover advantage and deter entry from other generic makers.

Reduce Price

This strategy leads to the lowest level of brand building, but narrows the price gap with generics. The equity of the brand can no longer sustain a large price differential and make doctors, pharmacists, and regulators indifferent between the two and may force the weakest generic makers out of business. However, price competition invites retaliation and can quickly degenerate into a price war that would kill all the profits in the category.

Chandon (Chandon, 2004) studied the strategies and conducted the case of GSK's antibiotic Clamoxyl in France after its patent expiration. Hong and colleagues (Hong et al., 2005) studied the product-line extensions and pricing strategies of brand-name drugs facing patent expiration. They studied (1) whether market entries of new-product extensions are associated with market success of original brand-name drugs before generic drug entry, and (2) whether original brand-name drugs exhibit price rigidity to generic entry only when they are extended. This retrospective follow-up study for total 27 prescription drug brands that lost their patents between 1987 and 1992 was limited to nonantibiotic, orally administered drugs containing only one active pharmaceutical ingredient. Information on patent expiration, entry of a product extension, and market success was determined from the U.S. Food and Drug Administration's Orange Book, First DataBank, and American Druggist, respectively. Market success was defined as whether an original drug brand was listed in the top 100 prescriptions most frequently dispensed before facing generic entry. Product-line extension was defined as the appearance of another product that a company introduces within the same market after its existing product.

Results from regression analyses show that achieved market success was 16 times more likely to be extended than were those that did not ($OR = 16.95\%$ confidence interval, $2.12-120.65$). The price rigidity to entry existed in drug brands with extensions ($b = 2.65\%$, $P < 0.033$), but not in those brands without extensions ($b = -2.40\%$, $P < 0.001$).

Open Technology Platform in EU Biotech

Business models as pictures of firms showing their position on the value chain form Research & Drug Discovery, Preclinical studies, Phase I, II, III, to Market, and the way they create and capture value.

Open Technology Platform (OTP) in EU Biotech challenges Brand Drug marketing. What 'open' means here is (1) no patent for licensing-in and licensing-out, (2) no one owns the technology, but can own the product, i.e., no exclusivity, (3) free access to a patented technology.

The question is: will OTP discourage technology innovation? OTP supporters argue that innovation can come from expired patents, programs of technological Research and Development previously developed from client projects, and scientific publications.

Value creation can come from a critical technological development for a client, improvement of knowledge, and re-use of technology development. The values captured include price of the service, milestones, royalties, time savings, cost savings, and new basis for a possible new activity.

8.3.3 *Stochastic Market Game*

A pharmaceutical company usually starts its marketing strategy research before the drug gets approval for marketing. There are several key factors to consider in making the strategy: (1) company marketing positioning, (2) characteristics of the prescription drug and its competitors, which include efficacy, safety, convenience, cost, (3) target patient segmentation and mapping to the drug characteristics in (2), (4) physician prescription behaviors of the drug class, (5) behavior characteristics of competitors, (6) financial condition of the company and its competitors, and (7) availability of marketing force.

Suppose we do marketing consulting for the company and have to decide marketing strategies. As an illustrative example, assume there are three patient segments (inferior, mixed, and prime) that are determined for the overall patient population. For each of the patient segments, we have to decide x \$ amount for advertising. If $x = 0$, it means no direct advertising at all for that segment; if $x = D_{\max}$, it reaches the financial constraint.

It is important to fully realize that the outcomes of advertising are not only dependent on the company's advertising strategy, but are also influenced by the behaviors of other game players (the competitors).

Let's build the Markov decision process (see Chapter 5) for the problem. Recall that a infinite horizon Markov decision process is a 4-tuple of four element $\{S, A, \Pr(S, A), g(S, A)\}$ with the following properties:

(1) Finite (N) set of states S

(2) Set of actions A (can be conditioned on the state s)

(3) Policy = action mapping to state s

(4) Immediate reward (utility or gain function) $g : S \times A \to \Re$

$g(s)$ = immediate fixed reward by reaching the state s and

$c(a)$ = an immediate cost by taking action a.

(5) Transition model (dynamics) $T : S \times A \times S \to [0, 1]$

$T(s, a, s')$ = probability of going from s to s' under action a.

$$T(s, a, s') = \Pr(s'|s, a) = P_{ss'}(a). \tag{8.10}$$

(6) Discount factor for future rewards $0 < \gamma < 1$.

(7) The goal is to find a policy $\pi^* = \{a_i^*, i = 1, ..., N\}$ that maximizes the total expected gain over a certain duration, which will be subject to some initial condition and other constraints, if any.

For the current problem (Figure 8.9), there are three states $S = \{s_1, s_2, s_3\}$ for each patient segment: (1) the inferior, who will mostly use the competitor's drug, the gain at this state is $g = g_1 = 0$, (2) the mixed, who will use both our client's and the competitors' drugs, so the gain at this state is $g = g_2(\xi)$, which is dependent on the patient segment ξ, (3) the prime, who will virtually use our client's drug only.

At each stage, we have to make a decision/action whether to launch a strong advertising campaign (SC), limited advertising (LA), or do nothing (DN), i.e., the action space $A = \{\text{SC, LA, DN}\}$. A cost associates to each action taken, specifically, $C = \{c_1, c_2, c_3\}$ in corresponding to $A = \{\text{SC, LA, DN }\}$. No discount γ will be considered.

The transition probabilities $p_{ij}(a)$ can be estimated using information about the competitor's possible strategies. We can use Table 8.6 to illustrate conceptually. The probability that both the sponsor and the competitor take strong marketing campaigns is $\tilde{p}_{ss}$ and the conditional transition probability from state i to state j under this companion condition is $\hat{p}_{ij}(ss)$. Therefore the transition probability is given by

$$p_{ij} = \sum_{a \in A \times A} \tilde{p}_a \hat{p}_{ij}(a).\tag{8.11}$$

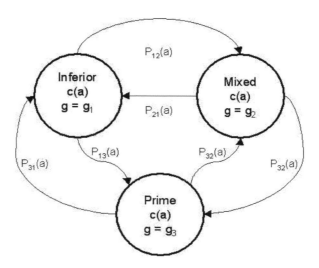

Figure 8.9:   Markov Decision Process for Marketing

Table 8.6: Probabilities of Strategy Matching

		Competitor		
		SC	LA	DN
Sponsor	SC	$\tilde{p}_{ss}$	$\tilde{p}_{sl}$	$\tilde{p}_{sd}$
	LA	$\tilde{p}_{ls}$	$\tilde{p}_{ll}$	$\tilde{p}_{ld}$
	DN	$\tilde{p}_{ds}$	$\tilde{p}_{dl}$	$\tilde{p}_{dd}$

Bellman's equation can be written as

$$V(s) = \max_{a \in A} \left(g(s') - c(a) + \gamma \sum_{s' \in S} \Pr(s'|s, a) \cdot V(s') \right).\tag{8.12}$$

The optimal policy $\pi^* = \{a_1^*, a_2^*, ..., a_N^*\}$ for the MDP is a vector whose i^{th} component is the optimal action taken state i and defined by

$$a_s^* = \arg\max_{a_s} \left\{ g\left(s'\right) - c\left(a\right) + \gamma \sum_{s' \in S} \Pr\left(s'|s, a_s\right) \cdot V\left(s'\right) \right\}. \qquad (8.13)$$

Equation (8.12) can be written in the matrix form:

$$\boldsymbol{V}_\pi = \boldsymbol{g}_\pi + \gamma \boldsymbol{P}_\pi \boldsymbol{V}_\pi. \qquad (8.14)$$

The solution to (8.12) can be written in a matrix form:

$$\boldsymbol{V}_\pi = \left(\boldsymbol{I} - \gamma \boldsymbol{P}_\pi\right)^{-1} \boldsymbol{g}_\pi. \qquad (8.15)$$

The problem now is ready to be solved by dynamic programming using Algorithm 5.1 in Chapter 5.

8.4 Compulsory Licensing and Parallel Importation

8.4.1 *Legal Complications of Drug Marketing*

Compulsory licenses are licenses that are granted by a government to use patents, copyrighted works, or other types of intellectual property. Compulsory licenses are an essential government instrument to intervene in the market and limit patent and other intellectual property rights in order to correct market failures. As concerns public health and compulsory licensing, the restrictions imposed by the intellectual property rights (IPR) system on access to (patented) drugs must be reasonable, not creating situations where entire populations are denied access to known therapies. Therefore, the 1994 World Trade Organization (WTO) TRIPs Agreement contains provisions on safeguards, exceptions, and mechanisms to protect essential public health interests. The TRIPs provide for compulsory licenses of patents, but also provide a number of restrictions on the use of compulsory licenses.

The propriety of parallel trade is a matter of intense policy debate in a number of countries and in the WTO. At present, WTO provisions allow member countries to establish their own rules for the "exhaustion" of IPR. If a country opts for national exhaustion of IPR, a rights holder there may exclude parallel imports, because intellectual property rights continue until such a time as a protected product is first sold in that market. If a country instead chooses international exhaustion of IPR, parallel imports cannot be blocked, because the rights of the patent, copyright, or trademark holder expire when a protected product is sold anywhere in the world. The United

States practices national exhaustion for patents and copyrights, but permits parallel imports of trademarked goods unless the trademark owner can show that the imports are of a different quality from goods sold locally or otherwise might cause confusion for consumers. The European Union provides for regional exhaustion of IPR whereby goods circulate freely within the trading bloc but parallel imports are banned from nonmember countries. Japanese commercial law permits parallel imports except when such trade is explicitly excluded by contract provisions or when the original sale is made subject to foreign price controls (Grossman and Lai, 2009).

When parallel trade comes into play, the regulated price cap becomes a strategic variable in an international setting. Parallel trade is an arbitrage mechanism through which the drugs produced in a low-price market flow into the high-price market, reestablishing nearly uniform prices in the presence of a large number of parallel traders. The price difference mainly results from the transportation and transaction costs for reimportation.

Public debate about parallel imports has been especially heated in the area of prescription drugs. In the United States, where consumers, public health officials, and politicians have become increasingly concerned about the high and rising cost of medicine, bills that would introduce international exhaustion of patent rights for prescription drugs have been introduced in one or both houses of Congress in each of the last three sessions. In fact, in 2000, Congress passed a bill to permit reimportation of medicines. President Bill Clinton signed the bill into law; his administration ultimately declined to implement it, citing concerns about consumer safety. New legislation was introduced to Congress in 2004 that would have forced deregulation of parallel imports of pharmaceuticals. In each case, the impetus for congressional action came from public pressures to step up imports from Canada, where regulations and price controls have generated prices for prescription drugs significantly lower than those across the border. Despite the continuing legal impediments to parallel imports, reimportation has been a growing source of pharmaceutical supply in the United States due to increased personal trafficking and the proliferation of Internet purchases (Grossman and Lai, 2009). By one estimate, parallel imports of prescription drugs from Canada amounted to $1.1 billion in 2004, or about 0.5% of the U.S. market (Cambridge Pharma Consultancy, 2004). Parallel trade in pharmaceuticals features prominently in Europe as well. Differences in price regulations have resulted in significant variation in pharmaceutical prices across member countries of the European Union and the European Free Trade Association.

Opponents of parallel trade are concerned that such trade undermines manufacturers' intellectual property rights. The prevailing wisdom, expressed, for example by, Barfield and Groombridge (1998, 1999), Chard and Mellor (1989), Danzon (1997, 1998), and Danzon and Towse (2003), is that parallel trade impedes the ability of research intensive firms such as those in the pharmaceutical industry to reap an adequate return on their investments in new technologies. Grossman and Lai (2009) challenged the prevailing wisdom that parallel trade is induced by different national price controls. They argue that the existing policy discussions and formal modeling overlook an important effect of national policy regarding the exhaustion of IPR. First, the admissibility of parallel trade introduces the possibility that a manufacturer will eschew low-price sales in the foreign market in order to mitigate or avoid reimportation. When arbitrage is impossible, the manufacturer is willing to export at any price above the marginal production cost. But when the potential for arbitrage exists, the manufacturer may earn higher profits by selling only in the unregulated (or high-price) market than by serving both markets at the lower, foreign-controlled price. Accordingly, a switch from a regime of national exhaustion to one of international exhaustion can induce an increase in the controlled price as the foreign government seeks to ensure that its consumers are adequately served. Second, the admissibility of parallel trade mitigates the opportunity for one government to free-ride on the protection of IPR granted by another.

8.4.2   Grossman-Lai's Game Model

In Grossman-Lai's game model, the flow of new products generated $\phi_j(t)$, in country j, by labor $L_j(t)$ and the fixed stock of research capital K_j at time t is assumed to be

$$\phi_j(t) = \frac{1}{\beta} K_j^{1-\beta} L_j^{\beta}(t). \tag{8.16}$$

Each new product has a useful economic life of length $\bar{\tau}$, which means that it can provide utility to consumers for a period of that duration. When $\bar{\tau}$ years have elapsed from the time of invention, the product ceases to be of economic value.

In the model, the world economy is divided into two sectors, North and South. Innovative products are consumed in both countries, whereas all innovation takes place in the North. In country j, $j = N$ (for North) or $j = S$ (for South), there are M_j (the size of market) consumers who demand the differentiated products of the innovating industry. Denote as $n(t)$ the number (measure) of differentiated products invented before time t that remains economically viable at t. Then the time derivative is $dn_j(t)/dt =$

$\phi_j(t) - \phi_j(t - \bar{\tau})$ because products invented at time $t - \bar{\tau}$ become obsolete at time t. In steady state, ϕ_j is constant and so $dn_j(t)/dt = 0$.

Denote by $\pi(p)$ the profits that a patent holder makes per consumer when it charges price p in some market and serves all local demand at that price. Note that consumers in both countries have identical demands, so these profits are the same (as a function of price) for sales in the North and South. Similarly, $C(p)$ is the surplus that a consumer in either country enjoys when the differentiated product i is available at price p. Let $C_C = C(c)$ be the surplus per consumer when a differentiated product is available at the competitive price c, and let $C_m = C(p_m)$ be the surplus per consumer when the patent holder charges the unconstrained monopoly price p_m. As usual, the monopoly price is such that the markup over marginal cost as a fraction of price is equal to the inverse demand elasticity

A Northern monopolist earns a flow of profits $M_n\pi(p_s) + M_s\pi(p_s)$ for a period of length τ, the present discounted value of which is

$$v = \Pi_n T, \qquad (8.17)$$

where $\Pi_n = [M_n\pi(p_n) + M_s\pi(p_s)]$ and $T \equiv (1 - e^{-r\tau})/r$ is the present value of a flow of one dollar from time zero to time τ with r being the future discount rate.

Grossman and Lai assume that firms in the North will continue to deploy labor in Research and Development until the marginal value product in this activity is equal to the wage:

$$v\frac{\partial\phi_n}{\partial L_n} = 1. \qquad (8.18)$$

In the North, aggregate welfare is the present value of spending plus consumer surplus, and spending is augmented by profit income but diminished by the savings that finance Research and Development. Accordingly, the government of the North will evaluate alternative trade regimes with an eye toward maximizing (without affecting final results, omitting the part for homogeneous products)

$$U_n = -\frac{L_n}{\rho} + \frac{\phi_n}{\rho}\left[TM_nC(p_n) + (\bar{T} - T)M_nC_C + T\Pi_n\right]. \qquad (8.19)$$

Considering that the number of Southern consumers is M_s, that innovation will be constant over time at rate ϕ_n, and that each newly invented good spends the first τ years of its economic life as a patented good with (endogenous) price p_s and the remaining $\bar{\tau} - \tau$ years as an unpatented good with price c, the South government's objective is to maximize the present discounted value of the sum of spending and consumer surplus,

$$U_s = \frac{L_s}{\rho} + \frac{M_s \phi_n}{\rho} \left[TC(p_s) + \left(\bar{T} - T \right) C_c \right], \qquad (8.20)$$

where T is defined analogously to T: $\bar{T} \equiv (1 - e^{r\bar{r}})/r$.

Compulsory licensing refers to covering the domestic market only or to exporting to countries unable to manufacture the drugs themselves, which is in accordance with the TRIPs Agreement. This means that those drugs licensed compulsorily are constrained by the South's boundaries and thus cannot be the object of parallel trade to the North, even if the northern region had decided for an international exhaustion regime and charges a higher price. As such, compulsory licensing represents a way to ensure southern consumers are served and incentives to northern firms are dulled only to the extent of the market size in the South, as compulsory licensing represents an exception to the rule of uniform pricing in a regime allowing parallel trade.

The maximizations of (8.19) and (8.20) are relatively straightforward under the national and international exhaustions, respectively.

8.4.3 *Sequential Game of Drug Marketing*

The sequential game consists of three-stages as follows.

Stage 1: The North decides to go for national exhaustion (ne) or international exhaustion (ie).

Stage 2: The South decides to exercise price control (pc), i.e., set up price cap p_c or compulsory license (cl).

Stage 3: The North decides the price for North and South, p_n and p_s.

The extended form of the sequential game is given in Figure 8.10.

Noncooperative Solution

The noncooperative solution is the solution to the game when the players take actions to maximize each individual gain (see Chapter 4). Let $U_{nij}(\cdot, \cdot)$ be the North utility when the North takes strategy i and the South takes strategy j; $U_{sij}(\cdot, \cdot)$ be the2 South utility when North takes strategy i and the South takes strategy j, as illustrated in Figure 8.10.

Using backwards induction, the South will take the action A_{sk} (price control or compulsory license) to maximize its utility U_{sk} such that $U_{sk} = \max(U_{skp}(p_n, p_s), U_{skc}(p_s))$, where the subscript $k = n$ for national exhaustion or $k = i$ for international exhaustion. After knowing the South will take action A_{sk}, the North will take the action A_{nk} to maximize its utility.

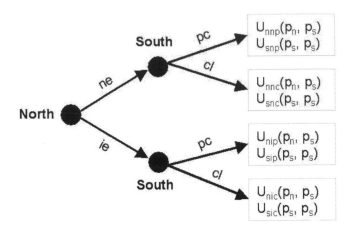

Figure 8.10: Extended Form of Drug Marketing Game

Example 8.1: Suppose $\max U_{nnp}(p_n, p_s) > \max U_{nnc}(p_n, p_s) > \max$ $U_{nip}(p_n, p_s) > \max U_{nic}(p_n, p_s)$, $\max U_{snp}(p_n, p_s) < \max U_{snc}(p_n, p_s)$, and $\max U_{sip}(p_n, p_s) > \max U_{sic}(p_n, p_s)$. In such a case, the South will decide to exercise compulsory license if the North opts for national exhaustion of IPR. On the other hand, the South will exercise price control if the North opts for international exhaustion, which implies the North either has utility $\max U_{nnc}(p_n, p_s)$ under national exhaustion or $\max U_{nip}(p_n, p_s)$ under international exhaustion. Knowing this fact and $\max U_{nnc}(p_n, p_s) > \max$ $U_{nip}(p_n, p_s)$, the North will exercise national exhaustion.

Cooperative Solution

As we have stated in Chapter 4, the noncooperative solution can often be improved. We use an example to illustrate how to find a Parato optimum to the cooperative game in Figure 8.10. Suppose $\max U_{nip}(p_n, p_s) = 10$ $> \max U_{nnp}(p_n, p_s) = 8 < \max U_{nnc}(p_n, p_s) = 5 < \max U_{nic}(p_n, p_s) = 1$, $\max U_{snp}(p_n, p_s) = 2 < \max U_{snc}(p_n, p_s) = 3 < \max U_{sip}(p_n, p_s) = 7 <$ $\max U_{sic}(p_n, p_s) = 10$. In such a case, the South will decide to exercise compulsory license regardless of the North's action (national or international exhaustion), which implies the North either has utility $\max U_{nnc}(p_n, p_s) = 4$ under national exhaustion or $\max U_{nic}(p_n, p_s) = 1$ under international exhaustion. It is obvious that North will exercise national exhaustion with a utility of 5 and the South will have a utility of 3. However, the result can be improved through an agreement that the North will use international exhaustion and the South will use price control. This is the only Pareto optimum for the game, which gives the North 10 and the South 7 for the utility.

Probabilistic Game Model

In calculating the utilities (8.19) and (8.20) or U_{kij}, the size of the market (SM) is fixed. In reality it is a random variable and depends on the drug price. The SM and other market uncertainties due to factors such as potential competitors and policy changes can be modeled using probability distribution and Monte Carlo simulation (Exercise 8.12).

8.5 Summary

There is critical public and political attention to high drug prices and large promotional budgets. In addition to price pressures, marketing for innovative therapies is also challenged from the following aspects: (1) evolving Medicare Part D drug benefits; an influx of generic therapies in costly therapeutic areas, (2) increasing involvement of consumers in healthcare decisions, (3) increased scrutiny of drug safety and off-label use, (4) the emergence of biosimilars, (5) declining marginal ROI for direct physician marketing, and (6) growing complexity in drug prescription and purchasing behaviors, due to trends such as formularies, Internet pharmacies, and DTC-driven demand.

Prescription drug marketing starts with a brand plan. A brand plan usually has both short (1–3 years) and longer term (over 10 years) objectives. The key outcome of the brand planning process is the brand positioning with respect to its target audience, its expected benefits, its key reasons for trial/usage, etc.

The financial projection and sales projection for an NCE are usually derived from analysis of product analogs, comparison of the NCE to existing treatment offerings in the marketplace, and team judgment regarding the level and type of marketing support for the compound. Econometric models and Monte Carlo simulation are often utilized. The projection includes three key concepts: (1) maximum or peak sales, (2) the average slope of revenue increase over time, and (3) the rate of falloff from peak sales.

The stock-flow dynamic model for brand planning represents an operational way to translate mental models from the implicit to the explicit, allowing for a set of specific business questions to be addressed and analyzed. The dynamic model includes three components: (1) patient flow, (2) doctor adoption, and (3) treatment attractiveness. These components are populated with data from epidemiology and a variety of physician and patient databases to ensure the entire model reflects actual market dynamics.

Paich's operating framework includes case, place, and pace, which provides a useful way to think about marketing strategy. The case for a new compound is the set of aggregate, macroeconomic market conditions of the indication being evaluated. The place for a new compound defines how it compares to the existing and future competition in terms of efficacy, safety, side effects, etc. The pace for the new compound relates to the speed at which it can reach peak share potential—the shape of the expected sales trajectory.

In stock flow, competitors are basically treated as static opponents, but that does not reflect the marketing reality. Competitive drug marketing strategy treats competitors as opponents in the game. The key to the marketing success of an NCE is to develop an adaptive (rather than static) strategy. This is because when your firm adopts a new and effective marketing mix, your competitors will detect that success quickly utilizing market data subscription services and respond with counter-strategies.

The strategies against generic pharmaceutical products can be summarized into five categories: divesting, innovating, providing more value for money, investing in generics, and reducing price. Divesting involves cutting all promotional and research expenses once the brand faces direct competition from generics and redirecting the savings toward other brands or new compound development. Innovating is to launch new forms and dosages or by demonstrating effectiveness for "new indications." Providing more value for the money is to introduce new and improved flavors, packaging, or delivery systems that can lead to additional emotional or functional consumer benefits (e.g., higher compliance). Investing in generics is to introduce the company's own generic and reduce the profitability of generic makers to deter them from entering the category. Reducing price leads to the lowest level of brand building, but narrowing the price gap with generics.

A pharmaceutical company usually starts its marketing strategy research before the drug gets approval for marketing. The key factors to consider are: (1) company marking positioning, (2) characteristics of the prescription drug and its competitors, which include efficacy, safety, convenience, cost, (3) target patient segmentation and mapping to the drug characteristics in (2), (4) physician prescription behaviors of the drug class, (5) behavior characteristics of competitors, (6) financial condition of the company and its competitors, and (7) availability of marketing force. A stochastic market process can be used to model the dynamics.

Compulsory licenses are licenses that are granted by a government to use patents, copyrighted works, or other types of intellectual property. Compulsory licenses are an essential government instrument to intervene in the market and limit patent and other intellectual property rights in order to correct market failures. Parallel trade is an arbitrage mechanism through which the drugs produced in a low-price market flow into the high-price market, reestablishing nearly uniform prices in the presence of a large number of parallel traders.

If a country opts for national exhaustion of IPR, a rights holder there may exclude parallel imports, because intellectual property rights continue until such a time as a protected product is first sold in that market. If a country instead chooses international exhaustion of IPR, parallel imports cannot be blocked, because the rights of the patent, copyright, or trademark holder expire when a protected product is sold anywhere in the world.

When compulsory licensing and parallel importation are options, Grossman-Lai's game model and sequential game model can be used in simulation for studying the optimal strategy in drug marketing.

8.6   Exercises

Exercise 8.1: What are the basic structures of a pharmaceutical market?

Exercise 8.2: What are the common pharmaceutical marketing strategies?

Exercise 8.3: Describe the traditional approach for the brand plan.

Exercise 8.4: Conduct research on the drug Feraheme™ or other drugs and construct a sensible patient flow of the stock-flow model for the indication.

Exercise 8.5: Do research on physician-adopt for the new drug Feraheme™ or other drugs and determine the model parameters in (8.5).

Exercise 8.6: Perform a treatment attraction analysis for the new drug Feraheme™.

Exercise 8.7: What are pricing and payer strategies?

Exercise 8.8: Construct a brand strategy for the brand drug Feraheme™, VELCADE®, or INTEGRILIN®.

Exercise 8.9: What are the challenges in brand drug marketing and what are the challenges in generic drug marketing?

Exercise 8.10: Divide students into two groups, representing innovating and generic drug makers, respectively, and discuss how the two companies compete against each other as in a noncooperative game and how they work together as described in cooperative game theory.

Exercise 8.11: Suppose you are the head of a sales department responsible for designing the sales strategy for a newly approved drug. In every state you must choose between saving money or advertising. The gains and transition probabilities are shown in Figure 8.11. The discount rate is 0.9. Develop and implement a Monte Carlo algorithm using value iteration or policy iteration to determine your optimal strategy. The first five value iterations are presented in Table 8.7 for you to validate your algorithm.

The calculations are presented in Table 8.7.

Table 8.7: Value Iteration

t	V(PU)	V(PF)	V(RU)	V(RF)
h	0	0	10	10
h-1	0	4.5	14.5	19
h-2	2.03	8.55	16.53	25.08
h-3	4.76	12.20	18.35	28.72
h-4	7.63	15.07	20.40	31.18
h-5	10.21	17.46	22.61	33.21

(Source: Pouport, 2005)

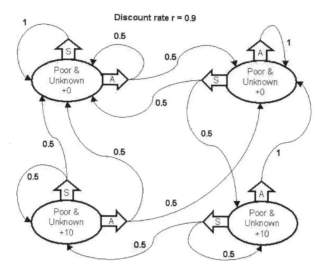

Figure 8.11: Stochastic Decision Making for Pharmaceutical Marketing
(Source: Moore, 2002)

Exercise 8.12: Construct the following probabilistic model for sequential games and devise a Monte Carlo algorithm for solving the game. The market size is a random variable.

Stage 1: The North decides to go for national exhaustion (ne) or international exhaustion (ie).

Stage 2: The South decides to exercise price control (pc), i.e., set up price cap p_c or compulsory license (cl).

Stage 3: The North decides the price for the North and South, p_n and p_s.

Chapter 9

Molecular Design and Simulation

This chapter will cover the following topics:

- Why Molecular Design and Simulation
- Molecular Similarity Search
- Overview of Molecular Docking
- Small Molecule Confirmation Analysis
- Ligand-Receptor Interaction
- Docking Algorithms
- Scoring Functions

9.1 Why Molecular Design and Simulation

9.1.1 The Landscape of Molecular Design

As mentioned earlier, pharmaceutical R & D expenses has increased dramatically over the past 15 years, while the number of NDAs approved is relatively flat. Innovative and cost-effective drug discovery approaches become inevitable for any pharmaceutical to stay competitive in the game. Molecular design and modeling is a new promising field that uses computer and chemical compound databases to screen, model, design NMEs to reduce discovery costs and accelerate the discovery process. The reasons why the computer can help in this aspect are (1) The numbers of compounds that can be examined by a human mind are limited compared to the capacity throughput of virtual, computer-based storage, modeling, and virtual screening systems. (2) Compound supply is also limited. Many different companies use blind screening for the same compound libraries even after many of the compounds have been proved structurally unfavorable, which often turns out to be a waste of time and resources. Computer-based design of activity enriched screening libraries can be of great value here. (3)

Traditional biochemical screening assays can be very expensive, especially for cell-based systems or when elaborate protein purification schemes are required. Costs have been estimated to fall somewhere between 0.02 and 10 dollars per well. Considering a screening library containing one million compounds with multiple measurements, the sums add up (Schneider and Baringhaus, 2008).

There are approximately 8000 drug targets, of which 5000 could be "hit" by small druglike molecules, only about 3000 targets out of the 5000 are of pharmacological interest, and only 200–500 targets are addressed by marketed drugs — there are many more targets to be explored in the future. It is estimated that, out of the 20,000–25,000 human genes supposed to code for about 3000 drugable targets, only a subset of the pharmacological space (about 800 proteins) has currently been investigated by the pharmaceutical industry (Paolini et al., 2006). Over 10 million nonredundant chemical structures cover the actual chemical space, out of which only about 1000 are currently approved as drugs. Chemogenomics is a new interdisciplinary field that attempts to fully match target and ligand space, and ultimately identify all ligands of all targets. The 8000 drug targets can be further categorized into seven difference classes: proteases (19%), kinases (12%), other enzyme (17%), G-protein coupled receptors (GPCR, 16%), ion channel (13%), nuclear receptor (4%), and other target (19%).

9.1.2 *The Innovative Drug Discovery Approach*

In Chapter 3, we discussed briefly the drug discovery process. The traditional drug discovery process is illustrated in Figure 9.1. Pharmaceutical companies purchase a large number of compounds from third party suppliers and synthesize combinatorial libraries of compounds with chemical diversity that covers a sufficient portion of the entire chemical space. The screening test is usually simple binding assays to answer the question if the compound binds to the target protein. A "hit" means that an interaction between the compound and the protein is found. There are two important stages in the process: lead generation and optimization. Lead generation is the process of finding the compound binds well, whereas lead optimization is finding a compound that binds better. The chemical similarity is critical at both stages.

When a "lead" has been identified, the next step is to find compounds that are similar to it, which might bind even better. This can be accomplished through similarity searching in an existing compound library. Chemists can also make specific changes to the lead compound to improve its binding affinity and other properties.

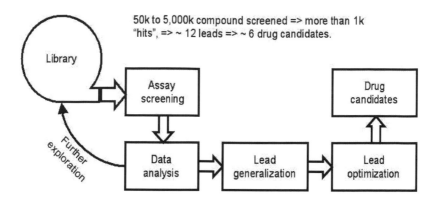

Figure 9.1:   Traditional Drug Discovery Paradigm

The steps in the standard drug lead-approach include (1) identifying a target (e.g., enzyme, receptor, ion channel, transporter), (2) determining DNA and/or protein sequence, (3) elucidating structures and functions of proteins, (4) proving therapeutic concept in animals ("knock-outs"), (5) developing assay for high-throughput screening (HTS), (6) mass screening, and (7) selecting lead structures.

Understanding structure-activity relationships (SAR) is essential for successful optimization of compound properties of a pharmacologically active substance. Once an SAR model is available, it is possible to perform rational drug design (Höltje et al., 2008). HTS of chemical libraries is a well-established method for finding new lead compounds in drug discovery. However, with the increase of available databases, the increase of such screenings, and the decreased hit rates, the problem cannot be effectively solved without the help of virtual screening (VS).

A goal of Monte Carlo molecular design is to identify novel substances that exhibit desired properties. This design certainly must include proper physicochemical and ADMET (absorption, distribution, metabolism, excretion, and toxicity) properties of the novel compounds (Schneider and Baringhaus, 2008).

A binding interaction between a small molecule ligand and an enzyme protein may result in activation or inhibition of the enzyme. If the protein is a receptor, ligand binding may result in agonism or antagonism. Docking is most commonly used in Monte Carlo drug design. Docking can be used for (1) virtual screening or hit identification, i.e., to quickly screen large databases of potential drugs in silico to identify molecules that are likely to bind to the protein target of interest and (2) lead optimization, i.e., to predict where and in which relative orientation a ligand binds to a protein — called the binding mode or pose.

9.1.3 The Drug-Likeness Concept

The term "drug-like" describes various empirically found structure characteristics of molecular agents, which are associated with pharmacological activities. It is not strictly defined but provides a general concept of what makes a drug a drug. Drug-likeness may be considered as an overall likelihood of a molecular agent that can be turned into a drug. Therefore, it is a measure of complex physicochemical and structural features of the compound which can be used to guide the rational design of lead structures that can be further optimized to become a drug. The construction of such a structure-property relationship (SPR) can be (1) substructure elements, (2) lipophilicity (hydrophobicity), (3) electronic distribution, (4) hydrogen-bonding characteristics, (5) molecule size and flexibility, or (6) pharmacophore features (Schneider and Baringhaus, 2008; Sadowski and Kubinyi, 1998).

The well-known QASR (quantitative structure-activity relationship), Lipinski's rule-of-five, is often used in rational drug design to reduce the risk of costly late-stage preclinical and clinical failures. The guidelines predict that poor passive absorption or permeation of an orally administered compound is more likely if the compound meets at least two of the following criteria (Lipinski et al. 1997):

(1) Molecular weight greater than 500Da
(2) High lipophilicity (expressed as clogP > 5)
(3) More than 5 hydrogen-bond donors, expressed as the sum of OHs and NHs
(4) More than 10 hydrogen-bond acceptors, expressed as the sum of Os and Ns
(5) Containing more than 5 rotatable bonds to limit its conformational freedom

These guidelines were developed based on an empirical pharmaceutical database. For example, Figure 9.2 is the distribution of the molecular weights of 4500 selected druglike molecules containing marketed drugs and drug candidates. We can see that most druglike molecules weigh between 300 and 600Da.

Other criteria include (1) possessing a polar surface area exceeding 120 $\overset{o}{A}$ to avoid potential bioavailibility problems of a compound and (2) having predicted aqueous solubility (logS) below -4 (solubility in mol/L).

Bioavailability, closely related to the partition coefficient and pKa, is an important component of drug-likeness. The partition coefficient is a measure of how well a substance partitions between a lipid (oil) and water. The pKa

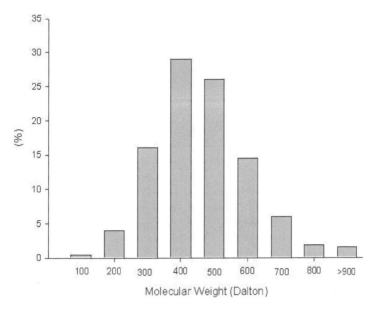

Figure 9.2: Weight Distribution of Druglike Molecules
(Source: Adapted from Schneider and Baringhaus, 2008)

or LogP is a measure of the strength of an acid or a base. The pKa allows you to determine the charge on a molecule at any given pH. The partition coefficient and pKa may be combined to predict the distribution of 'a drug compound in a biological system. Factors such as absorption, excretion, and penetration of the CNS may be related to the pKa value of a drug and in certain cases predictions can be made. Studies (Earll, 2006) found that the optimal values for LogP are around 2 ± 0.7 (CNS penetration), 1.8 (oral absorption), 1.35 (intestinal absorption), 5.5 (sublingual absorption), and 2.6 (percutaneous, and low molecule weight).

9.1.4 *Structure–Activity Relationship (SAR)*

From a set of compounds, we can model the QSAR to relate activity data (Y) with a set of molecular descriptors (X_i) using statistical methods such as linear regression (Hammett, 1939) and partial least-square (PLS) regression (Wold, et al. 1984). The types of molecular descriptors include 2D and 3D topological structures and quantum chemical properties (electronic and thermodynamic).

For structure analysis, molecules can be divided into scaffolds or frameworks, linkers, and side-chains that are attached to the ring systems (Figure 9.3).

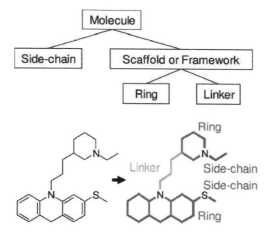

Figure 9.3:   Scaffold, Linkers, and Side-chains
(Source: Schneider and Baringhaus, 2008)

Substructure search is often the starting point for drugable candidates. Molecules with GPCR-privileged substructure motifs (Figure 9.4) may increase drug-ability, but keep in mind that the presence of a privileged motif in a molecule does not guarantee a desired binding behavior. In contrast, in Figure 9.5, examples of unfavorable motifs are listed; these are usually avoided in drug design because reactive or unstable groups tend to have poor aqueous solubility.

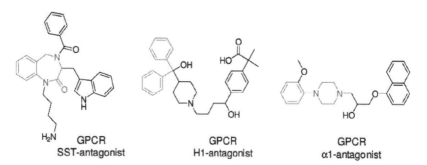

Figure 9.4:   Examples of GPCR-privileged Substructure Motifs
(Source: Schneider and Baringhaus, 2008)

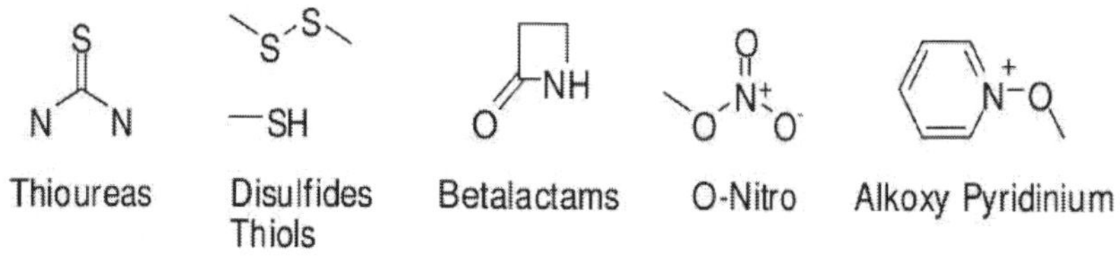

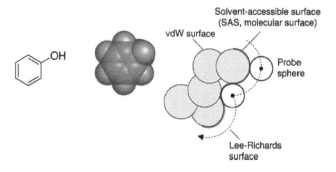

| Thioureas | Disulfides Thiols | Betalactams | O-Nitro | Alkoxy Pyridinium |

Figure 9.5: Examples of Unwanted Motifs in Drug Design
(Source: Schneider and Baringhaus, 2008)

9.2 Molecular Similarity Search

9.2.1 *Molecular Representation*

An adequate representation of molecular structure and physicochemical properties allows the extraction of molecular features that are responsible for a certain compound property or pharmacological behavior. Molecular structures can be represented graphically, where atoms are the vertices of the graph, and chemical bonds are the edges (Figure 9.6). Any given molecule may be drawn in topologically equivalent ways, e.g., as different mesomeric forms of aromatic systems, or as tautomers. However, millions of molecules in drug design require a fast computational differentiation and identification of molecular graphs. Therefore, it is desirable to have a unique way of representing each molecule so that computational efficacy remains.

Topological indices are instances of invariant graph properties of a molecule graph. The most common and basic invariants are the number of vertices and the number of edges, which have received wide attention in molecular modeling and design.

Figure 9.6: Molecular Representations

Among a large number of quantum mechanics (QM) and empirical descriptors that have been devised over the past decades, there are four main aspects of molecular structure and molecular recognition (Schneider and Baringhaus, 2008): (1) molecular distribution, (2) molecular shape, (3) directed interactions, and (4) nondirected interactions.

9.2.2 *Tanimoto Similarity Index*

The rationale behind a similarity search is the so-called similar property principle: structurally similar molecules are likely to have similar chemical/physiological properties. A variety of methods are used in these searches, including 2D and 3D shape similarity, graph theory, vector space model using 2D fingerprints, and machine learning methods.

Similarity searching can be achieved by comparing representations of molecules with respect to the substructure elements they contain. A popular similarity index is the Tanimoto (Jaccard) index defined by

$$T_{AB} = \frac{n_{AB}}{n_A + n_B - n_{AB}} \tag{9.1}$$

where n_A is the number of bits set to 1 in molecule A, n_B is the number of bits set to 1 in molecule B, and n_{AB} is the number of set bits common to both A and B (Figures 9.7 and 9.8). The possible value of T_{AB} ranges between 0 (maximal dissimilarity) and 1 (identical bitstrings). However, $T_{AB} = 1$ implies A and B have identical fingerprints, but does not necessarily mean that the two molecules A and B are identical.

Ligands A and B can be viewed as fingerprint vectors, and the quantity

$$D_{AB} = 1 - T_{AB} \tag{9.2}$$

is called the distance in vector space. For the distance, the following triangular inequality holds (Lipkus, 1999):

$$|D_{AB} - D_{AC} \leq D_{BC} \leq D_{AC} + D_{AB}. \tag{9.3}$$

From (9.3) we can obtain the following bound on the Tanimoto similarity index:

$$T_{BC} \leq 1 - |T_{AB} - T_{AC}|. \tag{9.4}$$

This bound (9.4) can be improved by the following theorem (Baldi and Hirschberg, 2009).

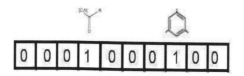

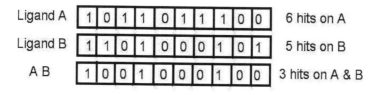

Binary Fingerprint:
code 1 if a substructure exists; otherwise 0.

Figure 9.7:   Binary Fingerprint with a Length of 10

Tanimoto Similarity:
AB/(A+B-AB) = 3/(5+6-3) = 0.375

Figure 9.8:   Tanimoto Similarity Between Ligands A and B

Theorem 9.1   *For any fingerprint A, B, and C, we have the inequality*

$$T_{BC} \leq \frac{\min(n_{AB}, n_{AC}) + \min(n_B - n_{AB}, n_C - n_{AC})}{n_B + n_C - \min(n_{AB}, n_{AC}) - \min(n_B - n_{AB}, C - n_{AC})}$$

$$\leq 1 - \left| \frac{n_{AB}}{n_A + n_B - n_{AB}} - \frac{n_{AC}}{n_A + n_C - n_{AC}} \right|. \tag{9.5}$$

The proof of this theorem is somewhat lengthy and is omitted here. One of the applications of (9.4) in similarity search is database pruning. The index bound given by (9.4) can also be used to measure the overall performance (interpretive power) of a library search method, i.e., measured by a "grand mean":

$$T_h = \frac{1}{nh} \sum_q \sum_k T_{qk}, \tag{9.6}$$

where h = number of hits considered, n = number of query compounds tested, T_{qk} = Tanimoto index for query structure q and hit k, T_h = grand mean of Tanimoto indices for h hits, ranging from 0 to 1. A set of thousands of general purpose substructures has been defined (Scsibrany et al., 2003) in a library for virtual screening.

9.2.3   *SimScore*

SimScore (Sakamoto, et al., 2007) was developed to evaluate quantitatively the structural similarity score of a target compound with the teratogenic drugs which are defined as serious human teratogens by the FDA. In SimScore, a molecular structure is divided into its skeletal and substituent parts in order to perform similarity comparison for these parts independently. The principle behind SimScore is that compounds with the same or similar skeleton show a similar biological activity, but their activity strengths depend on the variation of substituents.

The FDA uses five categories to classify teratogenic effects as follows: A (controlled studies show no risk), B (no evidence of risk in humans), C (risk cannot be ruled out), D (positive evidence of risk), or X (contraindicated in pregnancy) (Briggs et al., 2005). Positive evidence of fetal abnormalities for the drugs belonging to categories D and X have been confirmed by epidemiological studies in pregnant women (Sakamoto et al., 2007).

In SimScore, the atomic information in each molecule is expressed as an atom code array, which consists of the following eight atom codes: element, element group, hybridization type, ring, adjacent atom, hydrogen bonding, atomic charge, and stereo codes. The array $A(i, k)$ represents the kth atom code of atom i in the set of skeletal atoms. The array $B(i, j)$ denotes the number of bonds from atom i to an atom with the jth atomic number. The total similarity score S_{SS} is defined by the skeletal similarity scores S_{kSS} and the substituents similarity scores B_{SS}.

The skeletal similarity score is defined by

$$S_{kSS} = \left[\sum \sum S_s^2 \left(k, i\right) / \left(8 n_s\right) \right]^{1/2} \tag{9.7}$$

where $S_s(k, i)$ is the similarity score between the ith skeletal atom and its best matching atom i, k is the kth atom code, n_s is the number of skeletal atoms, and the summation is taken over all of the atom codes and matching atoms.

The substituents similarity score is defined by

$$B_{SS} = \left[\sum \sum S_b^2 \left(k, i\right) / \left(8 n_{bi}\right) \right]^{1/2} \tag{9.8}$$

where $S_b(k, i)$ is the similarity score between the substituent atoms attached to the ith skeletal atom, k is the kth atom code, n_{bi} is the number of substituent atoms attached to the ith atom, and the summation is taken over all of the atom codes and substituent atoms.

Total similarity score S_{SS} is defined as

$$S_{SS} = \frac{S_{kSS} + B_{SS}}{2 + S_{kSS}^2 + B_{SS}^2 - (S_{kSS} + B_{SS})}, \tag{9.9}$$

where S_{SS} ranges between 0 (dissimilarity) and 1 (perfect similarity between molecules).

Formulations (9.7) to (9.9) have been implemented in a knowledge-based system, SimScore^{MT} (Sakamoto et al., 2007).

9.2.4 *Bayesian Network for Similarity Search*

A bayesian network (BN) is a simple and popular way of doing probabilistic inference, which formalizes the way to synchronize the evidence using Bayes' rule:

$$P(H|E) = P(E|H)P(H)/P(E).$$

A bayesian network (Figure 9.9) is a directed acyclic graph and has the following properties:

- Nodes of the BN represent random variables; the parents of a node are those judged to be direct causes for it.
- The roots of the network are the nodes without parents.
- The arcs represent causal relationships between these variables, and the strengths of these causal influences are expressed by conditional probabilities.
- Let $X = \{x_1, ..., x_n\}$ be a set of parents of y (child node), where $x_i \cap x_j = \phi$ (empty) for $i \neq j$ and x_i is a direct cause of y. The influence of X on y can be quantified with the conditional probability $P(y|X)$.

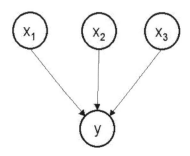

Figure 9.9: A Simple Bayesian Network

To use BN for molecular similarity search, the following steps are involved:

(1) Network model generation, i.e., representing the system using a suitable network form,
(2) Representation of importance of descriptors, i.e., determining the weighting schemes,
(3) Probability estimation for the network model, and
(4) Calculation of the similarity scores.

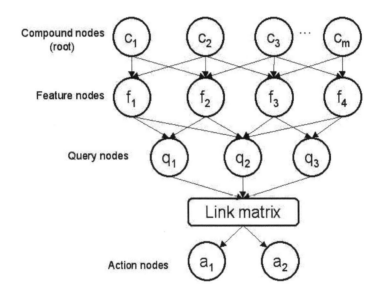

Figure 9.10:   Four-Layer Bayesian Network for Similarity Search

Figure 9.10 represents a BN with four layers: compound nodes (c_j), feature nodes (f_i), query nodes (q_k), and target nodes (A_m). The arcs or edges indicate the direct causality relationships. Abdo and Salim (2008) described the method as follows.

Random variable f_i is a binary variable indicating with (1) or without (0) the feature. $\{f_1, ..., f_n\}$ is an n-dimensional vector equivalent to a fingerprint with length n. Similarity, c_j is a binary variable with 0 indicating absence of the molecule and 1 indicating the existence of the molecule.

The retrieval of an active compound compared to a given target structure is obtained by means of an inference process through a network of dependences using conditional probability. Note that in BN, each variable is conditionally independent of all its nondescendants in the graph given the value of all its parents, i.e.,

$$P(X_1, ..., X_n) = \Pi_{i=1}^{n} P(X_i | \text{parents}(X_i)). \tag{9.10}$$

(1) If you conduct a random selection of molecules from a virtual molecular library, the prior probability associated with compound c_j can be estimated using the following flat distribution:

$$P(c_j) = \frac{1}{m}, \tag{9.11}$$

where m is the collection size, i.e., the number of different molecules in the virtual library.

(2) The conditional probability of feature nodes given compound c_j is given by

$$P(f_i | c_j) = \frac{P(c_j | f_i) P(f_i)}{P(c_j)}. \tag{9.12}$$

Practically, the following formulation can be used for the conditional probability:

$$P(f_i | c_j) = \frac{\hat{f}_{ij}}{\hat{f}_{ij} + 0.5 + 1.5 \left(\frac{L_j}{\bar{L}}\right)} \frac{\ln\left(\frac{m+0.5}{f_i^*}\right)}{\ln(m+1)}, \tag{9.13}$$

where $\hat{f}_{ij}$ = the frequency of the ith feature within the jth compound, f^* is the inverse compound frequency of the ith feature in the collection, L_j is the size of the jth compound, and $\bar{L}$ is the average length of the molecules in the collection $\bar{L} = 1/m \sum_{j=1}^{m} L_j$.

(3) The conditional probabilities in the third layer are given for the query nodes and are defined as

$$P(q_k | f_i) = \frac{\tilde{f}_{i,q_k}}{\sum_{i=1}^{n_f} \tilde{f}_{i,q_k}} \tag{9.14}$$

where n_f is the number of feature nodes and $\tilde{f}_{i,q_k}$ is the frequency of the query node q_k in the feature node f_i.

(4) The conditional probability $P(a_m | q_k)$ for the fourth layer (activity-need node) given a query node can only be defined empirically or based on beliefs.

We now can calculate the probability of activity a_m using the following equation:

$$P(a_m) = \sum_k \sum_i \sum_j P(A_m | q_k) P(q_k | f_i) P(f_i | c_j) P(c_j). \tag{9.15}$$

To select a list of the best compounds $\{c_j\}$, we can use the conditional probability such that

$$P\left(a_m|c_j\right) = \sum_k \sum_i \sum_j P\left(A_m|q_k\right) P\left(q_k|f_i\right) P\left(f_i|c_j\right) > \delta, \qquad (9.16)$$

where δ is a predetermined threshold.

9.3 Overview of Molecular Docking

9.3.1 *Concept of Molecular Docking*

Molecular docking can be thought of as a problem of "lock-and-key," where one is interested in finding the correct location and relative orientation of the "key" which will open up the "lock." The protein can be thought of as the "lock" and the ligand can be thought of as a "key." Each "snapshot" of the protein receptor-ligand pair in the fitting process is referred to as a pose (Figure 9.11). Molecular docking can also be treated as an optimization problem, which would describe the "best-fit" orientation of a ligand that binds to a particular protein of interest. However, since both the ligand and the protein are flexible, not right, in the fitting process, the ligand and the protein adjust their conformation to achieve an overall "best-fit," called

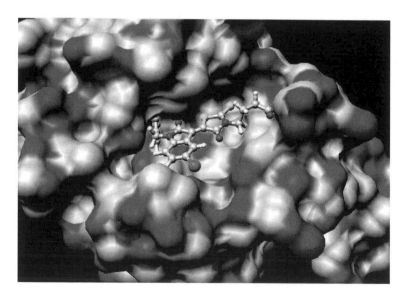

Figure 9.11: Molecular Docking

(Source: Wikipedia.com)

"induced-fit." The optimization of molecular docking can also be defined as the minimization of the free energy of the protein-ligand system. There are three commonly used virtual screening strategies: (1) ligand-based virtual screening, (2) structure (receptor)-based screening, and (3) combination approaches.

9.3.2 Database for Virtual Screening

Virtual screening can start with a known ligand 3D structure and the target binding pocket. In fact, virtual screening proceeds as a second step after HTS, using HTS activity data as the reference. Molecular geometries can be determined for gas-phase molecules by microwave spectroscopy and by electron diffraction. For solid state, the structure of a ligand is usually determined using a biophysical technique such as x-ray crystallography, or less often, NMR spectroscopy.

There are three basic design strategies. If you know the 3D structure of the target receptor (lock), use receptor-based design to build or find the key (ligand) that fits the lock. If you don't know the 3D structure of the target receptor, use homology modeling to build the lock and then find the key. If you don't know the 3D structure of the receptor, but know the structure of the ligand, use ligand-based design to infer the lock by inspecting the keys.

Ligand-based design of compound libraries requires known molecules (reference compounds) exhibiting the desired properties or pharmacological activities as a starting point. Based on the particular QSAR, novel structures having similar activities can be designed in silico or selected from collections of physically available compounds so that they exhibit similarities to the reference set. Of course, the choice of an appropriate similarity measure depends on the drug discovery project and is context dependent.

So far, combinatorial libraries contain only purified single compounds and a shift from random compound libraries to maximally diverse compound collections and targeted compound arrays is favored. There are numerous commercially available screening collections available both electron-

Table 9.1: Virtual Compound Libraries

Supplier	Size (k)	Website
ChemNavigator	24,000	http://www.chemnavigator.com/
PubChem	61,000	http://pubchem.ncbi.nlm.nih.gov/
Zinc	13,000	http://zinc.docking.org/index.shtml
ChemDB	10,000	http://www.chemdb.com/
ChemMine	6,000	http://bioweb.ucr.edu/ChemMineV2/

ically and physically. Table 9.1 presents some major virtual compound libraries available on the web. The size of the libraries is growing quickly. Therefore, the numbers of compounds in the table only reflect the information available at the time of writing this book.

In addition to the pick-the-winner approach based on desirable features or structures, we can also narrow the search by removing unsuitable molecules from the candidate database, i.e., pruning. To this end, we can either use a series of simple filters or classification models developed using artificial intelligence methods. When simple filters are used, each one excludes compounds with certain properties as described by (Rishton, 1997). Highly reactive and toxic compounds can be removed according to reactive moieties using the well-known filter, Lipinski 'Rule-of-Five,' as mentioned earlier. More complicated filters have been developed recently (Roche and Guba, 2005; Muresan and Sadowski, 2005).

9.3.3 *Docking Approaches*

There are two commonly used docking approaches: One approach uses a matching technique that describes the protein and the ligand as complementary surfaces using, e.g., a grid-based energy evaluation or a genetic algorithm (Meng et al., 2004) and an empirical binding free energy function (Morris et al., 1998). The second approach simulates the actual docking process in which the ligand-protein pairwise interaction energies are calculated (Feig et al., 2004). The protein structure and a database of potential ligands serve as inputs to a docking program, whereas the success of a docking program depends on the search algorithm and the scoring function.

Search Algorithm

The search space consists of all possible orientations and conformations of the protein paired with the ligand. It is impossible to exhaustively explore the search space because this would involve enumerating all possible distortions of each molecule and all possible rotational and translational orientations of the ligand to the protein. If the flexibility of the ligand and/or protein receptor is considered in a docking program, the computation task will be even more challenging. Therefore, many strategies for sampling the search space have been developed, e.g., using a QSAR, using a coarse-grained molecular dynamics simulation to propose energetically reasonable poses, using a linear combination of multiple structures determined for the same protein to emulate receptor flexibility, and using a genetic algorithm to evolve new poses that are successively more and more likely to represent favorable binding interactions.

Scoring Function

The scoring function takes a receptor-ligand pose as input and returns a number indicating the likelihood that the pose represents a favorable binding interaction. Most scoring functions are physics-based molecular mechanics force fields that estimate the energy of the pose; a low energy indicates a stable system and thus a likely binding interaction. Another approach is to derive a statistical potential for interactions from a large database of protein-ligand complexes with a similar structure, such as the Protein Data Bank, and evaluate the fitness of the pose according to this inferred potential. However, this approach is only an approximation meaning in the sense of averaging.

9.4 Small Molecule Confirmation Analysis

9.4.1 *Quantum Mechanics*

To conduct molecular modeling, we need to have a geometric model of the molecule in the computer by defining the relative positions of the atoms in space using a set of Cartesian coordinates. There are several methods to determine the geometric structure of a molecule.

The most accurate but costly (computation-wise) method is molecular quantum mechanics (QM) that is based on the Schrödinger equation:

$$H\Psi\left(\boldsymbol{r},t\right) = j\frac{h}{2\pi}\frac{\partial\Psi\left(\boldsymbol{r},t\right)}{\partial t} \tag{9.17}$$

where $\Psi\left(\boldsymbol{r},t\right)$ is the wavefunction, $j = \sqrt{-1}$, t, time, $\boldsymbol{r}$, location vector, and the Hamiltonian operator is defined as

$$H = -\frac{h^2}{8\pi^2 m}\left(\frac{\partial^2}{\partial x_1^2} + \frac{\partial^2}{\partial x_2^2} + \frac{\partial^2}{\partial x_3^2}\right) + U\left(\boldsymbol{r},t\right) \tag{9.18}$$

with $U\left(\boldsymbol{r},t\right)$ being potential energy.

The probability density of finding the particle at location $\boldsymbol{r}$ and time t is given by

$$\Psi^*\left(\boldsymbol{r},t\right)\Psi\left(\boldsymbol{r},t\right), \tag{9.19}$$

where $\Psi^*\left(\boldsymbol{r},t\right)$ is the complex conjugate of $\Psi\left(\boldsymbol{r},t\right)$.

When $\Psi\left(\boldsymbol{r},t\right)$ can be factored out as

$$\Psi\left(\boldsymbol{r},t\right) = \psi\left(\boldsymbol{r}\right)T\left(t\right), \tag{9.20}$$

we can substitute (9.20) into (9.17) and obtain

$$\frac{1}{\psi(r)} H\psi(r) = j\frac{h}{2\pi}\frac{dT(t)}{T(t)\,dt}. \tag{9.21}$$

The left-hand side of (9.21) is a function of r and the right-right side of (9.21) is a function of t. Therefore, they must equal a constant (the total energy E), i.e.,

$$j\frac{h}{2\pi}\frac{dT(t)}{T(t)\,dt} = E. \tag{9.22}$$

From (9.22), we can obtain

$$T(t) = A\exp\left(-\frac{2\pi jEt}{h}\right) \tag{9.23}$$

and

$$\Psi(r,t) = \psi(r)\exp\left(-\frac{2\pi jEt}{h}\right). \tag{9.24}$$

From (9.24), we conclude that the probability density of finding a particle at location r and time t is

$$\Psi^*(r,t)\,\Psi(r,t) = \psi^*(r)\,\psi(r). \tag{9.25}$$

In physics, $\psi^*(r)\,\psi(r)$ is the electron density at location r and time t.

Schrödinger equation (9.17) describes the relationship between the energy function and the location probability of an electron. One can imagine that a molecule is more complicated than an electron; larger protein molecules are more complicated than small ligand molecules. It is even more complicated to consider QM for a ligand-protein interaction system.

The commonly used HF-LCAO model is based on Hartree-Fock (HF) and the linear combination of atomic orbitals (LCAO) (see, e.g., Hinchliffe, 2008, Chapters 15 and 16), in which the so-called the Born-Oppenheimer approximation is also induced. In the calculation of potential energy with the Born-Oppenheimer approximation, a molecule is considered as a set of N point charges at N fixed locations.

We can see that QM is not feasible, at this moment, for the pharmaceutical industry to screen a vast number of molecules due to computational intensity. An alternative is to use molecular mechanics (MM) or molecular dynamics.

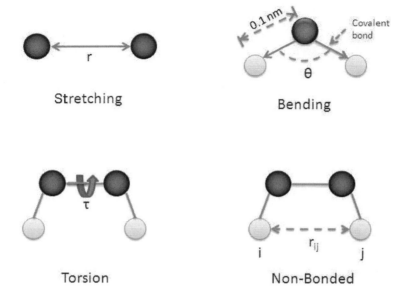

Figure 9.12: Molecular Displacements

9.4.2 Molecular Mechanics

Unlike QM approaches, MM treats the atomic composition of a molecule as a collection of masses interacting with each other via harmonic forces. This simplification in MM leads to a relatively fast computational method suitable for small and larger molecules, and even oligomolecular systems.

The term molecular mechanics was coined in the 1970s to describe the application of classical mechanics to determinations of molecular equilibrium structures, but the idea of treating molecules as balls joined by springs can be traced back to the 1930s (Hinchliffe, 2008). The basic equation for molecular interactions is expressed in terms of a potential energy function:

$$E = E_{Stretching} + E_{Bending} + E_{Torsion} + E_{Coulomb} + E_{Evdw} \qquad (9.26)$$

where $E_{Stretching}$, $E_{Bending}$, $E_{Torsion}$, $E_{Coulomb}$, E_{Evdw} are stretching, bending, torsion, Coulomb, and van der Waals energies, respectively (Figure 9.12).

The stretching energy can be expressed as

$$E_{Stretching} = \sum_{bonds} \frac{k_s}{2} (r - r_0)^2 . \qquad (9.27)$$

The bond stretching energy equation (9.27) estimates the bond vibration energy, where k_s is the elasticity of the bond "spring," r is the actual bound length, and r_0 is the equilibrium bond length. For different atom-pairs connected by a bond, unique parameter values are assigned.

The bending energy takes similar form as the stretching energy:

$$E_{Bending} = \sum_{angles} \frac{k_\theta}{2} (\theta - \theta_0)^2 \tag{9.28}$$

where k_θ reflects the "elasticity" of the bending "spring," θ is the actual, and θ_0 the equilibrium angle. The bending energy equation (9.28) is an estimate of the energy associated with vibration about the equilibrium bond angle.

The energy caused by torsion can be expressed as

$$E_{Torsion} = \sum_{Torsions} \frac{k_\tau}{2} [1 + \cos(n\tau - \tau_0)] \tag{9.29}$$

where k_τ = torsional barrier, τ = actual torsional angle, n = periodicity (number of energy minima within one full cycle), τ_0 = reference torsional angle (the value usually is $0°$ for a cosine function with an energy maximum at $0°$ or $180°$, but for a sine function, an energy minimum is expected at $0°$).

Coulomb potential energy and van der Waals dispersive energy are two nonbonded energies. Coulomb potential energy is the energy of the point charge interaction:

$$E_{Coulomb} = \sum_i \sum_j \frac{q_i q_j}{4\pi\varepsilon_0 r_{ij}}, \tag{9.30}$$

where q_i and q_j are localized charges of atoms i and j separated by a distance r_{ij} and ε_0 is the dielectricity constant.

van der Waals dispersive energy is induced by interactions between atoms that are not connected directly and is usually represented by a Lennard-Jones potential

$$E_{Evdw} = \sum_i \sum_j \left(\frac{B_{ij}}{r_{ij}^{12}} - \frac{A_{ij}}{r_{ij}^{6}} \right), \tag{9.31}$$

where parameters A_{ij} and B_{ij} define the depth and position of the potential energy wall for a given pair of nonbonded interacting atoms. The attractive interactions are expressed by the $1/r^6$ term, and repulsion by the stronger l/r^{12} dependency (Lennard-Jones potential). Repulsion occurs when the interatomic distance falls below the sum of the contact radii of the atoms, that is, in the case of collision.

The total energy is a measure of intramolecular strain relative to a hypothetical molecule with ideal geometry. By itself the total energy has no physical meaning.

9.4.3 Geometry Optimization

Pharmacophore is a 3D representation of a protein (or other) binding site. Most minimization algorithms can only find local minima on the potential energy surface, with no guarantee of finding the global minima. Energy-minimization methods can be the first derivative techniques like steepest descent and conjugate gradient, and second derivative methods like the Newton-Raphson.

It is found that a transformation from one conformation to another is primarily related to changes in torsion angles about single bonds. Only minor changes of bond lengths and angles are anticipated. Another important point to keep in mind is that it is widely accepted that the 'bioactive' conformation need not necessarily be identical with the lowest-energy conformation.

9.5 Ligand–Receptor Interaction

9.5.1 Concept of Energy Minimization

Biochemical processes within a cell or an organism are generally caused by molecular interaction and recognition events. It is critical to identify disease pathways and discover molecular structures that can be used to interfere with and slow down disease progression, or may eventually cure the disease. Due to efficacy and safety requirements for a drug, both high potency and specificity of action are important to NMEs.

Shape complementarity between a ligand and a binding pocket is believed to be a necessary attribute for a selective interaction. Proteins that have similar binding pockets or active sites are more likely to have similar biological (enzymatic) functions. All three methods, ligand-based, receptor-based, and combination methods, use analysis of complementary surface patches of receptor-ligand pairs.

Receptor–ligand complexes between drug molecules and their macromolecular targets are mostly based on noncovalent interactions. Covalent binders exist, but typically reversible binding causing reversible pharmacological effects is desirable, as covalent binding of drugs is often eventually responsible for various types of drug toxicity.

The design of ligands that interact with a target receptor always yields a low-energy ligand-receptor complex. The free energy (Gibbs energy) change ΔG for a receptor-ligand interaction was defined by Gibbs in 1873 as

$$\Delta G = \Delta H - T\Delta S \tag{9.32}$$

where ΔH and $T\Delta S$ are enthalpic and entropic terms, respectively, contributing to the change in the free energy of binding ΔG.

This ligand conformation is not necessarily the global minimum-energy conformation. However, typical bioactive ligand conformations are close to global minimum conformations in water, which might differ substantially from conformations in a vacuum.

Free energy differences between two states are almost independent of high-energy contributions. This allows approximation of each state by its mean partition function, taking into account only relevant low-energy conformations weighted by their Boltzmann probability. The energy differences between the two states can be quantified from Monte Carlo or molecular dynamics (MD) simulations (Schneider and Baringhaus, 2008).

Hydrogen-bonding interactions are considered as directed, and lipophilic (dispersive) interactions as undirected. This differentiation is important in selecting a ligand-receptor interaction. As discussed earlier, a protein-ligand interaction is comparable to the lock-and-key principle, in which the lock encodes the protein and the key is represented by the ligand. Therefore, protein surface cavities are the actual drug "targets." The biological activity of drugs requires binding of small molecules to receptors (e.g., GPCRs) or enzymes (e.g., proteases) yielding receptor modulation (activation or inhibition) or enzyme inhibition. Approximately 700–1000 distinct protein folds and 4000 structural protein superfamilies are believed to exist. There are only about five prominent folds among 1060 potential druglike ligands.

9.5.2 *Hard Sphere-Fitting Method*

Empirical studies have shown that often ligand binding sites coincide with the largest pocket of a protein's surface. A variety of computational methods exist for the location of possible ligand binding sites. Figure 9.13 shows a simple commonly used pocket detecting process. An initial gap sphere is placed midway between the van der Waals surfaces of a pair of receptor atoms. The radius of this gap sphere is reduced until there are no more clashes with any of the binding site atoms. More balls of different sizes fit into the space without any overlap. The pocket space can be estimated based on the balls fitting into the space. Pharnacophore-based pocket descriptors provide a possibility for functional pocket comparisons and ligand screening.

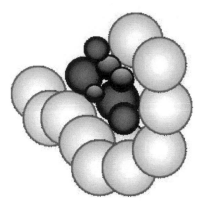

Figure 9.13: Hard Sphere-Fitting

9.5.3 *Method of Moments*

The method of moments, in statistics, is a method of estimation of population parameters, such as mean, variance, median, etc., by equating sample moments with unobservable population moments and then solving those equations for the quantities to be estimated. Here method of moments refers to a method of evaluating the difference of objects (ligand and protein pocket) in shape by equating sample moments about the pocket/ligand centers. Because the shape of an object is determined by the 3D coordinates of its surface, the method of moments is to compare the moments of the two data sets for the surfaces of the ligand and the pocket. In the method of moments outlined below, the key is to take proper sample data that can represent the surfaces of the ligand and protein. This will be achieved using initial sampling and second sampling. The other important steps are to find the center of the objects, i.e., the means of the samples, rotate the objects to the principal directions, and calculate the ith moments ($i = 1, ..., K$). The difference in moments between the two objects measures the similarity of the two objects.

The method of moments starts with selecting randomly a point in the pocket C_0 as the center of the coordinate system. The rest of the steps are as follows: (1) For a given pair $\left(\theta_i, \varphi_j\right)$, $0 \leq \theta_j \leq 180°$, and $0 \leq \varphi_i \leq 360°$ ($i = 1, .., m, j = 1, ..., n$), calculate the distance between C_0 and each sphere of the protein r_{ij}. (2) Find the minimum distance $r_{ij}^* = min\ \{r_{ij}\}$. This $\{\theta_i, \varphi_j, r_{ij}^*\}$ defines a pocket numerically. (3) To find the geometric center of the pocket, we use the transformation from a circular coordinate system to a Cartesian coordinate system:

$$\begin{cases} x_{ij} = r_{ij}^* \sin\theta_i \cos\varphi_j \\ y_{ij} = r_{ij}^* \sin\theta_i \sin\varphi_j \\ z_{ij} = r_{ij}^* \cos\theta_i \end{cases} \quad . \tag{9.33}$$

(4) Find the center of the pocket using the following formulation:

$$\begin{cases} x_c = \frac{1}{mn} \sum_{i=1}^m \sum_{j=1}^n x_{ij} \\ y_c = \frac{1}{mn} \sum_{i=1}^m \sum_{j=1}^n y_{ij} \\ z_c = \frac{1}{mn} \sum_{i=1}^m \sum_{j=1}^n z_{ij} \end{cases} , \tag{9.34}$$

where (x_c, y_c, z_c) are the Cartesian coordinates of the pocket center.

(5) In the circular coordinate system, the pocket center $(\theta_c, \varphi_c, r_c)$ is given by

$$\begin{cases} r_c = \sqrt{x_c^2 + y_c^2 + z_c^2} \\ \varphi_c = \tan^{-1} \frac{y_c}{x_c} \\ \theta_c = \tan^{-1} \frac{\sqrt{x_c^2 + y_c^2}}{z} \end{cases} . \tag{9.35}$$

(6) Consider the new coordinate center $(\theta_c, \varphi_c, r_c)$ and regenerate $(\theta_i, \varphi_j; i = 1, .., m; j = 1, n)$ and recalculate the distance r_{ij} from the center $(\theta_c, \varphi_c, r_c)$ to each sphere of the protein and find $r_{ij}^* = \min\{r_{ij}\}$. Note that $(\theta_c, \varphi_c, r_c)$ does not necessarily locate within the pocket.

For each optimized ligand, perform the same calculations as for the pocket. Rotate the ligand and pocket so that three principal directions coincide with the $x - y - z$ directions (Exercise 9.1). Then calculate the first K moments $\xi_i\, (i = 1, ..., K)$ for the pocket and each ligand and store them in the virtual library. A fitting score can be quickly calculated based on the difference between the ligand and the pocket in the ith moment (about the center of the ligand or pocket):

$$Score = 1/\sum_{i=1}^K w_i \Delta\xi_i, \tag{9.36}$$

where w_i is a weight function and $\Delta\xi_i$ is the ith moment difference.

9.5.4 *Ligand and Protein Flexibility*

The simplest docking procedure is rigid body docking, in which both protein and ligand are treated as rigid bodies. However, this approach is not accurate because both the actual ligand and the receptor are flexible. Semiflexible docking considers only ligand flexibility to reduce computation requirements. Fully flexible docking to consider both ligand and protein flexibility is computationally not very feasible at this time for VS with a large number of molecules in drug discovery.

To consider ligand flexibility, the simplest approach is to store multiple conformations of the ligands in the database, each conformation being regarded as rigid during the docking process, or dealing with ligand flexibility in real time using an incremental construction method during the docking process, in which the ligand is divided into fragments and incrementally built into the receptor binding site.

Recently, several advanced conformer generators (e.g., CATALYST, OMEGA, CORINA) have been developed, which usually produce among the set of proposed conformers one that is close to a bioactive conformation (Kirchmair et al., 2006).

Proteins are highly flexible molecules that exist in a range of conformational states, with low-energy barriers separating them. Protein motions are often decomposed into three components: (1) small-scale fast side-chain movements, (2) large-scale, slow hinge-bending movements, and (3) renaturation. Conformation analysis with flexible proteins is computationally challenging.

9.6 Docking Algorithms

9.6.1 *Incremental Construction Methods*

In an incremental construction algorithm, the ligand is divided into fragments and incrementally reconstructed inside the active site (Ewing et al., 2001). The interaction sites are assumed to be a sphere with an interaction type (hydrogen bond acceptor, hydrogen bond donor, etc.). The base fragment is oriented by searching for placements where the interactions between the protein and the ligand can occur. The remaining ligand components are then incrementally attached to the core. At each growing step, a list of preferred torsional angle values is read and the best conformation in terms of protein-ligand interactions is kept for further 'growing' of the ligand. All possible anchor placements are scored in terms of the dock scoring function, and the best ones are used for subsequent 'growing' of the ligand. Finally, the best-scored poses of the complete ligand are selected (Höltje et al., 2008).

9.6.2 *Genetic Algorithms*

Gold (Verdonk et al., 2003) used a genetic algorithm (GA) for docking a ligand to a protein. Each chromosome encodes a possible protein-ligand complex conformation. A chromosome is assigned a fitness score on the basis of the relative quality of that solution in terms of protein-ligand interactions. GA has been implemented in AutoDock 3.0.

Algorithm 9.1: Genetic Algorithm for Docking

(1) Choose a set of operators (crossing over, mutation, etc.).
(2) Define a fitness function.
(3) Generate randomly an initial population with individual fitness.
(4) Choose a genetic operator based on predetermined probabilities.
(5) Select randomly one or two chromosome parents based on their fitness scores.
(6) Apply the genetic operator to the parent(s) for generating children chromosomes.
(7) Compute fitness score for each new offspring(s).
(8) Stop if stopping criteria met; otherwise, go to (4).
§

In Algorithm 9.1, the mutation operator requires one parent and produces one child, while the crossover operator requires two parents and produces two children. Crossover thus combines features from two different chromosomes in one, whereas mutation makes a copy from the parent, for which random perturbations are made. The probability of selecting a parent chromosome is proportional to its fitness score, hence the population evolves toward a higher fitness score over time, i.e., better binding mode (see Chapter 13 for more about genetic programming).

9.6.3 *Monte Carlo Simulated Annealing*

In solid physics, annealing is known as a thermal process for obtaining lowest-energy states of a solid. The processes are governed by molecular dynamics, in which the system starts with a high temperature state with its particles being relatively free to move around. The temperature then slowly deceases and the particles are forced to line up to achieve local energy minimization. In this process, the system must be cooled down slowly; otherwise, if it decreases too fast, the particles will not have enough time to line up (Liu, 2003). In Monte Carlo simulated annealing, during each constant temperature cycle, random perturbations are made to the ligand's current orientation and conformation. The new state is accepted if its energy is lower than the energy of the preceding state. Otherwise, the configuration is accepted probabilistically based upon Boltzmann's equation

(Höltje et al., 2008). The probability of acceptance is given as

$$P_a = \exp\left(-\frac{\Delta E}{k_B T}\right), \tag{9.37}$$

where ΔE is the difference in energy from the previous step, T is the absolute temperature in Kelvin, and k_B is the Boltzmann constant.

From (9.37), we can see that the higher the temperature of the cycle, the higher the probability that the new state is accepted. When the energy change ΔE is negative, P_a will be larger than 1. Therefore, regardless of the direction of the energy change in Monte Carlo simulated annealing, the acceptance probability for a state can be written as

$$P_a = \min\left(1, e^{-\frac{\Delta E}{k_B T}}\right). \tag{9.38}$$

Keep in mind that the final state from Monte Carlo simulated annealing usually depends on the initial placement of the ligand because the algorithm does not explore the solution space exhaustively.

Algorithm 9.2: Simulated Annealing
Objective: Docking with simulated annealing
Set up initial ligand's coordinates.
Input temperature sequence $\{T_i\}$, k_B, and a small $\varepsilon > 0$.
For $i := 1$ **To** K
    Make random perturbations to the ligand's current orientation and conformation.
    Calculate the incremental energy ΔE
    Generate random number u from $U(0,1)$
    If $u < P_a = \min\left(1, e^{-\frac{\Delta E}{k_B T_i}}\right)$ **Then** accept new state
    If $\Delta E < \varepsilon$ **Then** **Exitfor**
Endfor
Return current state of the ligand
§

9.7 Scoring Functions

In the section on Molecular Similarity Search, we discussed the similarity measure of ligands. In this section, we study scoring functions. A scoring function is a measure of interaction between a ligand and a receptor; it is a measure of the drug-likeness of a ligand.

The free energy of binding is given by the Gibbs-Helmholtz equation:

$$\Delta G = \Delta H - T\Delta S, \tag{9.39}$$

where ΔG provides the free energy of binding, ΔH = the enthalpy, T = the temperature in Kelvin, and ΔS = the entropy. ΔG relates to the binding constant K_i through the equation:

$$\Delta G = -RT\ln K_i \tag{9.40}$$

where R is the gas constant.

The binding free energy difference between a ligand and a reference molecule can be accurately calculated using energy perturbation (Miyamoto and Kollman, 1993). However, such a time-consuming approach is not practical for virtual screening to compute energies for thousands of protein-ligand complexes. A less accurate but fast method is desirable. A scoring function, monotonic in ΔG, can be calculated quickly and the resulting conformation rankings based on a score function will be the same as with ΔG.

Höltje and colleagues (Höltje et al., 2008) categorize scoring functions into three groups: empirical scoring functions, force-field-based functions, and knowledge-based potential of mean force. Scoring functions can be used in two ways: (1) during the docking process, they serve a fitness function in the optimal placement of the ligand; (2) when the docking is completed, it is used to rank each ligand of the database for which a docking solution has been found.

9.7.1 *Empirical Scoring Functions*

Empirical scoring functions are usually functions derived from statistical models such as ANCOVA with significant terms that are found to be important in drug binding. These terms generally describe polar interactions such as hydrogen bonds and ionic interactions, apolar interactions such as lipophilic and aromatic interactions, loss of ligand flexibility (entropy), and eventually also desolvation effects (Eldridge et al., 1997, Rognan et al., 1999; Höltje et al., 2008).

Empirical scoring functions dissect the protein-ligand binding free energy into all its physically meaningful contributions and try to evaluate them explicitly, e.g.,

$$Score = \sum_i C_i F_i + C_0, \tag{9.41}$$

where C_i are regression coefficients and typical factor F_i can be van der Waals interaction, hydrogen bonding, solvation effects, electrostatic interaction, and conformational entropy.

9.7.2 Force-Field-Based Scoring Functions

Force-field scoring functions are usually based on the nonbonded terms of molecular mechanics, which include a Lennard-Jones potential representing van der Waals interactions (9.30) and Coulomb energy representing the electrostatic components of the interactions (9.31). Because these methods ignore the entropic component of the binding free energy, the approximation becomes inevitable for larger and most polar molecules that usually get the highest enthalpy interaction scores:

$$E_{nonbonded} = \sum_i \sum_j \frac{q_i q_j}{4\pi\varepsilon_0 r_{ij}} + \sum_i \sum_j \left(\frac{B_{ij}}{r_{ij}^{12}} - \frac{A_{ij}}{r_{ij}^6} \right). \tag{9.42}$$

9.7.3 Iterative Knowledge-Based Scoring Function

The theory behind the statistical potential approach is the assumption of Boltzmann-like energetics (9.37), i.e., the Boltzmann distribution law for a single closed system held at fixed temperature is applicable to a database of structures. Then we apply an inverse Boltzmann relation:

$$u(r) = -k_B T \ln \frac{\rho(r)}{\rho^*(r)}, \tag{9.43}$$

where k_B is the Boltzmann constant, and T is the absolute temperature; $\rho(r)$ is the number density of the protein-ligand atom pair at distance r, and $\rho^*(r)$ is the atom pair density in a "reference" state where the interatomic interactions are zero. Despite its efficiency, a limitation of (9.43) is that the reference states are usually not achievable. Therefore, extracted potentials by these methods are not equal to true potentials. Huang and Zou (2006) propose an iterative method to solve the problem, as described below.

The total energy score U is calculated as the sum of energies from all the ligand-receptor pairs:

$$U = \sum_{L-R \; pair} u(r), \tag{9.44}$$

where r is the atom pair distance.

The energy iteration algorithm is given by

$$u_{ij}^{(n+1)}(r) = u_{ij}^{(n)}(r) + \lambda k_B T \left(g_{ij}^{(n)}(r) - \hat{g}_{ij}(r) \right), \tag{9.45}$$

where $u_{ij}^{(n)}(r)$ is the nth iteration potential energy of the ith protein atom type and the jth ligand atom type; r is the atom pair distance. Without loss of generality, $k_B T$ can be set to unit 1; λ is a parameter to control the speed of convergence; $\hat{g}_{ij}(r)$ is the experimentally observed pair distribution function for the native binding modes of the training set. Mathematically,

$$\hat{g}_{ij}(r) = \frac{\hat{\rho}_{ij}(r)}{\hat{R}_{ij}} = \frac{\frac{1}{M}\sum_{m}^{M}\frac{n_{ij}^{m}(r)}{4\pi r^2 dr}}{\frac{1}{M}\sum_{m}^{M}\frac{N_{ij}^{m}}{4\pi R^3/3}}, \tag{9.46}$$

where the observed $\hat{\rho}_{ij}(r)$ and $\hat{R}_{ij}$ (given below) are the number densities of atom pair (i,j) occurring in a spherical shell of radius from $r - dr/2$ to $r + dr/2$ and in a reference sphere of radius R, respectively, where dr should be sufficiently small (e.g., $0.1\overset{o}{A}$) and R is relatively large (e.g., 10 $\overset{o}{A}$), where $n_{ij}^{m}(r)$ and $N_{ij}^{m} = \sum_{r} n_{ij}^{m}(r)$ are the numbers of atom pair (i,j) in the spherical shell and the reference sphere for the mth native complex structure, respectively. M is the number of protein-ligand complexes in the training database.

$$g_{ij}^{(n)} = \frac{\rho_{ij}^{(n)}(r)}{R_{ij}^{(n)}} = \frac{\frac{1}{ML}\sum_{m}^{M}\sum_{l}^{L}\frac{n_{ij}^{ml}(r)\exp(-\beta U_{ml})}{4\pi r^2 dr}}{\frac{1}{ML}\sum_{m}^{M}\sum_{l}^{L}\frac{N_{ij}^{ml}\exp(-\beta U_{ml})}{4\pi R^3/3}}, \tag{9.47}$$

where $\rho_{ij}^{(n)}(r)$ and $R_{ij}^{(n)}$ are the number densities of atom pair (i,j) occurring in a spherical shell of radius from $r-dr/2$ to $r+dr/2$ and in a reference sphere of radius R at the nth iterative cycle for the decoy complex structures, respectively. Here, $\rho_{ij}^{(n)}(r)$ and $R_{ij}^{(n)}$ are calculated as the Boltzmann-weighted pair frequencies over different decoy structures in (9.47) where $\beta = 1/k_B T$ can be set to 1 as mentioned above. $n_{ij}^{ml}(r)$ and N_{ij}^{ml} are the numbers of atom pair (i,j) in the spherical shell and the reference sphere for the lth decoy ligand orientation of the mth complex, respectively. U_{ml} is the energy score of this ligand orientation, defined as the sum over all interatomic interactions (9.44). L is the total number of putative ligand orientations generated for each complex (including the native binding mode).

The initial energy function can be defined as a piece-wise function combining the potential of mean force $w_{ij}(r)$ and the Lennard-Jones potentials $v_{ij}(r)$, as specified by

$$u_{ij}^{0}(r) = \begin{cases} -k_B T \ln \hat{g}_{ij}(r) & \text{for hydrogen-bond pairs,} \\ \frac{v_{ij}(r)\exp(-v_{ij}(r))+w_{ij}(r)\exp(-w_{ij}(r))}{\exp(-v_{ij}(r))+\exp(-w_{ij}(r))} & \text{otherwise.} \end{cases}$$
$$\tag{9.48}$$

This combination is necessary because potentials of mean force, $w_{ij}(r)$, are not true potentials and lack an effective short-distant repulsive component. A smooth function $F(\cdot)$ can be used to remove the fluctuations of the initial potentials at large distances.

$$F(r) = \begin{cases} \kappa \left(r_{\min} - r\right)^s - \varepsilon_0 & r < r_{\min} \\ \varepsilon_0 \left(e^{-\alpha(r-r_{\min})} - 1\right)^2 - \varepsilon_0, & r_{\min} \le r \le r_c \\ 0, & r > r_c. \end{cases} \qquad (9.49)$$

The determination of parameters in (9.49) has been addressed by Huang and Zou (2006) and Muryshev et al. (2003).

Before running the iterations, a series of putative ligand binding orientations (decoys) for each protein-ligand complex can be generated, which covers the space in the binding pocket as much as possible and serves as an approximation for an ensemble of structures.

Huang and Zou (2006) provide the following algorithm (Algorithm 9.3) using the iterative method and find it very efficient in convergence (within 20 cycles).

Algorithm 9.3: Iterative Knowledge-based Scoring Function
Objective: Iterative scoring function.

(1) Download protein-ligand complex structures from a virtual molecular library and prepare the database of native structures.

(2) Calculate the experimentally observed pair distribution functions $\hat{g}_{ij}(r)$ of the protein-ligand atom pairs for the native binding modes using (9.46); derive initial potentials $u_{ij}^{(0)}(r) = F\left(\hat{g}_{ij}(r)\right)$ using (9.48) and (9.49).

(3) For each protein-ligand complex, generate a series of putative ligand orientations around the binding site by using a molecular docking program, for the purpose of iterative calculations.

(4) Set the iterative step $n = 0$ and start iteration.

(5) Calculate the energy scores of different ligand orientations for each complex using (9.44) with the current interaction potentials $u_{ij}^{(n)}(r)$; identify the best-scored binding mode.

(6) If the convergence criterion or stopping rule is satisfied, skip to step 9; otherwise, continue.

(7) Calculate the current pair distribution functions $g_{ij}^{(n)}(r)$ of the structure ensembles by using a Boltzmann-weighted averaging method (9.47).

(8) Modify the current potentials $u_{ij}^{(n)}(r)$ according to (9.45) and obtain a set of improved potentials $u_{ij}^{(n+1)}(r)$; let $n := n + 1$ and return to step 5 for the next cycle.

(9) The iterative procedure is finished. Write out the final potentials.

§

9.7.4   *Virtual Screening of 5-Lipoxygenase Inhibitors*

Arachidonate 5-lipoxygenase (5-lipoxygenase, 5-LO or Alox5) is a human enzyme, a member of the lipoxygenase family. It transforms EFAs into leukotrienes. 5-LO is activated by 5-lipoxygenase activating protein (FLAP). Mutations in the promoter region of this gene lead to a diminished response to antileukotriene drugs used in the treatment of asthma and may also be associated with atherosclerosis and several cancers. Alternatively spliced transcript variants have been observed, but their full-length nature has not been determined. The 5-LO pathway has also been associated with atherosclerosis, cancer, and osteoporosis, so that 5-LO has become a current target for pharmaceutical intervention in a number of diseases. In fact, leukotrienes are important causes of pathological symptoms in asthma and 5-LO inhibitors were developed as asthma treatments.

The aim of a virtual screening campaign (Schneider and Baringhaus, 2008) was to search for potential novel 5-LO inhibitors in a natural product collection and natural product-derived compound libraries. Since there is lack of knowledge about the receptor structure, ligand-based virtual screening was used based on the similarity principle. A similarity search was conducted in the published 5-LO ligands literature. Virtual screening preceeded in the following two consecutive steps:

(1) In the first virtual screen, 42 5-LO pathway inhibitors were collected from the literature. The ten most similar compounds were retrieved for each of the 42 reference molecules. From this list of 420 candidates 17 molecules were manually selected by experienced medicinal chemists and tested in a cellular assay system for inhibition of 5-LO product synthesis. Then a topological pharmacophore descriptor was utilized to find new chemotypes in natural products and natural-product derived combinatorial compound collections.

(2) In the second virtual screening step, the two most active molecules from the first virtual screen served as the reference structures for similarity searching in a focused combinatorial library. Both charge-based and substructure-based molecular descriptors were used to find potentially more potent substances and to obtain a preliminary structure-activity relationship (SAR) model. As a result, 17 compounds were finally selected and tested for inhibition of 5-LO product synthesis in vitro.

A novel chemotype, as a result of the VS, exhibits nanomolar activity in a cellular assay. Chemists at AnalytiCon Discovery converted this natural product into a scaffold that is amenable to combinatorial library design. A

3D pharmacophore model was constructed that helped to explain the SAR of the combinatorial scaffold.

Schneider and Baringhaus (2008) concluded that natural product diversity can be exploited for virtual screening and in the identification of novel bioactive chemotypes with minimal experimental effort.

9.8 Summary

The failure rate of compounds in development is high: poor biopharmaceutical properties, 39%; lack of efficacy, 29%; toxicity, 21%; market reasons, 6%. Molecular design and modeling is a new promising field that uses computer and chemical compound databases to screen, model, and design NMEs so as to reduce the discovery cost and accelerate the discovery process. The reasons why computers can help in this aspect are (1) the numbers of compounds that can be examined by a human mind are limited compared to the capacity of VS and biochemical screening assays can be very expensive. Monte Carlo molecular design can be used to identify novel substances that exhibit desired properties. An example is a particular biological activity profile that includes proper physicochemical and ADMET properties of the novel compounds.

Molecular docking is commonly used in Monte Carlo drug design. Molecular docking can be used for virtual screening or fit identification and lead optimization. The four essential steps of any VS process are preparation, docking, scoring, and post-filtering.

Understanding structure-activity relationships (SAR) is essential for successful optimization of the compound properties of a pharmacologically active substance. Once an SAR model is available, it is possible to perform rational drug design.

The steps in the standard drug lead-approach include (1) identifying the target (e.g., enzyme, receptor, ion channel, transporter), (2) determining DNA and/or protein sequence, (3) elucidating structures and functions of proteins, (4) proving the therapeutic concept in animals ("knock-outs"), (5) developing an assay for HTS, (6) mass screening, and (7) selecting lead structures.

The term "drug-like" is a general concept of what makes a drug a drug by describing various empirically found structure characteristics of molecular agents, which are associated with pharmacological activities. Drug-likeliness is a measure of complex physicochemical and structural features of the compound, which can be used to guide the rational design of lead structures that can be further optimized to become a drug.

For structure analysis, molecules can be divided into scaffolds or frameworks, linkers, and side-chains that are attached to the ring systems. The rationale behind a structural similarity search is the so-called similar property principle: structurally similar molecules are likely to have similar chemical or physiological properties.

Similarity searching can be achieved by comparing representations of molecules with respect to the substructure elements they contain. A popular similarity index is the Tanimoto (Jaccard) index. SimScore was developed to evaluate quantitatively the structural similarity score of a target compound with teratogenic drugs which are defined as serious human teratogens by the FDA. The principle behind SimScore is that compounds with the same or similar skeleton show a similar biological activity, but their activity strengths depend on the variation of substituents. A Bayesian network is a simple and popular way of doing probabilistic inference in the similarity search.

The optimization of molecular docking can also be viewed as the minimization of the free energy of the protein-ligand system. There are three commonly used virtual screening strategies: (1) ligand-based virtual screening, (2) structure (receptor)-based screening, and (3) combination approaches.

There are two commonly used docking approaches: (1) a matching technique that describes the protein and the ligand as complementary surfaces using, e.g., grid-based energy evaluation or a genetic algorithm and (2) an empirical binding free energy function.

The scoring function takes a receptor-ligand pose as input and returns a number indicating the likelihood that the pose represents a favorable binding interaction. The score function is used in similarity ranking.

MQ and MM are commonly used methods for molecular confirmation analysis. Pharmacophore is a 3D representation of a protein (or other) binding site.

There is much docking software available. See http://www.bio.vu.nl/nbtb/Docking.html for such a list. Other useful sites are http://dock.compbio.ucsf.edu/ and www.agilemolecule.com/index.html.

9.9 Exercises

Exercise 9.1: Define the three principal directions in method of moments.

Exercise 9.2: How does molecular design and simulation accelerate drug development and reduce costs?

Exercise 9.3: What is Lipinski's rule-of-five and how is it used?

Exercise 9.4: What are the FDAs five categories used to classify teratogenic effects?

Exercise 9.5: What is a Bayesian network? What are the steps for Bayesian network modeling?

Exercise 9.6: What kind of database is needed for virtual screening?

Exercise 9.7: Describe the docking algorithms: incremental construction methods, genetic algorithm, and Monte Carlo simulated annealing.

Exercise 9.8: Explain the score functions: empirical scoring functions, force-field-based scoring functions, and Iterative knowledge-based scoring function.

Exercise 9.9: Try a molecular design software (commercial or freeware) you like.

Chapter 10

Disease Modeling and Biological Pathway Simulation

This chapter will cover the following topics:

- Computational Systems Biology
- Petri Nets
- Biological Pathway Simulation

10.1 Computational Systems Biology

10.1.1 *Cell, Pathway, and Systems Biology*

The cell is the structural and functional unit of all living organisms. It is the building block of life. There are two types of cells, prokaryotic and eukaryotic cells. Prokaryotic cells are singletons without a nuclear membrane, whereas eukaryotic cells contain membrane-bound compartments in which specific metabolic activities take place. All cells share the following activities: reproduction by cell division, use and production of enzymes and other proteins coded by DNA genes, and response to external and internal stimuli such as changes in temperature, pH, or nutrient levels. Living cells are composed of a wide array of compounds, and physiological or chemical reactions that occur simultaneously.

A *biological pathway* is a molecular interaction network in biological processes. The pathways can be classified into the fundamental categories metabolic, regulatory, and signal transduction pathways. There are about 10,000 pathways, nearly 160 pathways involving 800 reactions.

A *metabolic pathway* is a series of chemical reactions occurring within a cell, catalyzed by enzymes, resulting in either the formulation of a metabolic product to be used or stored by the cell, or the inhibition of another metabolic pathway. Pathways are important to the maintenance of homeostasis within an organism. Figure 10.1 is an illustration of major metabolic pathways.

A *gene regulatory pathway* or *genetic regulatory pathway* is a collection of DNA segments in a cell which interact with each other and with other substances in the cell, thereby governing the rates at which genes in the network are transcribed into mRNA. In general, each mRNA molecule goes on to make a specific protein or its particular structural properties. The protein can be an enzyme for breakdown of a food source or toxin. By binding to the promoter region at the start of other genes, some proteins can turn the genes on, initiating or inhibiting the production of another protein.

A *signal transduction pathway* is a series of processes involving a group of molecules in a cell that work together to control one or more cell functions, such as cell division or cell death. Molecular signals are transmitted between cells by the secretion of hormones and other chemical factors, which are then picked up by different cells. After the first molecule in a pathway receives a signal, it activates another molecule, and then another until the last molecule in the signal chain is activated. Abnormal activation of signaling pathways can lead to a disease such as cancer, and drugs are being developed to block these pathways.

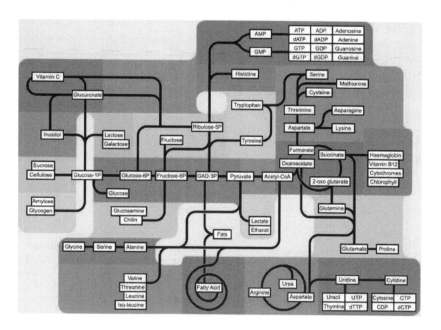

Figure 10.1:   Major Metabolic Pathways

(Source: Wikipedia.com)

Systems biology is a newly emerging, multi-disciplinary field that studies the mechanisms underlying complex biological processes by treating these processes as integrated systems of many interacting components (Materi and Wishart, 2007). Quantitative studies in systems biology require the utilization of computer modeling and simulation, which has given rise to a new discipline called computational systems biology (CSB). CSB can be a way to make drug discovery and drug testing better, faster, and cheaper. With this new approach, the pharmaceutical industry hopes to effectively identify the key points in a disease-related pathway, design a drug that targets those key points, and model organ specific metabolic stress responses or physiologically based pharmacokinetic models to rapidly and inexpensively characterize the toxicity profile of an NME — eventually leading to personalized medicine. However, CSB is often a tool to reduce experimental efforts, but it does not completely replace experiments. In fact, experimental data are often necessary to validate the simulation model.

The model and simulation can be carried out in different temporal and spatial scales, ranging from nanometers to meters, and milliseconds to days. Conventionally, "fine grain" models simulate events that concern short times (ms) or small (nm) dimensions and "coarse grain, models" simulate events that concern longer times (s) or larger (mm or cm) dimensions.

A fundamental challenge to CSB is how to develop models or modeling tools that can deal with this wide range of granularity. One approach is to use hierarchical object models, i.e., divide objects into subobjects, develop and valid the subsystems, and then integrate them into the integrated system.

In what follows, we will review the most commonly used techniques in CSB, including differential equations, cellular automata (CA), agent-based systems, and Petri nets (PN). In Section 10.2, we will elaborate on PN. The application of PN in biological pathways will be discussed in Section 10.3.

10.1.2 *Monte Carlo with Differential Equations*

The classical and most popular approach to model complex biological systems is the ordinal or partial differential equation systems (ODEs and PDEs), which are usually solved either analytically or numerically using standard numerical techniques. However, methods combining differential equations with Monte Carlo simulations can be very useful and will be discussed in PK and PD simulations in Chapters 11 and 12.

A simple example using ODEs and PDEs to model a biomolecular reversible conversion $(A_1 + A_2 \underset{k_b}{\overset{k_a}{\rightleftharpoons}} B_1 + B_2)$ is:

$$\begin{cases} \frac{d[A_i]}{dt} = -k_a[A_1][A_2] + k_b[B_1][B_2] \\ \frac{d[B_i]}{dt} = k_a[A_1][A_2] - k_b[B_1][B_2] \end{cases}. \tag{10.1}$$

There are two special cases of (10.1): (1) production (reaction: $A_1 + A_2 \overset{k_a}{\rightarrow} B_1$), where $[B_2] = 0$ and (2) degradation (reaction: $A_1 \overset{k_a}{\rightarrow} B_1 + B_2$), where $[A_2] = 1$ and $k_b = 0$ in (10.1).

If the container is not well stirred, the diffusion needs time and the governing equation for the diffusion-reaction process $(A + B \overset{k}{\rightarrow} C)$ is given by the following partial differential equation in the 3D Cartesian coordinate system $x - y - z$:

$$\begin{cases} \frac{\partial[A]}{\partial t} = D\nabla^2[A] - k[A][B] \\ \frac{\partial[B]}{\partial t} = D\nabla^2[B] - k[A][B] \\ -\frac{\partial[A]}{\partial t} = -D\nabla^2[C] + k[A][B] \end{cases}, \tag{10.2}$$

where D is the diffusion coefficient and the Laplace operator is given by

$$\nabla^2 = \frac{\partial^2}{\partial x^2} + \frac{\partial^2}{\partial y^2} + \frac{\partial^2}{\partial z^2}. \tag{10.3}$$

10.1.3   *Cellular Automata Method*

Cellular automata (CA) are a class of simple computer simulation methods used to model both temporal and spatiotemporal processes. CAs normally consist of large numbers of identical cells that form a lattice or drift (like a chessboard) with defined interaction rules. The formal definition of CA is given as follows.

Definition 10.1   A cellular automaton is a triple $CA = (S, f, s(0))$, where S is a set of double-infinite $0 - 1$ sequences, called the states of the automaton, a map $f : S \rightarrow S$ is called its transition rule, and $s(0) \in S$ is its initial state.

The collection of all consecutive states $s_0, s_1, s_2, ...$ of an automaton is called its evolution.

Cellula automata were invented in the late 1940s by von Neumann and Ulam (von Neumann, 1966) and have been used to model a wide range of artificial intelligence, image processes, virtual music creation, and physical sciences (Wolfram, 2002). Cellular automata also have a long history in biological modeling. Indeed, one of the first and most interesting CA simulations in biology is Conway's Game of Life (Berlekamp, Conway, and Guy, 1982). CA is simple but can virtually do anything that any computer can do. For example, there is a finite initial state such that any paragraph of English prose, when properly coded as a sequence of gliders, will result in a "spell-checked" paragraph of English prose (again coded as a sequence of gliders).

The rule of CA can be defined in many ways. Here are two simple examples.

Example 10.1: An occupant of a cell with less than two neighbors will, sadly, die of loneliness; with two or three neighbors, it will continue into the next generation; with four or more neighbors, it will die of over-excitement.

The objects (cells, proteins, or reagents) in a CA simulation usually do not move: they only appear, change properties, or disappear. Object properties, attributes, or information are the only things that "move" in CA simulations. Variations on the CA model, known as dynamic cellular automata (DCA), actually enable objects to exhibit motions (Wishart et al., 2005). We can apply random-walk or other stochastic processes to DCA. Depending on the implementation of the DCA algorithm, molecules can move one or more cells in a single time step. DCA models permit considerably more flexibility in simulating biological processes (Materi and Wishart, 2007).

There are CA applications in the pharmaceutical industry such as drug release in bio-erodible microspheres (Zygourakis and Markenscoff, 1996), lipophilic drug diffusion (Kier et al., 1997; Wishart et al., 2005) and drug-carrying micelle formation (Kier et al., 1996), the progression of HIV/AIDS and HIV treatment strategies (Peer et al., 2004), in simulation of different drug therapies or combination therapies. The CA model has the capacity to model efficiently extreme time scales (days to decades) and to simulate the spatial heterogeneity of viral infection.

10.1.4   *Agent-Based Models*

In an agent-based model (ABM) of a biological system, agents represent biological entities (molecule/drug, gene, cell, metabolites, proteins, tissue, organ, body, human ecosystem, etc.). The term "agent" is used to indicate a "conscious" computer program entity with potential learning capabilities, which is characterized by some degree of autonomy and asynchrony with regard to its interactions with other agents and its environment. An agent must be distinguishable from its environment by some kind of spatial, temporal, or functional attribute.

The first step in devising an agent-based model is to identify the entities to be modeled. There are many possible levels of entities, from molecule, cell, to human ecosystem, that can be chosen for modeling and simulation. An appropriate selection of entity level is important to the success of the simulation.

A quite interesting observation on agent-based simulation is that, by using simple agents, which interact locally with simple rules of behavior and actions limited to merely responding fittingly to environmental cues without necessarily striving for an overall goal, we have as a result a synergy which leads to a higher-level whole with much more intricate behavior than that of each component agent. Agents, though, as discrete, diverse, and heterogeneous entities, besides having their own goals and behavior, share the ability to adapt and modify their behavior to their environment, thus placing their autonomous characteristics on a more sophisticated level (Politopoulos, 2007). This shows again the general phenomenon called "micromotivated and macro-consequence."

In the medical field, ABMs have been used for real-time signaling induced in osteocytic networks by mechanical stimuli (Ausk et al., 2005), in studying social behavior of cells and understanding important clinical problems (Walker et al., 2006), investigating patterns in tumor systems and the dynamics of cell motility and aggregation (Mansury et al., 2002), studying the theory and approaches for stem cell organization in the adult human body (d'Inverno and Prophet, 2005), modeling the effect of exogenous calcium on keratinocyte and HaCat cell proliferation and differentiation (Walker et al., 2006), simulating bacterial chemotaxis (Emonet et al., 2005), modeling the calcium-dependent cell migration events in wound healing (Walker et al., 2004), developing optimal breast cancer vaccination protocols (Lollini et al., 2006), and predicting clinical trial outcomes of different anticytokine treatments for sepsis (An, 2004). In An's study an ABM model of the innate immune response was constructed using extensive literature data and information about all the relevant cell types, cell functions, and cell mediators (cytokines).

10.1.5 Network Models

There are thousands of biological and disease pathways or networks, e.g., metabolic, gene regulatory, and signal pathways. All these pathways can theoretically be modeled using mathematical networks such as Bayesian networks, artificial networks, and Petri nets (PN). Most of those networks can be solved using computer simulations. Bayesian networks, artificial neural networks, and genetic programming to automatically generate biological networks are discussed elsewhere in this book. In this chapter, we focus on Petri nets, discussing the topology and dynamics of PN, its simulations, and case studies.

10.2 Petri Nets

10.2.1 *Basic Concept of Petri Nets*

A Petri net (PN) is a mathematical network model for simulating a dynamic system such as an electronic signal process, a traffic system, biological pathways, etc. PN was proposed by Carl Adam Petri in 1962 in his PhD thesis in computer science. Petri nets are a graphical and mathematical formalism for the modeling and analysis of concurrent, asynchronous, and distributed systems. PNs have been in use for over 50 years, so their properties are well understood. Early problem domains included manufacturing systems and communication networks. PNs have gained increasing attention in biological science and drug development in the past ten years. PN research papers dominate the field in simulations of live science and PNs have been adopted more and more by the pharmaceutical industry.

A Petri net can be described either mathematically (graphic theory) or graphically (using a visual graph). The former is convenient for calculating the properties of PNs; the latter, however, can be easily used for conceptual studies. The combination of these two approaches will provide an effective tool for the simulation study of PNs.

The basic elements in PN include: *places* (or stelle) to symbolize the states or conditions of the system, *transitions* to symbolize the actions in the system, *tokens* to symbolize the resources responsible for the changes of the system, *directed arcs* to indicate the directions of token (resource) traveling, and *weights* for the directed arcs representing the minimum required tokens for firing (executing action). Graphically, a place is often denoted by a circle; a transition is denoted by a rectangle; tokens are allocated in places; places and transitions are connected by directed lines (arcs); and weights are values next to the corresponding arcs. When the numbers of tokens in places meet the minimum requirement for firing (execution), some of the tokens are moving from one place to another — the firing rules (see below for details). Before we explain the semantics of the places, transitions, tokens, and directed arcs in PNs, let's discuss a simple example of a PN.

Figure 10.2 represents a PN with three places (p_1, p_2, p_3), one transition (the square), two and five tokens (black dots) in places 1 and 2, respectively, and three arcs, with weights 2, 1, 2 (weight of one is often not shown in the graph for simplicity).

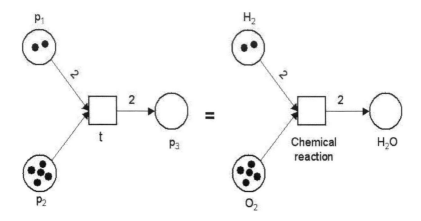

Figure 10.2:   PN Representing the Chemical Reaction of Water

The mathematical definition of PN can be described as follows.

Definition 10.2   A Petri net is a 5-tuple $PN = (P, T, F, W, M_0)$, where:

- $P = \{p_1, ...p_K\}$ is the set of K of places,
- $T = \{t_1, ...t_N\}$ is the set of N transitions, with $P \cap T = \emptyset$ and $P \cup T \neq \emptyset$,
- $F = I \subseteq (P \times T) \cup O \subseteq (T \times P)$ is the flow relation, defining the set of directed arcs,
- $W : F \to (\mathbb{N} \setminus \{0\})$ $(\mathbb{N} = \{0, 1...\})$ is the arc weight function, and
- $M_0 = \{m_{01}, ..., m_{0K}\} \in \mathbb{N}^K$ is the initial marking, i.e., an integer number of tokens associated to each place initially.

Note that the preset I corresponds to all the directed arcs from places to transitions, whereas postset O corresponds to all the directed arcs from transitions to places. $M(p)$ often denotes the number of tokens in place p in marking M.

The Petri net $PN = \langle P, T, F, W, M_0 \rangle$ in Figure 10.2 can be specified as follows: $P = \{p_1, p_2, p_3\}$, $T = \{t\}$, $I = \{\langle p_1, t \rangle, \langle p_2, t \rangle\}$, $O = \langle t, p_3 \rangle$, $F = \{\langle p_1, t \rangle, \langle p_2, t \rangle, \langle t, p_3 \rangle\}$, $W = \{\langle p_1, t \rangle \longmapsto 2, \langle p_2, t \rangle \longmapsto 1, \langle t, p_3 \rangle \longmapsto 2)\}$, and $M_0 = \{2, 5, 0\}$.

It is also convenient to introduce the input and output weight functions as follows. The input weight function $W_I(p_i, t_j) : P \times T \to \mathbb{N}$ defines the minimum number of tokens required from place p_i for firing (executing) the transition t_j as directed by the value next to the arc (if there is no arc from p_i to t_j, $W_I(p_i, t_j) = 0$). The output weight function $W_O\{\langle t_i, p_j \rangle\} : T \times P \to \mathbb{N}$ defines the number of tokens delivered to place p_j due to transition t_i as directed by the arc.

The state of a Petri system is characterized by the distribution of tokens in the places. The dynamics of PN is characterized by the firing mechanism. A place may contain zero or several tokens, which may be interpreted as resources. There may be several input and output arcs between a place and a transition. The number of these arcs is represented as the weight of a single arc. A transition is enabled if each input place contains at least as many tokens as the corresponding input arc weight indicates. When an enabled transition is fired, its input arc weights are subtracted from the input place markings and its output arc weights are added to the output place markings. Formally we have the following definition.

Definition 10.3 Petri Net Firing Rule: Let $\langle P, T, F, W, M_0 \rangle$ be a net and $M : P \rightarrow \mathbb{N}$ one of its markings. A transition $t \in T$ is M-enabled (firing condition), written as $M \xrightarrow{t}$, if and only if $\forall p \in I : M(p) \geq W_I$. An M-enabled transition t may fire (execute), producing the successor marking M', written as $M \xrightarrow{t} M'$, where

$$\forall p \in P : M'(p) = M(p) - W_I(p, t) + W_O(t, p). \qquad (10.4)$$

Example 10.2: Pre-markings $\{2, 5, 0\}$ and $\{3, 1, 1\}$ are $M \xrightarrow{t}$ enabled markings for the PN in Figure 10.2, with post-markings (successor markings) $\{0, 4, 2\}$ and $\{3, 0, 3\}$, respectively, whereas $\{1, 6, 0\}$ and $\{3, 0, 2\}$ are not enabled markings for the PN. Again, we can see that the PN state changes when enabled transitions are fired. When an enabled transition fires, tokens are removed from each of its pre-places and tokens (not necessarily the same number) are inserted in each of its post-places.

Petri nets can have different types: (1) place/transition PN (colored or noncolored) and (2) time-dependent PNs (discrete PN, continuous PN, hybrid PN for mixture of continuous and discrete systems, and stochastic PN).

10.2.2 *Why a Petri Net*

Biological networks or pathways are extremely complicated and it is difficult to understand the mechanics using the traditional representation of biological pathways as a two-dimensional pictorial drawing, without ambiguity. Using a Petri net, we can have a coherent presentation of the very diverse forms of information and solve the problem by means of computer simulation. A Petri net offers a general framework for analyzing the dynamic properties of large systems, from either a qualitative or a quantitative point of view. The mathematical properties of a standard Petri net have been well studied, which can be used for model validations. PNs can be used on an abstraction level with specification of limited resources possible and allow for combining all these different abstraction levels within one model. PNs allow for integration of qualitative and quantitative analyses. Petri nets have an executable graphical representation, supporting the intuitive understanding of the system modeled and communication between experimentally and theoretically working scientists. There are movable objects, the animation of which visualizes possible flows through the network. Model animation helps to experience the network behavior and allows us to test whether the model actually does behave in the desired manner (Koch and Monika, 2008). PNs can be used as both analysis and predictive tools. There exist many public-domain software tools such of as editors, animators, and analyzers. One of the nice features PN is its scalability to fit the constantly updated knowledge of systems biology. Any update to current knowledge can be easily implemented in the previous PN by simply modifying the relevant sub-structure of the PN without creating a completely new PN.

There are biological interpretations for most of the properties of a PN. For example, the reachability (see later in this section) of a marking from some other marking, in the PN model of a metabolic pathway, determines the possibility of formation of a specified set of product metabolites from another set of reactant metabolites, by some sequence of reactions which is dictated by the PN's firing sequence(s).

However, there are also some limitations and challenges in utilizing PNs; thus further efforts are required to overcome them. For example, at this time PNs are not designed to handle spatial events or spatial processes easily; the stochasticity in a PN is often "imposed," does not arise from biological or chemical interactions, and does not reproduce physical events that might be seen in a cell or bio-pathway. Data are important in PN validation and modeling improvement. However, data in biological pathways are diverse, grow fast, and have no unique standard to follow — integration is extremely challenging.

10.2.3   *Petri Net Dynamics*

PN dynamics include *reachability, coverability, liveness,* and *boundness.* They all relate to the initial marking. Reachability study concerns whether a marking under consideration can be reached from the initial marking; liveness study is to address if any transition will eventually be fired for the given initial marking, whereas boundness study is to investigate if the number of tokens at each place is bounded for any initial marking of the Petri net.

Recall that places can hold 0 or more tokens. The state of the system is represented by the distribution of tokens (markings) among the places. The initial marking is the initial allocation of tokens to places. A transition is said to be enabled if its input places contain at least the required number of tokens for its firing. The firing of an enabled transition will result in the consumption of tokens from the input places and production of tokens to the output places.

There are three different arc types in PNs: *weighted arc*: —>, *test arc*: <—>, *inhibitor arc*: —— ◯. Weighted arcs show how many tokens are consumed (if the arc points from a place to a transition) or created (if the arc points from a transition to a place). Test arcs connect places to transitions. No tokens are consumed by firing via a test arc. Inhibitor arcs check if the place has 0 tokens. If not, they disable the transition that they point to.

It is often interesting to know if a PN system will reach a specific (good or bad) state characterized by markings from a given initial marking M_0. This leads to the following definition.

Definition 10.4   Given the initial state M_0, the set of all possible states of a PN is called a reachability set and is denoted by $RS(M_0)$.

The purpose of a reachability study is to answer the following question: given a marking M, determine whether $M \in RS(M_0)$, i.e., check whether M is reachable via a firing sequence from the initial marking. It is obvious that for $M \in RS(M)$, and if $M' \to M''$ for some $t \in T, M' \in RS(M)$, then $M'' \in RS(M)$.

To visualize the $RS(M_0)$, we can draw all markings (if finite) and connect them using their associated transitions to form the reachability graph. A reachability graph of $PN = \langle P, T, F, W, M_0 \rangle$ is a rooted (at M_0), directed graph $G = \langle V, L, M_0 \rangle$, where $V = RS(M_0)$, $L = \{\langle M, t, M' \rangle \,|\, M, M' \in V \text{ and } M \to M'\}$.

A simple reachability graph is presented in Figure 10.3. The default weight is 1. The initial state is characterized by the initial marking $< 2, 1, 0, 0 >$. It's obvious that if t_1 is fired before t_2, t_3 can't be fired. This is often the case in biological systems. We will discuss timed PN later. Keep in mind that the total number of tokens in a PN is not always the same after a transition: some transition absorbs (produces) a net number of tokens.

To calculate the reachability graph, we can use Algorithm 10.1. The algorithm produces stack (or queue) E that contains pre-marking and post-marking that associate with every transition t and V that contains the

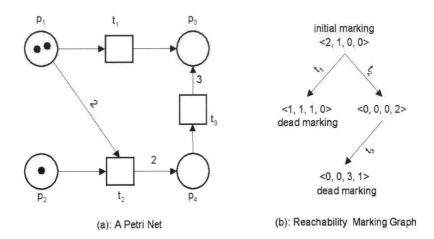

(a): A Petri Net   (b): Reachability Marking Graph

Figure 10.3:   Petri Net and Its Reachability Graph

sequence of markings associated with the transitions. v_0 is the initial marking vector M_0. RS(M) is the M-enabled set. The function fire(M, t) returns the post-markings M' based on the pre-markings M and the firing of the transition t. The function enabled(M) returns the enabled set of transitions by M.

Algorithm 10.1: Reachability Graph (P, T, F, W, M_0)
Objective: return reachability graph.
$< V, E, v_0 >:=< \{M_0\}, \emptyset, M_0 >$
workset $:= \{M_0\}$
While workset $\neq> \emptyset$:
     Select M from workset
     workset:=workset$\backslash\{M\}$
     For Each $t \in$ RS(M)
         $M' :=$fire($M, t_{(i)}$)
         If $M' \notin V$ **Then**
             $V := V \cup M'$
             workset:=workset $\cup \{M'\}$
         Endif
         $E := E \cup \langle M, t, M' \rangle$
     Endfor
Endwhile
Return $< V, E, v_0 >$

A reachability graph can be used to find a path: If M represents an error state, the firing sequence can be useful for debugging. If M is a desirable state, the shortest firing sequence to M is the optimal solution or fastest way to get the job done. Sometimes we want to check if the undesirable state M_U is reached before the desirable state M_D. This can be done by using a reachability graph or simulations. However, a reachability graph can't always be constructed because it can be infinitely large when there is a loop arc (test arc, bidirectional arc). In such a case, we have an approximate solution: coverability. Coverability has been studied using the coverability graph method.

Definition 10.5 Coverability: given a marking M, determine if there exists a reachable marking $M' \in RS(M_0)$ such that $M \le M'$; in other words, check whether a marking is reachable such that each place contains at least as many tokens as in M.

Let's introduce a new symbol ω to represent "arbitrarily many" tokens and extend the arithmetic on natural numbers with ω as follows. For all $n \in \mathbb{N}$, the arbitrarily many have the following properties:
$n + \omega = \omega + n = \omega$; $\omega + \omega = \omega$; $\omega - n = \omega$; $0 \cdot \omega = 0$; $\omega \cdot \omega = \omega$; $n \ge 1$ implies $n \cdot \omega = \omega \cdot n = \omega$; $n \le \omega$, and $\omega \in \omega$.

We also accordingly extend the notion of markings to ω-markings: in a ω-marking, each place p will either have $n \in \mathbb{N}$ tokens or ω tokens (infinitely many). The firing rule is as before. However, if a transition has a place with ω tokens in its preset, that place is considered to have sufficiently many tokens for the transition to fire, regardless of the arc weight. Also, if a place contains an ω-marking, then firing any transition connected with an arc to that place will not change its marking. An example of a coverability graph is presented in Figure 10.4.

Definition 10.6 Covering and Strictly Covering: An ω-marking M' covers an ω-marking M, denoted $M \le M'$, if and only if

$$\forall p \in P : M(p) \le M'(p).$$

Without an equal sign in the above equation, the ω-marking M' strictly covers the ω-marking M, denoted $M < M'$.

Let's now discuss the algorithm for coverability. The basic idea for constructing the coverability graph is to replace the marking M' with a marking for which all the places with increasing markings due to transitions are replaced by ω. The ω-marking replacement is accomplished using the function AddOmegas(M, t, M', V, E) in the following coverability algorithm

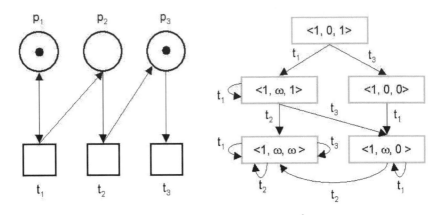

Figure 10.4:   PN with a Loop and Its Coverability Graph

(Algorithm 10.2). The rest of the steps in the algorithm are similar to reach-ability Algorithm 10.1.

Algorithm 10.2: Coverability Graph (P, T, F, W, M_0)
Objective: Return coverability graph.
$\langle V, E, v_0 \rangle := \langle \{M_0\}, \emptyset, M_0 \rangle$
workset $:= \{M_0\}$
While workset $\neq \emptyset$:
    Select M from workset
    workset:=workset$\backslash\{M\}$
    For Each $t \in \text{RS}(M)$
        $M' := \text{fire}(M, t_{(i)})$
        $M' := \text{AddOmegas}(M, t, M', V, E)$
        If $M' \notin V$ **Then**
            $V := V \cup M'$
            workset:=workset $\cup \{M'\}$
        Endfor
        $E := E \cup \langle M, t, M' \rangle$
    Endfor
Endwhile
Return $\langle V, E, v_0 \rangle$

The coverability graph is an approximation of the answer. When looking for 'bad' states, this analysis is conservative in the sense that bad states will not be missed, but when looking for a desired state, the analysis might be anti-conservative in the sense that the desired state may never be reached.

Reachability implies coverability, but coverability does not guarantee reachability.

Note that if the reachability graph is finite, the algorithm AddOmegas(M, t, M', V, E) will return M', i.e., the function has no effect and the coverability graph algorithm will return the reachability graph.

To prove the termination of coverability graph Algorithm 10.2, we need to use Dickson's lemma.

Lemma 10.1   *Dickson's lemma: Every infinite sequence $u_1, u_2, \ldots$ of n-tuples of natural numbers contains an infinite subsequence $u_{i_1} \leq u_{i_2} \leq u_{i_3} \leq \ldots$.*

Proof.   We will use mathematic induction.

For $n = 1$, let u_{i_1} be the smallest of $u_1, u_2, \ldots$, let u_{i_2} be the smallest of $u_{i_1+1}, u_{i_1+2}, \ldots$ etc. Thus the Lemma is true.

For $n > 1$, consider the projections $v_1, v_2, \ldots$ and $w_1, w_2, \ldots$ of $u_1, u_2, \ldots$ onto the first $n - 1$ components and the last component, respectively. By induction hypothesis, there is an infinite subsequence $v_{j_1} \leq v_{j_2} \leq v_{j_3} \leq \ldots$. Consider the infinite sequence $w_{j_1} \leq w_{j_2} \ldots$. By the induction hypothesis, this sequence has an infinite subsequence $w_{i_1} \leq w_{i_2} \ldots$. So we have $u_{i_1} \leq u_{i_2} \leq u_{i_3} \ldots$. $\qquad\square$

Theorem 10.1   *Theorem: The Coverability Graph Algorithm Terminates.*

Proof.   (Biining, Lettmann, and Mayr, 1988) Assume that the algorithm does not terminate. We derive a contradiction. If the algorithm does not terminate, then the coverability graph is infinite. Since every node of the graph has at most $|T|$ (the number of elements in T) successors, the graph contains an infinite path $\sqcap = M_1 M_2 \ldots$. If an ω-marking M_i satisfies $M_i(p) = \omega$ for some place p, then $M_{i+1}(p) = M_{i+2}(p) = \ldots = \omega$.

So $\sqcap$ contains an ω-marking M_j such that all markings $M_{j+1}, M_{j+2}, \ldots$ have ω's at exactly the same places as M_j. Let $\sqcap'$ be the suffix of $\sqcap$ starting at M_j. Consider the projection $\sqcap'' = m_j m_{j+1} \ldots$ of $\sqcap'$ onto the non-ω places. Let n be the number of non-ω places. $\sqcap''$ is an infinite sequence of distinct n-tuples of natural numbers.

By Dickson's lemma, this sequence contains markings M_k, M_l such that $k < l$ and $M_k \leq M_l$. This is a contradiction, because, since $M_k \neq M_l$, when executing AddOmegas(M_{l-1}, t, M_l, V, E) the algorithm adds at least one ω to M_{l-1}. $\qquad\square$

We now discuss two other important properties of Petri nets: boundness and liveness. Boundness can be used to check if there are enough resources available for operation of the networks.

Definition 10.7   Boundness: A PN is said to be bounded (or *k-safe*) if, in each place during the evolution of the net, the number of tokens will never exceed a finite number k, formally, if for all $M \in RS(M_0)$ and $p_i \in P$, there exists $k \in \mathbb{N}$ such that $m_i \leq k$, where m_i denotes the ith component of the marking vector M.

Liveness is often used to check if a desired state may not be reached because of a deadlock in the PN.

Definition 10.8   Liveness: A PN is called live if, starting from any reachable marking, any transition in the net can be fired, possibly after some further firings. Formally, for all $M \in RS(M_0)$ and $t_i \in T$, there exists $M_0 \in RS(M)$ such that t_i is enabled at M_0. A net has a deadlock (or dead state) if it is possible to reach a marking in which no transition is enabled.

A Petri net is nonlive if there exists at least one sequence of rings which leads to a dead marking (i.e., a marking for which no transition is enabled). This situation denotes the existence of steady states.

Often, we want to know if there is a deadlock, which usually indicates errors. Formally, a marking M of a $PN = \langle P, T, F, W, M_0 \rangle$ is called a deadlock if no transition $t \in T$ is enabled in M. A net PN is deadlock-free if no reachable marking is a deadlock. To check if there is a deadlock, inspect whether there is a vertex without an outgoing edge in the reachability graph.

10.2.4   *Petri Net Static Properties*

PN static (structural) properties include P-invariance (or S-invariance) and T-invariance. A P-invariant refers to a set of places for which the weighted sum of tokens is constant, independent of the sequence of firings. A T-invariance refers to a firing sequence that reproduces a marking, i.e., the firing sequence starting from a marking to reproduce the same marking. Both properties are only dependent on the net topology (independent of initial marking) and they can be generally studied through the incidence matrix of the net. P-invariance and T-invariance can be used to check the validity of the PN. However they are necessary but not sufficient conditions of a valid PN.

The incidence matrix and state equation of PN are important in studying the structure properties of the net.

Definition 10.9   State Equation: Let $PN = (P, T, F, W, M_0)$ be a Petri net. The state equation defines the transition firing rules:

$$M = M_0 + A^T U \tag{10.5}$$

where the $N \times K$ incidence matrix A has component $a_{tp} = W_O(t, p) - W_I(p, t)$, and U is the firing vector of N elements.

We can see that the state equation defines the firing rule globally for the whole PN, whereas in Definition 10.3, we define the firing rule based on individual place p.

If a place p (e.g., representing an enzyme) and transition t are connected by two oppositely directed arcs (loop), the firing of transition t removes the token in place p and restores it afterwards. In the absence of the loop, the Petri net is said to be pure and its incidence matrix A fully describes its topology.

From the state equation, we can prove that decomposition of firing vector $U = U_1 + U_2$ will lead to

$$M = M_0 + A^T U = M_0 + A^T (U_1 + U_2) = M_0 + A^T (U_1) + A^T (U_2).$$

In other words, the effect of a firing sequence is additive.

Example 10.3: Given

$$M_0 = \begin{bmatrix} 1 \\ 1 \\ 0 \end{bmatrix}, \ U = \begin{bmatrix} 1 \\ 0 \\ 1 \\ 0 \end{bmatrix}, U_1 = \begin{bmatrix} 1 \\ 0 \\ 0 \\ 0 \end{bmatrix}, U_2 = \begin{bmatrix} 0 \\ 0 \\ 1 \\ 0 \end{bmatrix},$$

$$W_I = \begin{bmatrix} 1 & 0 & 0 \\ 1 & 0 & 0 \\ 0 & 2 & 1 \\ 0 & 0 & 1 \end{bmatrix}, \ \text{and } W_O = \begin{bmatrix} 1 & 0 & 2 & 0 \\ 0 & 0 & 0 & 1 \\ 0 & 1 & 0 & 0 \end{bmatrix},$$

we can calculate the incidence matrix as

$$A = W_O^T - W_I = \begin{bmatrix} 0 & 0 & 0 \\ 1 & 0 & -1 \\ -2 & 2 & 1 \\ 0 & -1 & 1 \end{bmatrix}.$$

Based on this incidence matrix A, the post-marking can be calculated as follows:

$$M_1 = M_0 + A^T U = \begin{bmatrix} -1 \\ 3 \\ 1 \end{bmatrix} = M_0 + A^T (U_1 + U_2).$$

Definition 10.10   T-invariant: a T-invariant of a PN is an N-dimensional vector X that satisfies:

$$A^T X = 0, \ X \neq 0, \ x_i \in \mathbb{N}, \tag{10.6}$$

where A^T denotes the transposed incidence matrix.

The existence of a T-invariant implies that the system can potentially recycle on M. However, starting from a generic state, we can't guarantee that there will be a firing sequence that allows the PN to recycle.

If X is a T-invariant representing a firing sequence, then the following holds:

$$M = M_0 + A^T X = M_0. \tag{10.7}$$

In other words, the firing sequence X doesn't change the marking M, i.e., invariant. Therefore, the result can also be explained as: each component x_i of T-invariance X represents the number of times (not necessarily the minimum required) that a transition should fire to take the net from a state M back to state M itself (recycling).

Definition 10.11   The support of a T-invariant X is the set of transitions corresponding to nonzero entries of X and is denoted by $\|X\|$. A T-invariant X is minimal if there is not any other T-invariant X' such that $x_i' \leq x_i$ for all $i = 1, ..., N$. A support is minimal if no proper nonempty subset of the support is also a support of a T-invariant. The minimal support T-invariant is the unique minimal T-invariant corresponding to a minimal support.

The second structure property of PNs we are going to discuss is place-invariance or P-invariance.

Definition 10.12   P-invariant or S-invariant: Let $PN = (P, T, F, W, M_0)$ be a Petri net with an $N \times K$ incidence matrix A. A P-invariant is a K-dimensional vector which can be calculated as a solution of the following equation:

$$AY = 0. \tag{10.8}$$

If a P-invariant $Y = (y_1, ..., y_K)$ with all positive components exists, then the net is called conservative since the weighted sum of the tokens remains constant during the evolution of the net, i.e., it is constant for each marking of its reachability set:

$$M \in RS(M_0) \Rightarrow \sum_{i=1}^{K} y_i m_i = c, \tag{10.9}$$

where c is a constant.

Let M be marking reachable with a transition sequence whose firing count is expressed by U, i.e., $M = M_0 + AU$. Let Y be a P-invariant. Then, the following holds:

$$M^T Y = (M_0 + A^T U)^T Y = M_0^T Y + U^T (AY) = M_0^T Y = \sum_{i=1}^{K} y_i m_i = c.$$

In other words, the "product" of marking by Y is unchanged (invariant). The property can be used to check the validity of a PN.

Note that multiplying an invariant by a constant or component-wise addition of two invariants will again yield a P-invariant. That is, the set of all invariants is a vector space. Another important point is when there are test arcs that cancel each other out in the incidence matrix, the incidence matrix can be used to show that a marking M is unreachable if $M_0 + A^T U = M$ has no natural solution for U. However, a solution of U does not ensure the marking is reachable.

The support of an S-invariant is the set of places whose token count does not change with any firing sequence. The support of an S-invariant is analogous to the set of pathways that do not undergo any net change in the course of a biotransformation. The supports to T-invariants give an insight into the direct mechanisms which are necessary to form a cyclic pathway (Reddy et al., 1993).

There are different algorithms for calculating the p-invariants. The Farkas algorithm (Farkas, 1902) can be used to compute a set of so-called minimal P-invariants. These are positive place invariants from which any other positive invariant can be computed by a linear combination.

The Farkas algorithm is an iteration/recursive process. Let $B = (A|I)$ denote the augmentation of the $N \times K$ incidence matrix A (N transitions and K places) by an $N \times N$ identity matrix I at the last N columns and denote B_i the ith iteration of matrix B. Denote gcd greatest common divider.

Algorithm P-invarince (Farkas, 1902)

Objective: Compute P-invariance

$B_0 := (A|I)$

For $i := 1$ To N

    For each pair of rows $(b_1, b_2) \in B_{i-1}$ where $b_1 b_2 < 0$

        $b := |b2(i)| \cdot b1 + |b1(i)| \cdot b2;$ (* b(i) = 0 *)

        $\tilde{b} := b / \gcd(b(1), b(2), ..., b(N+K))$

        Augment B_{i-1} with $\tilde{d}$ as last row

    EndFor

Delete all rows of B_{i-1} whose i^{th} component is different from 0, the result is B_i

EndFor

Delete the first N columns of B_N

Return B_N

10.3   Biological Pathway Simulation

10.3.1   *Introduction*

In this section, we discuss the standard Petri net, its extensions, and their applications in biological networks or pathway simulations. The first step in simulation using a PN is to determine the abstract level and then choose the places and transitions accordingly. To determine the abstract level, we should start with the biological questions to be addressed, the applicability of the method, and the nature and quality of available data. The simulation can be performed stagewise with progressive abstract levels. There are three commonly used abstract levels: (1) molecular level: biochemical network, (2) gene cross-regulation level: genetic network, and (3) tissue level: intercellular network, in which the biological cells are believed to operate with a steady state of the internal metabolites. Note that the same compound can be presented using multiple places in the same network if they play different biological roles.

Large Petri nets can be reduced by the substitution of certain combinations of places and transitions with smaller units without sacrificing the original properties of the net. This is particularly useful because metabolic pathways are complex networks and any concession in the structure leads to a simpler analysis (Reddy et al., 1993).

The first applications of Petri nets in biological networks were published in the 1990s (Reddy et al., 1993; Hofestädt, 1994; Reddy, 1994). Since then Petri nets have been used to model a wide range of biological processes, including qualitative modeling of apoptosis (Heiner et al., 2004), iron homeostasis and the yeast mating response (Sackmann et al., 2006), modeling and biomedical profiling of metabolic disorders (Chen and Hofestädt, 2006), building a hybrid Petri net that qualitatively modeled metabolite levels, transcription factor activity, and signaling pathway changes (Chen and Hofestädt, 2006), and modeling biological regulatory networks (Chaouiya et al., 2008). PNs have been used successfully for modeling various biological pathways, including metabolic networks (Matsuno et al., 2003; Koch et al., 2005; Oliveira et al., 2003; Voss et al., 2003), signal transduction networks (Heiner et al., 2004; Matsuno et al., 2003; Sackmann et al., 2006), gene regulatory networks (Srivastava, 2001; Matsuno et al., 2003; Steggles, 2006), and combinations of them (Chen and Hofestädt, 2003, Marwan et al., 2005; Matsuno et al., 2003; Simao et al., 2005).

The Petri net structure can mimic the biochemical topology, and dynamics produced by the repeated firing of transitions can model partial order sequences of chemical reactions (i.e., some reactions must occur in a certain sequence, others can occur concurrently in the network). The four basic structures of biological Petri nets are logic OR, logical AND, activator, and inhibitor (Figure 10.5).

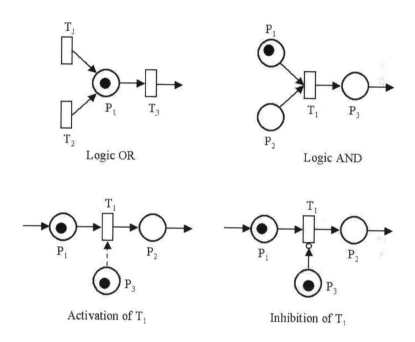

Figure 10.5: Elemental Nets in PNs for Biological Pathways

Different Petri nets have been applied to metabolic, signal transduction, and gene regulatory pathways. The main difference in modeling the three pathways with a PN is that metabolic networks are related to substance flows (mass flows, continuous values), which are determined by the stoichiometry of the underlying chemical reaction equations. The arc weights correspond to the stoichiometric factors. In signaling networks, the signal flow is realized by activation and deactivation (binary values) of proteins or protein complexes building signal cascades without stoichiometry (Figure 10.6). Thus an arc weight of one is usually used in the PN (Koch and Heiner, 2008).

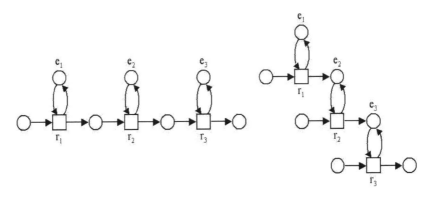

Figure 10.6:   Essential Difference Between Metabolite Networks (left) and Signal Transduction Networks (right) (Source: Koch and Heiner, 2008)

10.3.2   *Modeling of Metabolic Networks*

A metabolic pathway is a series of enzymatic reactions consuming certain metabolites and producing others. These metabolites usually participate in more than one metabolic pathway, forming a complex network of reactions.

S-transformation of a biochemical reaction (Figure 10.7) can be modeled using PNs, in which (1) places can be metabolites, reactants, products, genes, cells, enzymes, (2) transitions can be reactions, catalysis, activation, inhibition, and (3) weighted arcs can be stoichiometries. The pathway for glycolysis, which generates high-energy molecules, ATP and NADH, is illustrated in Figure 10.7.

Stoichiometric Analysis of Metabolic Networks (Structural Analysis):

Stoichiometry is the calculation of quantitative (measurable) relationships of reactants and products of chemicals based on the law of conservation of mass (elements), the law of constant composition, and the law of multiple proportions. In general, chemical reactions combine in definite ratios of chemicals. Stoichiometry is often used to balance chemical equations. For example, the two diatomic gases, hydrogen and oxygen, can combine

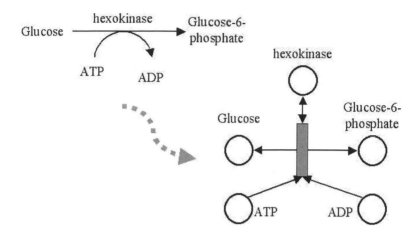

Figure 10.7:   S-Transformation of a Biochemical Reaction

to form a liquid, water, in an exothermic reaction, as described by the following equation:

$$2H_2 + O_2 \rightarrow 2H_2O. \tag{10.10}$$

Stoichiometry concerns the reaction directionality, i.e., reversible or irreversible reaction, catalyzing enzymes (e.g., hexokinase), but the dynamics (time) are neglected.

For the example shown in Figure 10.7, hexokinase is the name of the enzyme (protein) that catalyzes the first reaction in the glycolysis pathway. The reaction involves transferring a phosphate group from adenosine triphosphate (ATP) to glucose to produce glucose-6-phosphate and adenosine diphosphate (ADP).

Let K be the number of metabolites, N the number of reactions, and A the $(N \times K)$ stoichiometric matrix (element a_{ij} = stoichiometric coefficient of i in reaction j).

$$\frac{dC(t)}{dt} = AR(t), \tag{10.11}$$

where K-dimensional vector $C(t)$ = vector of current metabolite concentrations, N-dimensional vector $R(t)$ = a flux vector. Note that the stoichiometric matrix A corresponds to the incidence matrix in PN representation.

At the steady state, metabolite concentrations C and reaction rates are constant, i.e.,

$$\frac{dC(t)}{dt} = AR(t) = 0. \tag{10.12}$$

Clearly, the flux vector $R(t)$ corresponds to T-invariants in the PN with incidence matrix A.

The law of conservation of mass can be stated as the weighted sums of metabolite concentrations, which remain constant in the system because of

$$A^T C = 0. \tag{10.13}$$

A simple biological example of T-invariants is ADP+ATP = constant in a normal cell.

Most of the reactions in a pathway are reversible. When the reaction is reversible, the PN cannot be fully determined by the incidence matrix A. In other words, A is not a full-ranked matrix and most T-invariants of the net are not useful/meaningful — just reflect the cell keeps looping in producing and destroying the same substance.

Glycolysis features excellent examples of the problem of reaction reversibility: (1) As glucose enters a cell it is immediately phosphorylated by ATP to glucose-6-phosphate in the irreversible first step. This is to prevent the glucose from leaving the cell. (2) In times of excess lipid or protein energy sources glycolysis may run in reverse (gluconeogenesis) in order to produce glucose-6-phosphate for storage as glycogen or starch (Marin, 2006).

Definition 10.13 Reversibility: A Petri net is reversible, if the initial marking can be reached again from each reachable marking.

An irreversible system can behave predictably, such as burning out or accumulation of certain compounds. Most metabolic pathways are not literally reversible, due to the thermodynamic reversibility of many reactions. However, an alternate set of reactions may reproduce the precursor metabolites. This constitutes a regulatory function which can shift the metabolism in either direction, with the aid of pertinent enzymes, depending on the need for the compounds (Reddy et al., 1993).

Case Study 10.1: Petri Net for a Metabolic Pathway

Koch et al. (2005) investigated the metabolic network concerning the main carbon metabolism in potato (*Solanum tuberosum*) tubers. The conversion of sucrose through hexose phosphates to starch is the major flux in potato tuber metabolism, in which enzymatic reactions are well characterized.

They developed an unbounded Petri net (Figure 10.8) which is not ordinary, not homogenous, and not conservative. It is pure, but not static conflict free. The Petri net includes 17 places and 25 transitions describing the main carbon metabolism in potato tubers. The Petri net represents an open system or unbounded model.

The reachability graph in the PN is unbounded because of the test arcs. Computation of the coverability graph was also not successful because of the huge amount of possible states. Therefore, they constructed a smaller and bounded net version by summarizing the hexoses into one place, in which the set of reachable states consists of more than 10^{10} states. Based on this reachability set, they studied the liveness and reversibility for the bounded model.

The three minimal p-invariants were identified. Two of them comprise the metabolites containing uridine and adenosine residues, respectively. As the synthesis and degradation of nucleotides was not included in the model, and the sum of these metabolites is not variable, which is likely to reflect the actual biological system behavior. The turnover in utilization and regeneration of adenylates as energy donors is much higher than its biosynthesis and degradation. The third invariant represents the set of all compounds, which provide directly or indirectly a phosphate group. If the phosphate group is transferred from one compound to another, the sum of the phosphorylated metabolites is unchanged. If no phosphate is taken up or secreted by a cell, the sum of phosphate groups in all metabolites, including the inorganic phosphate itself, will not change (Koch et al., 2005). Among 19 minimal T-invariants, 7 of them are trivial ones because they reflect reversible reactions and 12 are nontrivial T-invariants representing biologically meaningful subnetworks for the different possibilities of sucrose breakdown through invertase or sucrose synthase producing hexoses, which further result in starch production, glycolysis, ATP consumption, and also futile cycles. In the model, they also identified a transition, involved only in a trivial T-invariant, which means that this transition has no effect in the steady state and deletion of this transition will not affect steady state behavior.

10.3.3 *PN for a Signal Transduction Pathway*

Case Study 10.2: PN for a Signal Transduction Pathway

Apoptosis is the process of programmed cell death in organisms. Programmed cell death involves a series of biochemical events leading to a characteristic cell morphology and death. Apoptosis confers advantages during an organism's life cycle. For example, the differentiation of fingers and toes in a developing human embryo occurs because cells between the fingers apoptose. About 60 billion cells die each day due to apoptosis in the av-

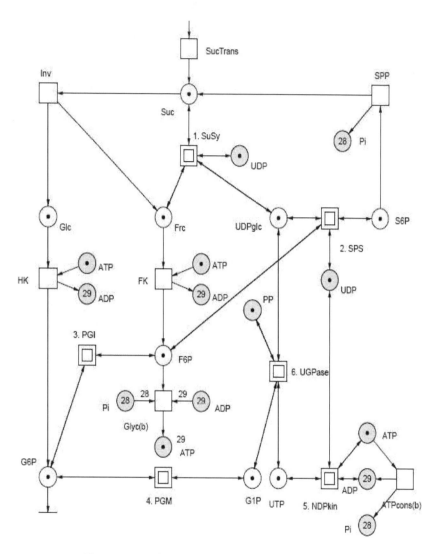

Figure 10.8:   *Solanum Tuberosum* Metabolic Network
(Source: Koch et al., 2005)

erage human adult. Defective apoptotic processes have been implicated in an extensive variety of diseases: If a cell is unable to undergo apoptosis because of mutation or biochemical inhibition, it continues to divide and develop into a tumor. Apoptosis also plays an important role during neural development. It is estimated that at least half of the original cell population is removed as a result of apoptosis during the development of the nervous system. Neurodegenerative diseases (e.g., Alzheimer's, Huntington's, and Parkinson's disease) often exhibit disturbances in apoptosis or its regulation (Heiner et al., 2004).

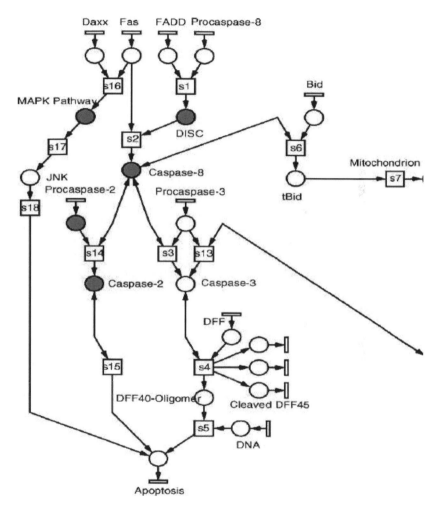

Figure 10.9:   Petri Net of Apoptosis Induced by Fas Receptor
and Intrinsic Apoptotic Stimuli
(Source: Heiner et al., 2004)

Heiner et al. (2004) developed a PN model for signal transduction in apoptosis. In their model (Figure 10.9), apoptosis inhibitors are excluded from the system or considered as the system environment. The tokens for all input nodes are generated by input transitions (source nodes, having no predecessors), whereas the tokens of all output places are consumed by output transitions (sink nodes, having no successor nodes). The input and output nodes are drawn as flat hollow bars in Figure 10.9. The list of the abbreviations in the figure can be found in the appendix of their paper.

Note that the computation of T-invariants requires only structural reasoning; the state space need not be generated. Analysis of the PN leads to the following results.

There are two receptors (Fas, TNFR-1) and three basic apoptotic pathways per receptor (caspase-8, JNK, caspase-2) as well as an apoptotic stimuli-induced pathway in the model. Altogether, there are ten T-invariants, excluding the sources and sinks for simplicity. This case study confirms that Petri net based model validation with the focus on T-invariant analysis can also be applied to a signal transduction pathway.

10.3.4   *Stochastic PN for Regulatory Pathways*

Case Study 10.3: Stochastic PN for Regulatory Pathways

Regulation of gene expression (or gene regulation) includes the processes (amount and timing) turning the information in genes into gene products (RNA or protein). The majority of known mechanisms regulate protein coding genes. Any step of the gene's expression may be modulated, from DNA-RNA transcription to the post-translational modification of a protein. The stages where gene expression is regulated are chromatin domains, transcription, post-transcriptional modification, RNA transport, translation, mRNA degradation, and post-translational modifications. Gene regulation is essential for viruses, prokaryotes, and eukaryotes as it increases the versatility and adaptability of an organism by allowing the cell to express protein when needed. The first example of a gene regulation system discovered (by Jacques Monod) was the lac operon, in which protein involved in lactose metabolism is expressed by *E. coli* only in the presence of lactose and the absence of glucose.

The kinetics or the speed of reactions is not reflected in a standard PN. The reaction speed may rely on sufficient substance present in a cell. There are random variabilities in the data, environmental noise, and intrinsic noise. Also, the actual network states are dependent on the firing sequence and timing of the firing associated with each transition. All these are not considered in the standard PN. Thus there is need for PN model extension. We will discuss two forms of extensions, i.e., stochastic PN (SPN) and hybrid PN (HPN). Keep in mind that at any given moment t, stochas-

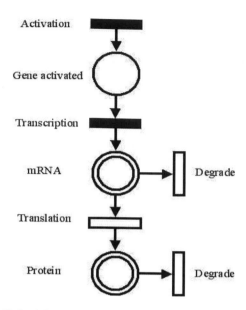

Figure 10.10: Hybrid Petri Nets: Simplified Gene Regulation Model. Gene is activated, activation is "consumed" by producing mRNA, protein is produced depending on mRNA concentration, both mRNA and protein degrade over time.

tic NP (SPN) can be analyzed the same way as static PN. Thus theory for the standard PN can be applied.

Marwan et al. (2005) studied SPN for the regulatory network controlling commitment and sporulation in *Physarum polycephalum* using SPN modeling and simulation. *P. polycephalum* is typically yellow in color, and eats fungal spores, bacteria, and other microbes. *P. polycephalum* is one of the easiest eukaryotic microbes to grow in culture, and has been used as a model organism. *Plasmodium* is a genus of parasitic protozoa. Of the over 200 known species of *Plasmodium*, at least 10 species infect humans (Wikipedia.com, June, 10, 2009).

Marwan et al. (2005) modeled the regulatory network controlling commitment and sporulation of *P. polycephalum* using a hierarchical stochastic Petri net and experimental results. The stochastic Petri net describes the structure and simulates the dynamics of the molecular network as analyzed by genetic, biochemical, and physiological experiments within a single coherent model.

Commitment of *P. polycephalum* plasmodia to sporulation is tightly regulated by environmental conditions and can be experimentally triggered by exposing a starving plasmodium to a few minutes, pulse of visible light.

After the inductive pulse, it takes several hours until the plasmodial cell suddenly becomes committed and several hours later a cascade of differentially regulated genes is triggered and morphogenesis of the fruiting bodies and the spores contained therein follows (Marwan et al., 2005)

In the stochastic Petri net model, the probability of firing is p that associates the first order rate constant k of a monomolecular reaction. Firing occurs if the generated (from $U(0,1)$) random number is less than or equal to p. Visible light or heat shock only induce sporulation in *P. polycephalum* if plasmodia are starved for glucose. This mechanism is modeled using the model in Figure 10.11. The presence or absence of glucose as well as the physiological states (fed or starved) are represented as places. Marwan et al. then combined the Petri net of glucose consumption and starvation using the logic elements shown in Figure 10.11 into a model that can control sporulation by light and starvation (see Marwan et al., 2005 for details). The Petri net for modeling time-resolved somatic complementation experiments fulfills three requirements: (1) the activity of transitions that represent a gene-dependent step should depend on the presence of the respective gene product; (2) the flow of signaling intermediates and of gene products between the two halves of a fused plasmodial cell should be accounted for by linking the corresponding places of the two Petri nets by transitions, which are disabled until the moment of fusion; (3) the flow of tokens must have a time basis in order to allow kinetic analyses (Marwan et al., 2005). The effects of time to starvation and delay time on sporulated plasmodia were studied as well as other behaviors of the PN.

10.3.5   *Hybrid PN for Regulatory Pathways*

Case Study 10.4: Hybrid PN for Regulatory Pathways

In many cases, molecular concentration is considered as continuous rather than discrete. How do we deal with actual molecule numbers? If we represent each molecule by one token, it is not feasible for simulations; if one token stands for, e.g., 1 mol of a substance, it might be not accurate enough. The solution is to allow continuous values for certain places, which leads to so-called hybrid Petri nets (HPN). The basic elements in HPN are presented in Figure 10.12.

An HPN can have continuous and discrete tokens in places. Discrete places have tokens, whereas continuous places contain real variables. Discrete transitions fire after a certain delay. Continuous transitions fire continuously at a given rate.

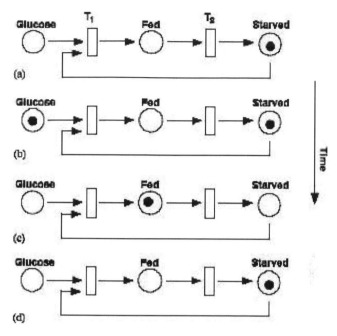

Figure 10.11:   Glucose Consumption and Starvation of a *Physarum plasmodium*
Represented by a Petri Net
(Source: Marwan et al., 2005)

Chen and Hofestädt (2003) conducted a case study on the urea cycle disorder, a genetic disease caused by a deficiency of one enzyme in the urea cycle which is responsible for removing ammonia from the bloodstream. In urea cycle disorders, nitrogen, a metabolic waste product, is not removed from the body. Ammonia then reaches the brain through the blood, where it causes irreversible brain damage, coma, and/or death.

Metabolic behavior is modeled using continuous places and transitions, whereas gene regulations are modeled by discrete net elements. Regulation of both genomic and metabolic levels can be simulated. A generalization of hybrid Petri nets (hybrid function Petri nets) was developed by Matsuno et al. (2003). Typical examples they studied include a metabolic pathway (glycolysis) and a signaling pathway (Fas ligand induced apoptosis). The effectiveness of PN based biopathway modeling was demonstrated in the circadian rhythm *Drosophila* and apoptosis induced by Fas ligand. The simulations of these models were performed with the software tool Genomic Object Net.

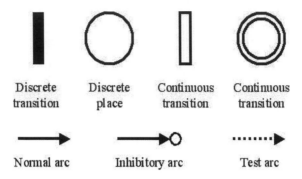

Figure 10.12:   Symbols in HPN

10.3.6   *General Stochastic PN and Algorithm*

Definition 10.14   A general stochastic Petri net (GSPN) is a tuple defined as: GSPN $= (P, T, I(\cdot, \cdot), O(\cdot, \cdot), F(\cdot, \cdot), M_0)$, where:

- $P = \{p_1, ... p_M\}$ is the set of M places;
- $T = \{t_1, ... t_N\}$ is the set of N transitions (both immediate and timed), with $P \cap T = \emptyset$ and $P \cup T \neq \emptyset$;
- $W_I(p_i, t_j) : P \times T \to \mathbb{N}$ is the input function, defining weighted arcs between places and transitions, where $1 \leq i \leq M, 1 \leq j \leq N$;
- $W_O(t_i, p_j) : T \times P \to \mathbb{N}$ is the input function, defining weighted arcs between transitions and places, where $1 \leq i \leq N, 1 \leq j \leq M$;
- $F(S, S', \tau) : P \times P \times t \to \Re$ is the transition rule defining the transition between two states at time τ;
- $M_0 = \{m_{01}, ..., m_{0M}\} \in \mathbb{N}^M$ represents the initial state of GSPN, i.e., the number of tokens in each place at the initial state.

To implement the general stochastic PN, we can use object-oriented programming (OOP). OOP is a programming paradigm based on the concept of "objects." An object-oriented program may be viewed as a collection of objects that work together as a team: each object is capable of certain tasks such as receiving messages, processing messages, and sending messages to other objects. Each of these objects can be viewed as an independent 'machine' with a distinct role or responsibilities. In OOP, a generic version (class) of an object is created first and stored in an object library. The actual objects of this type (class) can be instantiated as many as necessary at running time.

A class usually includes (static) properties to indicate the current state of an object and (dynamic) behaviors or methods to determine how the object responds (output) once it receives an input (stimuli). A main advantage of OOP is the reusability of the code: a class doesn't have to be created from scratch. Instead, the inheritance capability allows one to use all the features of a parent object (class) using a single line of code and then modify or enhance the inherited object. An important OOP feature that is often used in biological pathways is the capability of event awareness — the object can fire events and recognize events fired by others automatically. This feature is available for any OOP language with the capabilities of timing (synchronization and asynchronization) and multiple threads. There are many OOP languages available such as Java, Ruby, C#, Visual Basic.net, etc. A typical structure of class in OOP is presented below with the class name BioPnLet that is inherited from the parent class PnLet.

Class BioPnLet inherited PnLet;

{

Property A

Property B

.....

Method A { ...... }

Method B { ...... }

......

Event A { ...... }

Event B { ...... }

......

Event_Listener { ...... }

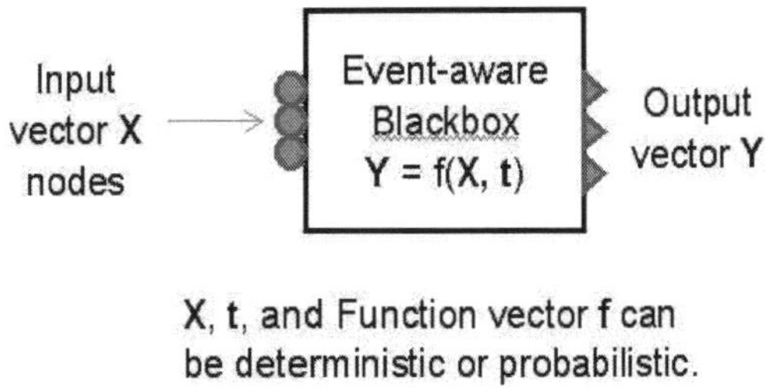

}

Figure 10.13:   Event-Aware Object in OOP General Networks

The OOP can have visual objects. In fact, most simulation software in biology has visual objects. The event-aware object can fire the events automatically, e.g., output a value (rate) over a duration of time (continuously or discretely). This can be easily accomplished using visual simulation software such as ExtendSim^{TM} or using the built-in timer object in VB.net.

Figure 10.13 is a visual representation of the event-aware BioPnLet class. The BioPnLet object can detect any environmental changes and take input vector X, process it, and output resulting vector Y. The outputs are determined by the current states Z (properties) of the object, current inputs X, current time t, and the vector-valued function (reflecting the biological mechanisms) $f(Z, Y, t)$. Note that $f(Z, Y, t)$ for BioPnLet can be very simple, but a PN as a collection of simple BioPnLets can be very complicated, particularly when $f(Z, Y, t)$ is a probabilistic function.

With this BioPnLet, we can build PNs for complicated biological pathways, and properties such as coverability and reachability graphs can be constructed over time using simulations. Practically, if a state can not be reached for a very long time in the simulation, it can be considered as non-reachable. A PN with event-aware objects can be considered as an agent-based model.

Validation of the simulation software is important. The strategy can be a stagewise approach: develop and validate lower level modules first; simplify them using a property analysis and other methods such as genetic programming; then move up to the next level, and so on. There are also dozens of fast growing software products available. See http://systems-biology.org/software/simulation/ for such a list.

10.4   Summary

A biological pathway is a molecular interaction network in biological processes. Pathways can be classified into the fundamental categories metabolic, regulatory, and signal transduction pathways. There are about 10,000 pathways, nearly 160 pathways involving 800 reactions.

Commonly used methods for biological pathway modeling and simulation include differential equation systems, cellular automata, agent-based models, and network models. The traditional differential equation systems for biological pathways can be solved using Monte Carlo method as illustrated in Chapter 1.

Cellular automata are a class of simple computer simulation methods used to model both temporal and spatiotemporal processes. Cellular automata normally consist of large numbers of identical cells that form a lattice or drift with defined interaction rules. The aggregative behavior of the individual rules of each cell can be complicated enough to model the complex biological system.

In an agent-based model of a biological system, agents represent biological entities (molecule/drug, gene, cell, metabolites, proteins, tissue, organ, body, human ecosystem, etc.). The term "agent" is used to indicate a "conscious" computer program entity with potential learning capabilities, which is characterized by some degree of autonomy and asynchrony with regard to its interactions with other agents and its environment.

Biological and disease pathways or networks can be modeled using mathematical networks such as Bayesian networks, artificial networks, and Petri nets (PN).

Biological pathways are extremely complicated and it is difficult to understand the mechanics. Using a Petri net, we can have a coherent presentation of the very diverse forms of information and solve the problem by means of computer simulation. A Petri net offers a general framework for analyzing the dynamic properties of large systems.The mathematical properties of standard Petri nets are well studied, which can be used for model validations. One of the nice features with PN is its scalability to fit the constantly updated knowledge of systems biology. Any update to current knowledge can be easily implemented in the previous PN by simply modifying the relevant substructure of the PN without recreating a completely new PN.

The first step in simulation using a PN is to determine the abstract level; then choose the places and transitions accordingly. To determine the abstract level, we should start with the biological questions to be addressed, the applicability of the method, and the nature and quality of available data. The simulation can be performed stepwise with progressive abstract levels. There are three commonly used abstract levels to model: (1) molecular level modeled by a biochemical network, (2) gene cross-regulation level modeled by a genetic network, and (3) tissue level modeled by an intercellular network.

To reduce the complexity and computational burden, large Petri nets can be reduced by the substitution of certain combinations of places and transitions with smaller units without sacrificing the original properties of the net.

Different Petri nets have been applied to metabolic, signal transduction, and gene regulatory pathways. The main difference in modeling the three pathways with PN is that metabolic networks are related to substance flows (mass flows, continuous values), which are determined by the stoichiometry of the underlying chemical reaction equations. The arc weights correspond to the stoichiometric factors. In signaling networks, the signal flow is realized by activation and deactivation (binary values) of proteins or protein complexes building signal cascades without stoichiometry.

The topological and dynamic properties of a PN, such as reachability, coverability, liveness, boundness, P-invariance, and T-invariance, are important in biological pathway simulations. These terms have meaningful biological interpretations (Exercise 10.2).

10.5   Exercises

Exercise 10.1: What is a metabolic pathway, a gene regulatory pathway, and a signal transduction pathway?

Exercise 10.2: Give mathematical definitions and biological interpretations of terms in a Petri net: reachability, coverability, liveness, boundness, P-invariance, and T-invariance.

Exercise 10.3: What is the usefulness of the state equation of a PN?

Exercise 10.4: What are the different types of arcs in Petri nets?

Exercise 10.5: Compute the reachability marking graph for the PN in Figure 10.14.

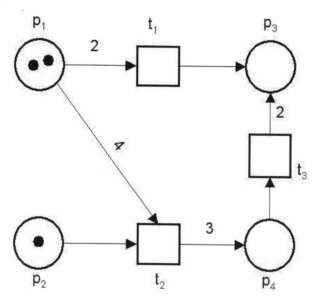

Figure 10.14:   A Petri Net

Exercise 10.6: Compute the coverability graph for the PN in Figure 10.14.

Exercise 10.7: Construct the incidence matrix A for the PN in Figure 10.14 and find a T-invariance and a P-invariance.

Exercise 10.8: Implement Algorithms 10.1 and 10.2.

Chapter 11

Pharmacokinetic Simulation

This chapter will cover the following topics:

- ADME
- Absorption Modeling
- Distribution Modeling
- Metabolism Modeling
- Excretion Modeling
- Physiologically Based PK Model

11.1 Overview of ADME

As pointed out by Shargel et al. (2005), the objectives of pharmacokinetic modeling and simulation are to:

(1) Predict plasma, tissue, and urine drug levels with any dosage regimen
(2) Calculate the optimum dosage regimen for each patient individually
(3) Estimate the possible accumulation of drugs and/or metabolites
(4) Correlate drug concentrations with pharmacologic/toxicologic activity
(5) Evaluate differences in the rate or extent of availability between formulations (bioequivalence)
(6) Describe how changes in physiology or disease affect the absorption, distribution, or elimination of the drug
(7) Explain drug interactions

As we discussed in Chapter 9, for a drug to interact with a target, it is necessary for the drug to present a sufficient concentration in the fluid medium surrounding the cells with receptors. Pharmacokinetics is the study of the kinetics of absorption, distribution, metabolism, and excretion (ADME) of a drug. It analyzes the way the human body works with a drug after it has been administered, and the transportation of the drug to the specific site for the drug-receptor interaction.

In what follows, we will discuss the ADME mechanisms to guide our PK modeling and simulation. There are two schools of modeling and simulation approaches. One is to directly model the complex ADME, treating the whole body as one entity — the macro-approach. The mixed effect population PK model is an example of this type of statistical modeling. There are nearly 100 commercial software products available (see, e.g., www.boomer.org/pkin/soft.html for such a list) for this type of modeling and most PK specialists are familiar with the approach and software. I am not going to discuss this approach. Alternatively, we can use low-level modeling, which either models the four components of ADME separately or models the mechanisms at the organ level such as the physiologically based model; then integrated the low level components into an integrated model. The integration is accomplished through simulation and will be discussed extensively in this chapter.

11.2   Absorption Modeling

The systemic absorption of a drug is dependent on (1) the dosage form, (2) the physicochemical properties of the drug, (3) the nature of the drug product, and (4) the anatomy and physiology of the drug absorption site. All of these are important to consider in the manufacture and biopharmaceutic evaluation of drug products. Proper drug product selection requires a thorough understanding of the physiologic and pathologic factors affecting drug absorption to assure therapeutic efficacy and to avoid potential drug–drug and drug-nutrient interactions (Macheras and Iliadis, 2006; Shargel et al., 2005).

A drug in the body experiences complicated processes: moving between tissues and fluids, binding with plasma or cellular components, or being metabolized. The biological nature of drug distribution and disposition is complex, and drug events often intervene. Statistical and Monte Carlo simulations are useful in handling the inherent and infinite complexity of these events and predicting the time course of drug efficacy for a given dose — simulating the rate processes of drug absorption, distribution, and elimination to describe and predict drug concentrations in the body as a function of time.

Drug absorption will be affected by the dose and route of drug administration (the site, form, rate, and duration of drug administration). There are several routes for administering drugs, including oral, intravenous, buccal, sublingual, rectal, subcutaneous, intramuscular, transdermal, topical, nasal, and inhalational. All the routes of administration, with the exception of intravenous, require the drug to be absorbed before it can enter the bloodstream for distribution to target sites (Figure 11.1).

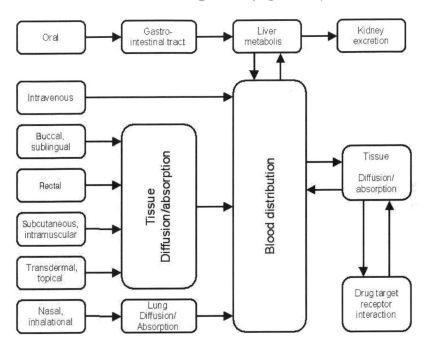

Figure 11.1: Drug Administration (Adapted from Ng, 2005)

11.2.1 *Formulations and Delivery Systems*

The ADME process means that most drugs have tortuous paths to reach their targets after they are administered, and their bioavailability is usually gradually reduced over the course of ADME. A commonly used approach to overcome the vagaries of ADME is to have larger doses or more frequent administrations. The oral route for drug administration is convenient and does not normally require a physician's intervention. Most protein-based drugs are, however, not administered via the oral route because they are destroyed by the low pH medium in the stomach. Alternatively, we can use certain enteric coatings for some drugs; e.g., drugs coated with cellulose acetate phthalate can withstand the acid environment in the stomach and yet readily dissolve in the slightly alkaline environment of the intestine. In this way, protein-based drugs can have a safe passage to the intestine for absorption to take place. To reduce the frequency of drug administration, people also put encapsulation over a drug using polymer matrices to prolong the release of the drug in the bloodstream. These are known as microspheres, polymer micelles, and hydrogels. The polymers are made with biodegradable materials and, through processes of hydrolysis, drug molecules are released at controlled rates as the polymer is degraded.

Drugs come in various forms such as tablets, capsules, injections, ointments, suppositories, solutions, and others. A single active substance can sometimes be administered in various drug forms. A drug form can have a significant impact on ADME characteristics and eventually therapeutic effects.

Reasons to add excipients to the active substance(s) in a drug, according to the US Pharmacopoeia and National Formulary definition, can be to:

- Control the release of a drug substance in the body
- Improve the assimilation process and bioavailability
- Enhance drug dissolution as disintegration promoters
- Extend the stability and shelf life of the drug as antioxidants or preservatives
- Aid in the manufacturing processes in the form of fillers, lubricants, wetting agents, and solubilizers
- Mask an unpleasant taste of the active pharmaceutical ingredient
- Use as an aid for identification of the product

11.2.2   *Drug Dissolution*

According to Macheras and Iliadis (2006), the term drug dissolution encompasses several processes that contribute to the transfer of drugs from the dosage form to the bathing solution such as gastrointestinal fluids, dissolution medium. Depending on the release mechanism, controlled release systems can be classified into (1) diffusion-controlled, (2) chemically controlled, and (3) swelling controlled. Diffusion is the principal release mechanism, whereas chemically controlled release is mainly controlled by the degradation of the hydrolytic or enzymatic cleavage of the drug-polymer chemical bond in pendant chain systems. In swelling-controlled systems, after the inward flux of the liquid bathing, the drug molecules diffuse toward the bathing solution.

Drug dissolution testing is a quantitative method for assessing drug release from pharmaceuticals, in particular solid oral dosage forms such as tablets and capsules. In this sense, a dissolution test can be viewed as a surrogate marker of the availability of a drug (bioavailability) for systemic circulation. Gamma scintigraphy is commonly used to track drug dosage form movement from one region to another within the GI tract after oral administration. In the formulation, a nonabsorbable radionuclide that emits gamma rays is generally included as marker. The image of the capsule breaking up in the stomach or the GI tract is monitored using a gamma camera and blood levels or urinary excretion of the drug may be measured. Gamma scintigraphy has also been widely used for formulation studies including the mechanism of drug release from a hydrophilic matrix tablet (Abrahamsson et al., 1998).

In this section, we study mathematical models for the effect of dosage forms on drug release, including hydroxypropyl methylcellulose (HPMC) controlled-release dosage forms, the most widely used hydrophilic polymer for oral drug delivery systems.

Powder Drug

Assumption: The drug release rate is proportional to the amount of drug undissolved. Drug release is governed by the differential equation:

$$\frac{dV(t)}{dt} = -k_v V(t), \tag{11.1}$$

where $V(t)$ is the drug volume left (undissolved) and k_v is a constant.

Solving the differential equation (11.1) for $V(t)$ using the initial conditional $V(0) = V_0$, we have

$$V(t) = V_0 \exp(-k_v t). \tag{11.2}$$

After we obtain $V(t)$, the drug substance dissolved at any time t can be easily obtained:

$$V_{drug}(t) = C_0 (V_0 - V(t)), \tag{11.3}$$

where C_0 is the concentration of the drug in the dosage form.

Arbitrary Finite Shape

Assumption: The drug release rate is proportional to the surface area of the drug left.

$$\frac{dV(t)}{dt} = -k_s S(t), \tag{11.4}$$

where k_s is a constant, $V(t)$ and $S(t)$ are the volume and surface area of the drug dosage.

Sphere:

For a sphere, the volume $V(t) = \frac{4}{3}\pi r^3(t)$ and surface area $S(t) = 4\pi r^2(t)$, where $r(t)$ is the radius of the sphere at time t. Substituting these relationships into (11.4), we obtain

$$\frac{dr(t)}{dt} = -k_s. \tag{11.5}$$

Solving the differential equation (11.5) for $r(t)$ using initial condition $r(0) = r_0$, we arrive at

$$r(t) = r_0 - k_s t. \tag{11.6}$$

Therefore, the undissolved volume at time t can be written as

$$V(t) = \frac{4\pi}{3}(r_0 - k_s t)^3, \ t \leq r_0/k_s. \tag{11.7}$$

Cube:

Similarly, for a cube, $V(t) = a^3(t)$ and $S(t) = 6a^2(t)$, where $a(t)$ is the length of each side; substituting into (11.4), we can obtain the volume as a function of time t:

$$\frac{da(t)}{dt} = -2k_s. \tag{11.8}$$

Therefore , the volume function is given by

$$V(t) = (a_0 - 2k_s t)^3, \ t \leq \frac{a_0}{2k_s} \tag{11.9}$$

where $a_0 = a(0)$.

Cylinder or Disk:

For a cylinder, $V(t) = \pi r^2(t) h(t)$. From previous examples, we can see the linear relationship of each dimension of the object to time t. We can immediately obtain the volume function:

$$V(t) = \pi(r_0 - k_s t)^2 (h_0 - 2k_s t), \ t < \frac{\min(r_0, h_0)}{k_s} \tag{11.10}$$

Ellipse:

The volume of an ellipse with three axes a, b, and c has volume $V = \frac{4\pi}{3}abc$. At time t, each dimension reduces $k_s t$. Therefore, at time t the volume of the dosage is given by

$$V(t) = \frac{4\pi}{3}(a_0 - k_s t)(b_0 - k_s t)(c_0 - k_s t), \ t < \frac{\min(a_0, b_0, c_0)}{k_s}, \tag{11.11}$$

where a_0, b_0, c_0 are the initial values of the axes.

Higuchi Model and Power Law

In 1961 Higuchi analyzed the kinetics of drug release from an ointment, assuming that the drug was homogeneously dispersed in the planar matrix and the medium into which drug was released acted as a perfect sink. The cumulative amount $q(t)$ of drug released at time t is:

$$V_0 - V(t) = b\sqrt{t}, \tag{11.12}$$

where b is a constant.

The empirical power law was also proposed:

$$V_0 - V(t) = bt^{\alpha}, \tag{11.13}$$

where α is a constant. Note that the power law is suitable for infinite volume.

The models discussed so far are based on the volume of the drug. However, models can also be in terms of concentrations as the following two models.

Noyes–Whitney Model

The rate at which a solid substance dissolves in its own solution is proportional to the difference between the concentration of that solution and the concentration of the saturated solution (Noyes and Whitney, 1897).

$$\frac{dC(t)}{dt} = k(C_s - C(t)), \tag{11.14}$$

where the rate $C(t)$ is a concentration of dissolved species and C_s is saturation solubility.

Solving for $C(t)$, (11.14) leads to

$$C(t) = C_s(1 - \exp(-kt)). \tag{11.15}$$

Hixson–Crowell Model

Hixson and Crowell (1931) considered the effect of reduction in drug surface area and proposed the following so-called cube-root law:

$$q_0^{1/3} - q^{1/3}(t) = k_{1/3}t, \tag{11.16}$$

for sphere particles with a mono-dispersed size distribution under sink conditions. If sink conditions do not apply, they proposed the following:

$$\frac{1}{q^{2/3}(t)} - \frac{1}{q_0^{2/3}} = k_{2/3}t. \tag{11.17}$$

The dissolution process can be interpreted stochastically since the accumulated fraction of amount dissolved from a solid dosage form gives the probability of the residence times of drug molecules in the dissolution medium as described below:

$$\frac{q(t)}{q_\infty} = \Pr[\text{leave the formulation prior to } t] = \Pr[T \leq t] \qquad (11.18)$$

and

$$1 - \frac{q(t)}{q_\infty} = \Pr[\text{survive in the formulation prior to } t] = \Pr[T > t],$$

where $q_\infty = q(\infty)$.

The mean dissolution time (MDT) is given by

$$MDT = \int_0^\infty \frac{t}{q_\infty} dq(t) = \frac{1}{k}. \qquad (11.19)$$

Practically, the MDT is usually calculated using this reciprocal relationship.

11.3   Distribution Modeling

Except for intravenous injection, drug molecules have to cross cell membranes to reach target sites. The transport of drugs can be classified into diffusion (including passive and facilitated diffusion) and perfusion (including active and vesicular transport). Diffusion is due to the difference in drug concentration between the two locations and perfusion is due to the difference in hydrostatic pressure between the two locations. Perfusion of drugs is usually carried out by a drug carrier, i.e., blood flow and the gradient of pressure are the driving forces for perfusion. Perfusion is usually much faster than diffusion.

11.3.1   *Darcy's Law for Perfusion*

Drug substances transversing capillary membranes can experience passive diffusion and perfusion, but passive diffusion is the main process for most drugs. Active transport is a carrier-mediated transmembrane process that plays an important role in gastrointestinal absorption and in renal and biliary secretion of many drugs and metabolites. The active transport mechanism requires energy to drive the transportation of drugs against the concentration gradient, from low to high. The active transportation rate is dependent on the availability of carriers and energy supply via a number of biological pathways.

Hydrostatic pressure is responsible for penetration of water-soluble drugs into spaces between endothelial cells and possibly into lymph. In the kidneys, high arterial pressure creates a filtration pressure that allows small drug molecules to be filtered in the glomerulus of the renal nephron. Blood flow-induced drug distribution is rapid and efficient, but requires blood pressure. As blood pressure gradually decreases when arteries branch into the small arterioles, the flow slows down and transits from perfusion to concentration-driven diffusion into the interstitial space where the flow is facilitated by the large surface area of the capillary network. According to Shargel et al. (2005), the average pressure of the blood capillary is higher (+18 mm Hg) than the mean tissue pressure (−6 mm Hg). This pressure difference (24 mm Hg) is offset by an average osmotic pressure in the blood of 24 mm Hg. Thus, on average, the pressures in the tissue and most parts of the capillary are equal, with no net flow of water. At the arterial end, as the blood newly enters the capillary, however, the pressure of the capillary blood is slightly higher (about 8 mm Hg) than that of the tissue, causing fluid to leave the capillary and enter the tissues. This pressure is called hydrostatic or filtration pressure. This filtered fluid (filtrate) is later returned to the venous capillary due to a lower venous pressure.

Because of the difference between arterial and venous blood pressures, (Chiou 1989; Mather 2001) the validity of the well-stirred assumption is questionable. According to Shargel et al. (2005), differences ranging as high as several hundred-fold for Griseofulvin due to differences in arterial and venous blood levels have been reported. Forty compounds have been shown to exhibit marked site dependence in plasma or blood concentration after dosing in both humans and animals. In some cases, differences are due mostly to large extraction of drugs in poorly perfused local tissues, such as with nitroglycerin (3.8-fold arteriovenous difference) and procainamide (234% arteriovenous difference, venous being higher). Recognizing the difference in concentration, most pharmacokinetic studies are modeled based on blood samples drawn from various venous sites after either intravenous or oral dosing.

The rate of perfusion can be modeled using Darcy's law:

$$\frac{dQ}{dt} = kdH, \tag{11.20}$$

where Q is the mass of the flow, k is the perfusion coefficient, and H is the total head which includes blood pressure and the elevation difference between the flow-in and flow-out locations. If the elevation difference is negligible (e.g., at a lay down position), dH can be the difference between $H_{diastolic} - H_{systolic}$.

11.3.2   *Fick's Law for Diffusion*

Fick's law of diffusion is a macro result of Brownian motion (random motion) of particles at the microscopic level. Keep in mind that the term diffusion has been used loosely. Diffusion is sometimes called passive diffusion; sometimes diffusion means flow through porous media.

In PK analysis, we usually consider one-dimensional flow. Denote the location of a particle by $z(t)$ at time t. The starting position of the particle is $z(0) = 0$. At time t_{i-1}, the particle randomly moves from $z(t_{i-1})$ to either $z(t_{i-1}) - \delta$ or $z(t_{i-1}) + \delta$ with a probability of 0.5, where δ is a small (relative to the macro scale) positive constant. In other words,

$$z(t_i) = z(t_{i-1}) + \varepsilon, \tag{11.21}$$

where ε is a binary random variable taking value $\varepsilon = \pm\delta$ with an equal probability of 0.5.

The square of the displacement (11.21) is given by

$$z^2(t_i) = z^2(t_{i-1}) + \varepsilon^2 + 2\varepsilon z(t_{i-1}). \tag{11.22}$$

Take the expectation, we have

$$E\left(z^2(t_i)\right) = E\left(z^2(t_{i-1})\right) + \delta^2. \tag{11.23}$$

We arrange (11.23) and sum over t_0 to t_n; it leads to the following result:

$$\sum_{i=1}^{n} E\left(z^2(t_i)\right) - E\left(z^2(t_{i-1})\right) = \sum_{i=1}^{n} \delta^2, \tag{11.24}$$

i.e.,

$$E\left(z^2(t_n)\right) = n\delta^2. \tag{11.25}$$

Assume it takes time τ for a particle to travel randomly δ distance. We can write (11.25) as

$$E\left(z^2(t_n)\right) = \frac{t_n}{\tau}\delta^2. \tag{11.26}$$

This result is also true for two and three dimensional random-walk or Brownian motion. Here we can see that random motion at the microscopic level leads to a macro consequence

$$E\left(z^2(t)\right) = 2Dt, \tag{11.27}$$

which implies that it would take four times as long to get twice as far. Therefore, transport by diffusion is very slow in terms of distance. The constant

$$D = \frac{\delta^2}{2\tau} \tag{11.28}$$

is called a diffusion coefficient. It has the dimension of area/time and takes different values for different solutes in a given medium at a given temperature. Hence, the value of D is characteristic for a given solvent (or better, medium structure) at a given temperature of the diffusing tendency of the solute. According to Macheras and Iliadis (2006), a small drug molecule in water at 25°C has $D \approx 10^{-5} cm^2/s$, while a protein molecule like insulin has $D \approx 10^{-7} cm^2/s$. Using these values one can roughly calculate the time required for the drug and protein molecules to travel a distance of 1 mm; it takes $(0.1)^2/10^{-5} \approx 1000a \approx 16.6$ min for the drug and 1667 min for insulin. Hence, the value of D is heavily dependent on the size of the solute molecules. More examples of molecular permeability are listed in Table 11.1.

Table 11.1: Permeability of Various Molecules

Molecule Name	Molecular Weight	Radius of equivalent sphere A (0.1 mm)	Diffusion coefficient in water $(cm^2/sec) \cdot 10^5$
Water	18		3.20
Urea	60	1.6	1.95
Glucose	180	3.6	0.91
Sucrose	342	4.4	0.74
Raffinose	594	5.6	0.56
Inulin	5500	15.2	0.21
Myoglobin	17,000	19	0.15
Hemoglobin	68,000	31	0.094
Serum albumin	69,000		0.085

(Source: Adapted from Goldstein et al., 1974.)

In addition to the distance traveled in time, the amount of substance transported per unit time or the rate of diffusion is also important, which leads to the concept of "flux" at the macroscopic level. Fick's laws of diffusion describe the flux of solutes undergoing classical diffusion.

Flux J is defined as the net amount of flow through an area per unit time per unit area at location z (Figure 11.2). Consider a cube at left and right sides of location z. Because of small δ, we approximate the concentrations in the two cubes by $C\left(z - \frac{\delta}{2}\right)$ and $C\left(z + \frac{\delta}{2}\right)$, respectively. Denote by A the area of the cross-section at location z. Noticing that there is

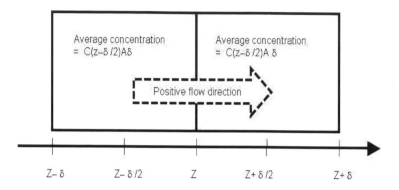

Figure 11.2:   Flux of a Solute

$C\left(z - \frac{\delta}{2}\right)A\delta$ flow in the positive direction and $C\left(z + \frac{\delta}{2}\right)A\delta$ flow in the negative direction, the flux can be calculated as

$$J \approx -\frac{1}{2A\tau}\left(C\left(z - \frac{\delta}{2}\right)A\delta - C\left(z + \frac{\delta}{2}\right)A\delta\right)$$
$$= -\frac{\delta^2}{2\tau\delta}\left[C\left(z - \frac{\delta}{2}\right) - C\left(z + \frac{\delta}{2}\right)\right], \tag{11.29}$$

where the negative sign indicates the particles move from the location with a higher concentration to the location with a lower concentration, and the constant 2 in the denominator is due to the fact that there is a 1/2 probability of each particle moving in an opposite direction.

Because of (11.28), we can write (11.29) as

$$J \approx -\frac{D}{\delta}\left[C\left(z - \frac{\delta}{2}\right) - C\left(z + \frac{\delta}{2}\right)\right]. \tag{11.30}$$

Taking the limit $\delta \to 0$, we can obtain Fick's first law

$$J(z,t) = -D\frac{\partial C(z,t)}{\partial z}. \tag{11.31}$$

Further, based on the mass conservation law, duration of the time interval τ, the molecule increment within the cube of fluid between $z - \frac{\delta}{2}$ and $z + \frac{\delta}{2}$ (Figure 11.2), is equal to the amount of molecules flowing into the cube. Therefore we have the equality:

$$A\delta\left[C(z,t+\tau) - C(z,t)\right] = A\tau\left[J\left(z - \frac{\delta}{2},t\right) - J\left(z + \frac{\delta}{2},t\right)\right]. \tag{11.32}$$

Dividing both sides by $A\delta\tau$ and letting $\delta \to 0$ and $\tau \to 0$, we obtain

$$\frac{\partial C(z,t)}{\partial t} = -\frac{\partial J(z,t)}{\partial z}. \tag{11.33}$$

Substituting Fick's first law (11.31) into (11.33), we can immediately obtain Fick's second law:

$$\frac{\partial C(z,t)}{\partial t} = D\frac{\partial^2 C(z,t)}{\partial z^2}. \tag{11.34}$$

In practice, Fick's first law of diffusion (11.31) is often written as (Shargel et al., 2005, p. 252)

$$\frac{dQ}{dt} = \frac{-DKA(C_p - C_t)}{\delta} \tag{11.35}$$

where $C_p - C_t$ is the difference between the drug concentrations in the plasma (C_p) and in the tissue (C_t), respectively; A is the surface area of the membrane; δ is the thickness of the membrane; K is the lipid-water partition coefficient; and D is the diffusion constant. The negative sign denotes net transfer of drug from inside the capillary lumen into the tissue and extracellular spaces. Diffusion is spontaneous and temperature dependent.

As mentioned earlier, passive diffusion is the random movement of molecules in fluid usually due to a concentration difference. If a fluid is separated by a semi-permeable membrane, more dissolved molecules will diffuse across the membrane from the higher concentration side to the lower concentration side than in the reverse direction. Because of the lipid bilayer construction of the membrane, nonpolar (lipid soluble) molecules are able to diffuse and penetrate the cell membrane. However, polar molecules cannot penetrate the cell membrane readily via passive diffusion. Lipid solubility determines the readiness of drug molecules to cross the gastrointestinal tract, blood-brain barrier, and other tissues. Molecular size is another factor that determines the diffusion of drugs across a membrane, with the smaller molecules the easier to diffuse (Ng, 2003).

In facilitated diffusion, the transportation of a drug substance across the cell membrane is facilitated by transmembrane carriers such as proteins. Facilitated diffusion is also from a region of high concentration to low concentration and it's diffusion rate is faster than passive diffusion. However, these carriers may become saturated at high drug concentrations, reaching rate plateaus.

For facilitated transport, the mechanism is similar to enzyme dynamics. Hence we will discuss its modeling at the end of the enzyme dynamics discussion.

11.4   Metabolism Modeling

11.4.1   *Metabolic Process*

Metabolism may precede distribution to the site of action, resulting in a decline in plasma concentrations. A decline in plasma concentration after drug administration can also be due to renal excretion or removal by the body. For most drugs, the principal site of metabolism is the liver, although metabolism can occur in other tissues or organs (e.g., lung, skin, gastrointestinal mucosal cells, microbiological flora in the distal portion of the ileum, kidney, and large intestine). Figure 11.3 depicts the main ADME network in the human body, grouped by tissue and organ.

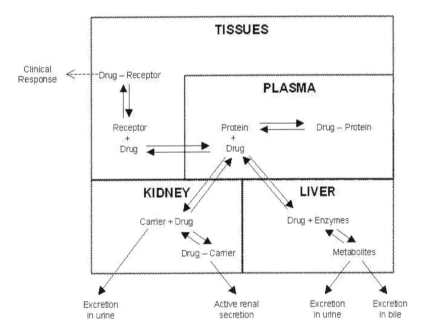

Figure 11.3:   Main ADME Network
(Source: Adapted from Shargel et al., 2005)

To predict whether a change in drug elimination is likely to be affected by renal disease, hepatic disease, or a drug–drug interaction, it is helpful to know the fraction of the drug that is eliminated by metabolism and the fraction of drug that is eliminated by excretion. Renal drug excretion is highly dependent on the glomerular filtration rate (GFR), which varies slightly among individuals with normal renal function. For this reason, intersubject variability in elimination half-lives is small for drugs that are eliminated primarily by renal drug excretion. In contrast, drugs that are highly metabolized demonstrate larger intersubject variability in elimination half-lives. This is because drug metabolism is dependent on the intrinsic activity of biotransformation enzymes, which are highly influenced by genetic and environmental factors.

11.4.2 *Enzyme Dynamics*

The rate process for drug metabolism is commonly modeled by the Michaelis-Menten equation, in which the rate of an enzymatic reaction is assumed to be dependent on the concentrations of both the drug and the enzyme. In the process, the drug and an energetically favored drug-enzyme intermediate is initially formed, followed by the formation of the product and regeneration of the enzyme (Figure 11.4).

$$\frac{d[ED]}{dt} = k_1[E][D] - k_2[ED] - k_3[ED] \qquad (11.36)$$

where $[ED]$ is the amount of enzyme in the enzyme-drug complex, rate of intermediate $[ED]$ formation $= k_1[E][D]$, rate of intermediate $[ED]$ decomposition $= k_2[ED] + k_3[ED]$.

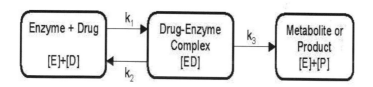

Figure 11.4:   Enzyme Dynamics

Assume that the total enzyme is unchanged and equal to the initial enzyme $[E_0]$, which is the sum of the free enzyme and the drug-enzyme complex; therefore, we have

$$[E] = [E_0] - [ED]. \qquad (11.37)$$

At equilibrium, $\frac{d[ED]}{dt} = 0$; (11.36) can be written as the Michaelis–Menten equation:

$$[ED] = \frac{[E_0][D]}{K_m + [D]}, \qquad (11.38)$$

where

$$K_m = \frac{k_2 + k_3}{k_1}. \tag{11.39}$$

Letting $V_{\max} = k_3 E_0$, and $V = k_3[ED]$, (11.38) can be written as

$$V = \frac{V_{\max} C_d}{K_m + C_d}, \tag{11.40}$$

where V is the rate of conversion, $V_{\max}$ is the maximum rate of conversion, $C_d = [D]$ is the substrate concentration or drug concentration, and K_m is the Michaelis constant, the substrate concentration at which the rate of conversion is half of $V_{\max}$.

If the reaction is slow, i.e., $\frac{d[ED]}{dt}$ is small, we can use (11.40) for a non-equilibrium condition at time t:

$$\frac{dC_{ed}}{dt} = \frac{V_{\max} C_d(t)}{K_M + C_d(t)}, \tag{11.41}$$

where C_{ed} is the concentration of enzyme in the enzyme-drug complex. We will use (11.41) in building a physiologically based pharmacokinetic simulation model.

The liver is the major organ responsible for drug metabolism. However, intestinal tissues, lung, kidney, and skin also contain appreciable amounts of biotransformation enzymes, based on the metabolic marker CYT P-450 from rat data: the CYT P-450 are 0.73, 0.5, 0.135, 0.012, 0.046, 0.042, and 0.016 nmole/mg microsome protein for liver, adrenal gland, kidney, skin, lung, small intestine, colon, respectively (Shargel et al., 2005).

11.5   Excretion Modeling

Drug clearance or elimination is important in determining the frequency of maintenance dose administration and influences the dosing interval necessary to maintain therapeutic drug levels and intended efficacy response and prevent cumulative overdosing.

In addition to drug elimination by the metabolism as discussed in the previous section, excretion is another important elimination process. The main function of the liver biliary system is to drain waste products from the liver into the duodenum and help in digestion with the controlled release of bile (a greenish-yellow fluid consisting of waste products, cholesterol, and bile salts), which includes the secretion of bile and the excretion of drugs. Larger molecule drugs are excreted mainly in the bile; medium size molecule drugs (molecular weights between 300 and 500) are excreted both in urine and in bile; small molecule drugs (molecular weights < 300) are excreted almost exclusively via the kidneys into urine.

The term clearance is a measure of drug elimination from the body without identifying the mechanism or process. Clearance (drug clearance, systemic clearance, total body clearance) considers the entire body as a single unit undergoing elimination processes, both drug metabolism and excretion. In this way, collectively, drug elimination from the body is quantitated using the simple concept of drug clearance, despite the complex mechanisms of drug elimination. Drug clearance refers to the volume of plasma fluid that is cleared of drug per unit time (e.g., mg/min or mg/hr). For a zero-order elimination process, expressing the rate of drug elimination as mass per unit time is convenient because the rate is constant. In contrast, the rate of drug elimination for a first-order elimination process is not constant and changes with respect to the drug concentration in the body. For first-order elimination, drug clearance expressed as volume per unit time (e.g., L/hr or mL/min) is convenient because it is a constant. For many drugs, first-order elimination is applicable, mathematically,

$$\frac{dC}{dt} = kC, \tag{11.42}$$

where C is the plasma concentration of the drug and k is a constant.

Traditionally, people use the term clearance defined by

$$Cl = \frac{dC}{dt}\frac{V_a}{C} = kV_a, \tag{11.43}$$

where V_a is the apparent volume dependent on each individual.

V_a is not an actual volume, but an equivalent volume when converting the heterogeneous body to an equivalent homogeneous body for the purpose of PK calculation. Therefore, drug Cl represents the sum of the clearances for many drug-eliminating organs.

The clearance concept may also be applied to any organ and is used as a measure of drug elimination by the organ, e.g., hepatic clearance may be defined as the volume of blood that perfuses the liver and is cleared of drug per unit of time.

So far, we have discussed all four aspects of the ADME process. The overall kinetics of ADME can be summarized by percent of dose over time, as shown in Figure 11.5.

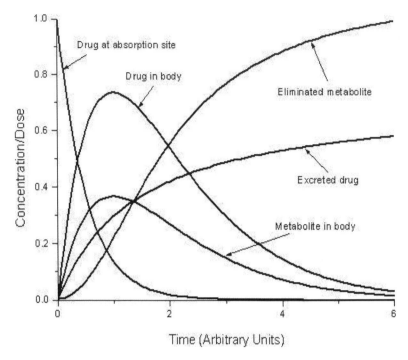

Figure 11.5:   Time Course of Oral Drug and Metabolite
(Source: Adapted from Rowland and Tozer, 1995)

11.6   Physiologically-Based PK Model

11.6.1   *Classic Compartment Model*

There are basically three types of compartment models: mammillary, catenary, and physiologically based models. The mammillary model consists
of one central compartment and several attached compartments. The central compartment is assigned to represent plasma and highly perfused tissues that rapidly equilibrate with the drug. The drug is gradually eliminated from the central compartment through primarily kidney and liver
are well-perfused tissues. The mammillary model consists of one or more
compartments around a central compartment like satellites. In contrast,
the catenary model consists of compartments joined to one another like
the compartments of a train. In reality, it is a mixture of mammillary and
catenary models — physiologically based PK models.

A one-compartment model (sometimes also called a noncompartment
model) with a "drug supply source" can be described by the following

ordinal differential equation:

$$\frac{dC}{dt} = -kC. \tag{11.44}$$

Solving for C by integration, it leads to

$$C = C_0 e^{-kt}, \tag{11.45}$$

where C_0 is the initial concentration.

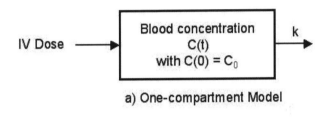

a) One-compartment Model

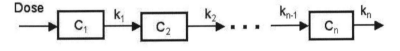

b) Multi-compartment Model

Figure 11.6: Compartment Models

The mathematical description of the catenary model (Figure 11.6) is based on the mass conservation law, i.e., the mass flows into a compartment must be equal to the sum of mass increase in the compartment and mass flow out of that compartment.

Given the initial condition:

$$C_1(0) = C_2(0) = \ldots = C_n(0) = 0, \tag{11.46}$$

and an intravenous (IV) bolus (or IV uniform injection) dose, we suspect the concentration in the compartment takes the form

$$C_1(t) = \sum_{i=1}^{n} b_k \exp(-k_i t), \ \alpha > 0. \tag{11.47}$$

We let students find out if (11.47) is the solution for the catenary model (Exercise 11.3).

We are interested in the asymptotic form of (11.47) when $n \to \infty$, which turns out to be a power function:

$$t^{-\alpha} = \frac{1}{\Gamma(\alpha)} \int_0^\infty x^{\alpha-1} \exp(-xt)\, dx. \qquad (11.48)$$

That explains why the power function is widely used in PK modeling. Beard and Bassingthwaighte (1998) showed that a power function can be represented as the sum of a finite number of scaled basis functions. Any probability density function may serve as a basis function. They considered as a basis function a density corresponding to the passage time of a molecule through two identical tanks in series. Power functions can arise if the administered molecules undergo random walks with drift, as in the well-known Wiener process (Norwich, 1997).

It is interesting that the power law can also be derived from the *fractal* structure of the biological material. One of the most interesting properties of fractals is geometric self-similarity, which means that the parts of a fractal object are smaller exact copies of the whole object. The replacement rule used to generate the fractal structures is in the form of

$$z_{i+1} = g(z_i) \qquad (11.49)$$

where z_i and z_{i+1} are the input and output, respectively, at two successive steps.

A binary tree is an example of a fractal object. In the biological world, fractal structures like the venular and arterial tree cannot be characterized by geometric self-similarity; rather they possess *statistical self-similarity*. The fractal is statistically self-similar since the characteristics (such as the average value or the variance or higher moments) of the statistical distribution for each small piece are proportional to the characteristics that concern the whole object (Macheras and Iliadis, 2006).

Scaling laws for fractal objects state that if one measures the value of a geometric characteristic $\theta(w)$ on the entire object at resolution w, the corresponding value measured on a piece of the object at finer resolution $\theta(rw)$ with $r < 1$ will be proportional to $\theta(w)$:

$$\theta(rw) = k\theta(w) \qquad (11.50)$$

where k is a proportionality constant that may depend on r.

The above-delineated dependence of the values of the measurements on the resolution applied suggests that there is no single true value of a measured characteristic. A function satisfying (11.50) is the power law:

$$\theta(w) = \beta w^\alpha \qquad (11.51)$$

where β and α are constants for the given fractal object or process studied. From (11.50) and (11.51), we can see that $k = \beta r^{\alpha}$.

We proved earlier the diffusion law in regular geometric space:

$$E\left(Z\left(t\right)^{2}\right) \propto t^{1/2}. \tag{11.52}$$

In fractal space, the dimension can be any positive real number (not necessarily an integer) and the corresponding diffusion law is given by

$$z\left(t\right) \propto t^{2/d_{f}} \tag{11.53}$$

where d_{f} = fractal dimension can be any positive real number.

From (11.53), we can expand the scaling-law for fractal materials to other properties such as concentration, leading to the power law for the concentration:

$$C\left(t\right) = \beta_{c}t^{\alpha_{c}}. \tag{11.54}$$

According to Macheras and Iliadis (2006), the exponential model is applicable to homogeneity and the power law is applicable to heterogeneity. They elaborate this further: most drug substances intermix rapidly within their distribution spaces, and the rate-limiting step in their removal from the system is biochemical transformation or renal excretion. Substances of this nature are best described by compartmental models and exponential functions. Conversely, some substances are transported relatively slowly to their site of degradation, transformation, or excretion, so that the rate of diffusion limits their rate of removal from the system. Substances of this nature are best described by noncompartmental models and power functions. Power-laws have an important application in intraspecies and interspecies parameter scaling.

11.6.2 *Description of the PBPK Model*

PBPK model structures are based on the actual physiological and biochemical structure of the species being described, allowing for the physiological and biochemical parameters in the model to be changed from those for the test species to those appropriate for humans to perform animal to human extrapolations and predicting drug effects over a wide range of conditions. The improved dose metric can then be used in place of traditional dose metrics (e.g., administered dose) or can be generated as a time-dependent input for a more biologically based response model to simulate the time course of the drug. Figure 11.7 is an illustration of a PBPK model.

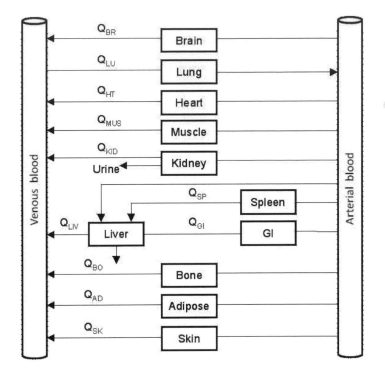

Figure 11.7: PBPK Model

(Source: Adapted from Shargel et al., 2005)

In building a PBPK model, it is essential to have good knowledge of the organs and tissues you are dealing with for the drug under consideration. Simulation performers should work with physiologists, physicians, and/or PK specialists whenever it is necessary.

In general, disease is a major source of variability in drug response and for many diseases this variability is due primarily to differences in pharmacokinetics. The pharmacokinetics, as well as the pharmacodynamics, of some drugs have been shown to be influenced by the presence of concurrent diseases other than the one for which the drug is used (Rowland and Tozer, 1995).

Brain

Drug deposition and accumulation in tissue are generally controlled by the diffusional barrier of the capillary membrane and other cell membranes. The brain is well perfused with blood, but many drugs with good aqueous solubility have high kidney, liver, and lung concentrations and yet little or negligible brain drug concentration. The brain capillaries are surrounded by a layer of tightly joined glial cells that act as a lipid barrier to impede the diffusion of polar or highly ionized drugs (Shargel et al., 2005).

Lung

The lung or pulmonary system is the essential respiration organ. Lung perfusion is unique because the pulmonary artery returns venous blood flow to the lung, where carbon dioxide is exchanged for oxygen and the blood becomes oxygenated. The blood from the lungs flows back to the heart (into the left atrium) through the pulmonary vein, and the quantity of blood that perfuses the pulmonary system ultimately passes through the remainder of the body. In describing drug clearance through the lung, perfusion from the heart (right ventricle) to the lung is generally considered as venous blood (Figure 11.7).

In normal adults, both blood flow and ventilation are distributed preferentially to the dependent lung zones. After intravenous drug administration, drug uptake in the lungs may be very significant if the drug has high affinity for lung tissue. If actual drug clearance is at a much higher rate than the drug clearance accounted for by renal and hepatic clearance, then lung clearance of the drug should be suspected, and a lung clearance term should be included in the equation in addition to lung tissue distribution (Shargel et al., 2005).

Lung diseases such as asthma, chronic bronchitis, COPD (chronic obstructive pulmonary disease), emphysema, pulmonary fibrosis, and sarcoidosis can significantly affect ADME characteristics by reducing lung function.

Heart

The heart, as the pump for blood flow, needs energy from different fuels, glucose, or fatty acids depending on availability, according to recent research reported by ScienceDaily (May 10, 2007). Two closely related nuclear receptors known as ERRa and g play essential roles in coordinating the expression of a set of proteins that the heart requires to produce the energy it needs to pump effectively. A person with congestive heart failure has decreased cardiac output, resulting in impaired blood flow, which may reduce renal clearance through reduced filtration pressure and blood flow. Other circulation disorders such as shock and malignant hypertension are generally characterized by diminished vascular perfusion to one or more parts of the body and reduce the rate of drug delivery to the site.

Muscles

Blood flow is important in determining how rapid and how much drug reaches the receptor site. About 20% of the cardiac output at rest goes to skeletal muscle and skeletal muscle blood flows may be 1–4 ml/min per 100 g. During extreme physical exertion, more than 80% of cardiac output can be directed to contracting muscles, resulting in maximal blood flows of 50–100 ml/min per 100 g depending upon the muscle type. For this reason, changes in skeletal muscle resistance and blood flow can greatly influence arterial pressure. Diabetic patients receiving intramuscular injection of insulin could change the onset of drug action during exercise. The accumulation of carbon dioxide may lower the pH of certain tissues and may affect the level of drugs reaching those tissues.

Kidney

The human kidneys are two bean-shaped organs, one on each side of the backbone, representing only 0.5% of total body weight, but receiving 20–25% of the total arterial blood pumped by the heart. In 24 hours the kidneys reclaim 1,300 g of NaCl, 400 g $NaHCO_3$, 180 g glucose, and 180 liters of water.

The kidney is the major site for excretion of an unchanged active ingredient of a drug and its metabolites. In patients with compromised renal function, urinary excretion of drugs is diminished. The degree of reduction in renal elimination depends on the reduction in renal function. Diabetes insipidus is characterized by excretion of large amounts of a watery urine, 8 gallons per day.

Dose adjustment may be needed for patients with kidney disease, especially hemodialysis patients. A general guideline (Rowland and Tozer, 1995) is as long as the fraction excreted is unchanged (in a typical patient it is 0.30 or less) and the metabolites are inactive, no change in regimen is called for, based on renal function.

Liver

The liver is the largest glandular organ of the body (1.36 kg), consisting of four lobes of unequal size and shape. Blood is carried to the liver via two large vessels called the hepatic artery and the portal vein. The hepatic artery carries oxygen-rich blood from the aorta (a major vessel in the heart). The portal vein carries blood containing digested food from the small intestine. These blood vessels subdivide in the liver repeatedly, terminating in very small capillaries. Each capillary leads to a lobule. Liver tissue is composed of thousands of lobules, and each lobule is made up of hepatic cells, the basic metabolic cells of the liver.

This organ plays a major role in metabolism and has a number of functions in the body, including glycogen storage, decomposition of red blood cells, plasma protein synthesis, hormone production, and detoxification. It produces bile, an alkaline compound which aids in digestion, via the emulsification of lipids. It also performs and regulates a wide variety of high-volume biochemical reactions requiring highly specialized tissues, including the synthesis and breakdown of small and complex molecules, many of which are necessary for normal vital functions. The liver is also responsible for producing cholesterol. It produces about 80% of the cholesterol in the body.

Table 11.2: Blood Flow to Human Tissues

Tissue	Percent body weight	Percent cardiac output	Blood flow*
Adrenals	0.02	1	550
Kidneys	0.40	24	450
Thyroid	0.04	2	400
Liver			
Hepatic	0.20	5	20
Portal		20	75
Heart (basal)	0.40	4	70
Brain	2.00	15	55
Skin	7.00	5	5
Muscle (basal)	40.0	15	3
Connective tissue	7.00	1	1
Fat	15.0	2	1

* Unit = (ml/100g tissue/min)

(Source: Adapted from Butler, 1972)

Several diseases states can affect the liver. Some of the diseases are Wilson's disease, hepatitis (an inflammation of the liver), liver cancer, and cirrhosis (a chronic inflammation that progresses ultimately to organ failure). Alcohol alters the metabolism of the liver, which can have overall detrimental effects if alcohol is taken over long periods of time. The most significant effect of hepatic diseases is, from an ADME perspective, a reduction in the metabolic function of the body.

Because invasive methods are available for animals, tissue/blood ratios or partition coefficients can be determined accurately by direct measurement. Using experimental pharmacokinetic data from animals, physiologic pharmacokinetic models may yield more reliable predictions. For humans, the average blood flows to tissues are listed in Table 11.2.

11.6.3   *Probabilistic PBPK Model*

Most physiologic pharmacokinetic models assume rapid drug distribution between tissue and venous blood. Rapid drug equilibrium assumes that drug diffusion is extremely fast and that the cell membrane offers no barrier to drug permeation. In reality one can consider the entire course of a drug in the body as consecutive and/or concurrent processes of diffusion and perfusion.

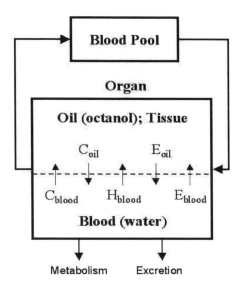

Figure 11.8:   Organ PK Model

     The challenge is to figure out R, the ratio of drug concentration in the organ tissue to drug concentration in the blood. In a typical organ compartment, drug substances can travel from blood to tissue in three ways: passive diffusion due to concentrations in the blood C_{blood}, perfusion due to hydrostatic pressure H_{blood}, and active facilitated transport due to carriers and energy E_{blood}. In contrast, drug molecules travel from tissues to blood in two ways: passive diffusion due to concentrations in oil C_{oil} and passive facilitated diffusion by a carrier such as protein and energy E_{oil}. Furthermore, the drug may be eliminated from the organ through metabolism or excretion (Figure 11.8).

     (1) If drug molecule movement is treated as a random walk, then the amount of molecules entered into tissue due to C_{blood} during time t to $t + dt$ (dt is very small) is proportional to $C_{blood}(t)\,dt$. Hence the increase

of concentration is

$$dC_{oil}(t) = k_b C_{blood}(t) dt, \tag{11.55}$$

where k_b is a constant for a given organ. We can see that (11.55) is a special case of Fick's first law.

(2) Similarly, $C_{oil}(t)$ change due to drug concentration in oil C_{oil} is given by

$$dC_{oil}(t) = -k_o C_{oil}(t) dt, \tag{11.56}$$

where k_o is a constant.

(3) From Darcy's law, the concentration increase in tissue due to the difference in blood pressure $H = H_{Arterial} - H_{Ventricular}$ is

$$dC_{oil}(t) = k_h H dt, \tag{11.57}$$

where k_h is a constant.

(4) When there are enough drug carriers, the concentration increase due to E_{blood} is proportional to $C_{blood}(t)$. However when $C_{blood}(t)$ increases there may not be enough carriers available (saturated) and the concentration eventually reaches a plateau, exhibiting saturation kinetics. Because of the similarity of the enzyme dynamics and carrier-mediated transport, the Michaelis-Menten equation can be used for carrier-mediated transport (Macheras and Iliadis, 2007):

$$\frac{dC_{oil}(t)}{dt} = \frac{R_{b\max}C_{blood}(t)}{K_{bm} + C_{blood}(t)} = k_{bR}(t) C_{blood}(t), \tag{11.58}$$

where $R_{b\max}$ is the maximum transport rate due to carrier saturation and K_{bm} is a constant.

(5) Similarly, the concentration reduction due to energy E_{oil} is assumed to be

$$\frac{dC_{oil}(t)}{dt} = \frac{R_{o\max}C_{oil}(t)}{K_{om} + C_{oil}(t)} = k_{oR}(t) C_{oil}(t), \tag{11.59}$$

where $R_{o\max}$ is the maximum transport rate due to energy constraint and K_{om} is a constant.

(6) The change $C_{oil}(t)$ due to metabolism is as previously discussed (see (11.40) in Section 11.4.2)

$$\frac{dC_{oil}(t)}{dt} = \frac{V_{o\max}C_{oil}(t)}{K_{om}^* + C_{oil}(t)} = k_V(t) C_{oil}(t), \tag{11.60}$$

where $R_{o\max}$ is the maximum rate of conversion due to the limit in enzyme availability and K_{om}^* is a constant.

(7) The concentration reduction due to excretion is, in normal conditions, given by

$$dC_{oil}(t) = -k_{ex}C_{oil}(t)\,dt. \tag{11.61}$$

So far we have not used the condition that the same amount of fluid flows in and out for incompressible material. We may not need the constraint unless the steady state is considered.

Assume the additive model, i.e., the total amount of increase in concentration is the sum of all 7 dC_{oil}s, which leads to the following form for the concentration change:

$$dC_{oil} = (k_{oil}(t)\,C_{oil}(t) + k_{blood}(t)\,C_{blood}(t) + k_h H)\,dt, \tag{11.62}$$

where $k_{oil}(t)$ and $k_{blood}(t)$ have the form of

$$k_i(t) = a + \frac{b}{d + C_i(t)} \tag{11.63}$$

with a and b being constants and i = oil or blood.

Equation (11.63) is the nonlinear differential equation governing the concentration in a typical organ. The parameters $k_1(t)$ and $k_2(t)$ vary in time and from person to person, but k_3 varies from person to person. Note that k_i do not directly relate to the size of the tissues or organs unless K^*_{om} and $V_{o\,max}$ are related to the size of the tissue.

The determination of $k_i(t)$ can be based on other physiological or biochemical factors and the elasticity of tissues and veins. In using Darcy's law for perfusion, we have ignored the elevation difference between the arterial network (inflow) and the venular network (outflow) of a compartment.

Due to a heterogeneity consideration (non-well-stirred condition), other forms of $k_i(t)$ such as power function

$$k_i = \beta_i t^{-\alpha_i}, \ \beta_i > 0, \alpha_i > 0, i = \text{oil or blood} \tag{11.64}$$

may also be used, which will greatly simplify the model.

11.6.4   *Relationship to MCMC*

In general, a compartment model can be viewed as a stochastic network, where the transition probability distribution is the permeability matrix

$$\begin{bmatrix} k_{11} & k_{12} & \cdots & k_{1n} \\ k_{21} & k_{22} & \cdots & k_{2n} \\ \vdots & \vdots & \ddots & \vdots \\ k_{n1} & k_{n2} & \cdots & k_{nn} \end{bmatrix}, \tag{11.65}$$

where $k_{ij} =$ the k between the ith and j^{th} compartment. If k_{ij} are constants, the network is a Markovian process; if k_{ij} are time dependent, the model is a time-dependent Markovian chain. In general, the model is not necessarily a Markovian process. The convergence of the simulation may be dependent on the size of Δt. Although mathematically even a small Δt doesn't guarantee convergence, practically it should be convergent if Δt is sufficiently small; otherwise the model has a validity issue.

11.6.5 *Monte Carlo Implementation*

Implementation of the PBPK model can follow the steps outlined in Algorithm 11.1. If you know any OOP and visual simulation tools such as ExtentSim, building a PBPK is a straightforward job programming-wise. However, determining the parameters and validating the model are still challenging.

Algorithm 11.1: Physiologically Based Pharmacokinetics

(1) Construct a typical compartment model using object-oriented programming (any OOP computer language or visual simulation tool)
(2) Make copies of the typical compartment model (TCM) and customize based on PBPK model
(3) Connect the TCMs based on the PBPK diagram
(4) Input parameters for each TCM:
    The model parameters can be assumed fixed values, from data, or validated by data. The model parameters can also be chosen as random variables. In such cases, one can generate parameter distributions for each compartment using the technical information in Chapter 2.
(5) Determining output parameters:
    Many different PK outputs can be easily obtained to the model for each compartment (organ) or the body as a single entity. The PBPK simulation model can also output the traditional PK parameters such as $C_{\max}$, AUC, $t_{1/2}$, etc., as described below.
    §

Common Output Parameters

Blood flow, tissue size, and tissue storage are also important in determining the time course of distribution. Table 11.2 lists the blood flow and tissue mass for different tissues in the human body. The single most commonly used measure regarding the time course is the distribution half-life $t_{1/2}$, i.e., the time for 50% distribution. Drug affinity for a tissue or organ refers to the partitioning and accumulation of the drug in the tissue:

$$k_d = \frac{Q}{VR},$$ (11.66)

where k_d = first-order distribution constant, Q = blood flow to the organ, V = volume of the organ, R = ratio of drug concentration in the organ tissue to drug concentration in the blood (venous).

For a one-compartment exponential model, the half-life can be easily calculated: $t_{1/2} = ln(2)/k_d$. The ratio R is determined experimentally from tissue samples. To determine the tissue distribution of a drug, the partition coefficient $P_{o/w}$ is introduced, which is defined as a ratio of the drug concentration in the oil phase divided by the drug concentration in the aqueous phase measured at equilibrium under a specified temperature in vitro in an oil/water two-layer system.

Areas under concentration curves (AUCs) are important measures of drug exposure. The three commonly used AUCs are 24-hour AUC after dosing, steady-state AUC, and total AUC as defined by:

$$AUC_{24h} = \int_0^{t_{24h}} C(t)\, dt; \;\; AUC_{ss} = \int_0^{t_{ss}} C(t)\, dt; \;\; AUC = \int_0^{\infty} C(t)\, dt.$$ (11.67)

Another similar measure for drug exposure is area under the moment curve defined by

$$AUMC = \int_0^{\infty} tC(t)\, dt.$$ (11.68)

Mean residence time (MRT) is a marker of drug safety and efficacy. After an intravenous bolus drug dose, the drug molecules distribute throughout the body. These molecules stay (reside) in the body for various time periods. Some drug molecules leave the body almost immediately after entering, whereas other drug molecules leave the body at later time periods. The term mean residence time (MRT) describes the average time for all the drug molecules to reside in the body.

$$MRT = \frac{\int tC(t)\, d}{\int C(t)\, dt} = \frac{AUMC}{AUC}.$$ (11.69)

For mixed exponential concentration, the corresponding formulations are

$$C(t) = \sum_{i=1}^{n} a_i \exp(-\lambda_i t),$$

$$AUC = \sum_{i=1}^{n} \frac{a_i}{\lambda_i}, \tag{11.70}$$

$$AUMC = \sum_{i=1}^{n} \frac{a_i}{\lambda_i^2}, \tag{11.71}$$

where the initial concentration $C(0) = \sum_{i=1}^{n} a_i$. In simulation, we use $\sum$ to replace the integral $\int$.

Clearance rate is an indirect measure of drug availability, which is defined as

$$Cl = \frac{\text{Elimination rate}}{\text{Concentration in blood}}. \tag{11.72}$$

It can be shown that

$$Cl = \frac{\text{DrugDose}}{\text{AUC}}, \text{ and } \frac{V}{C} \frac{dC}{dt} = -kV = -Cl, \tag{11.73}$$

where V = apparent volume (volume of distribution), constant Cl = clearance, but Cl may not be a constant for PBPK.

Sampling of Biological Specimens

Sampling of biological specimens is important in PK modeling and simulations, especially for parameter determination and model validation.

Invasive methods such as sampling blood, spinal fluid, synovial fluid, tissue biopsy, and any biologic material that requires parenteral or surgical intervention in the patient can be used extensively in animals other than humans. In contrast, noninvasive methods that include sampling of urine, saliva, feces, and expired air are much easy to conduct. The measurements of drug and metabolite concentration in each of these biologic materials yield critical information regarding the amount of drug retained in or transported into that region of the tissue or fluid, and provide the likely pharmacological or toxicological outcome of drug dosing and drug metabolite formation or transport.

The most direct approach to assessing the pharmacokinetics of a drug in the body is to measure drug concentration in the blood, serum, or plasma. To obtain serum, whole blood is allowed to clot and the serum is collected from the supernatant after centrifugation using an anticoagulant. Plasma perfuses all the tissues of the body, including the cellular elements in the blood. Under the assumption that a drug in the plasma is in dynamic equilibrium with the tissues, changes in the drug concentration in plasma will reflect changes in tissue drug concentrations.

Measurement of a drug in urine is an indirect method to ascertain the bioavailability of a drug. The rate and extent of drug excretion in the urine reflects the rate and extent of systemic drug absorption. However, there are challenges in obtaining valid urinary excretion data because: (1) the assay technique must be specific for the unchanged drug and must not include interference due to drug metabolites that have similar chemical structures; (2) sampling time points must be sufficient for capturing the time course; (3) urine samples should be collected periodically until almost all of the drug is excreted.

Case Studies

There are plenty of published case studies in PK modeling and simulations. We especially recommend the book "Physiologically Based Pharmacokinetic Modeling" by Readdy, Yang, Clewell, and Adersen (2005), where a broad array of case studies with PBPK simulations are collected. In the book, Tami McMullin has classified PBPK models into (1) emphasizing factors that influence the distribution of drugs, (2) emphasizing metabolism/clearance of drugs, (3) developed for drugs incorporating altered physiological states, (4) describing drug stereospecificity, (5) describing kinetics of drugs under non-steady-state conditions, (6) developed for drug–drug interactions, (7) emphasizing in vitro to in vivo extrapolation.

11.7   Summary

Pharmacokinetics is the study of the kinetics of absorption, distribution, metabolism, and excretion (ADME) of a drug. It analyzes the way the human body works with a drug after it has been administered, and the transportation of the drug to the specific site for drug-receptor interaction.

The ultimate goal of pharmacokinetic modeling and simulation is to determine the optimum dosage regimen for each patient individually since the time course (ADME) of a given NME will determine its efficacy and safety profile.

The systemic absorption of a drug is dependent on (1) the dosage form, (2) the physicochemical properties of the drug, (3) the nature of the drug product, and (4) the anatomy and physiology of the drug absorption site. Proper drug product selection requires a thorough understanding of the physiologic and pathologic factors affecting drug absorption to assure therapeutic efficacy and to avoid potential drug–drug and drug-nutrient interactions.

Except for intravenous injection, drug molecules have to cross cell membranes to reach target sites. The transport of drugs can be classified into perfusion and diffusion. Perfusion of drugs is usually carried out by a drug carrier, i.e., the blood flow and the gradient of pressure are the driving forces for perfusion. Perfusion is usually much faster than diffusion. Diffusion is due to the difference in drug concentration between two locations and perfusion is due to the difference in hydrostatic pressure.

The rate of perfusion can be modeled using Darcy's law (11.20), i.e., the mass of the flow is proportional to the gradient of blood pressure or hydrostatic pressure.

From the random-walk model, we know that in diffusion, the distance traveled is proportional to the square root of time, which implies that it would take four times as long to get twice as far. Therefore, transport by diffusion is very slow in terms of distance.

Fick's first law (11.31) or (11.35) is important in studying drug diffusion, which states that the rate of concentration decrease over time is equal to the rate of flux increase over a distance.

Metabolism may precede distribution to the site of action, resulting in a decline in plasma concentration. The decline in plasma concentration after drug administration can also be due to renal excretion or removal by the body. For most drugs, the principal site of metabolism is the liver.

Drug clearance or elimination is important in determining the frequency of maintenance dose administration and influences the dosing interval necessary to maintain therapeutic drug levels and intended efficacy response and prevent cumulative overdosing.

For many drugs, first-order elimination is applicable, mathematically, $\frac{dC}{dt} = kC$. Traditionally, people use the term clearance defined by

$$Cl = \frac{dC}{dt}\frac{V_a}{C} = kV_a.$$

PBPK models are based on the actual physiological and biochemical structure of the species being described, allowing for the physiological and biochemical parameters in the model to be changed from those for the test species to those appropriate for humans to perform animal to human extrapolations and predicting drug effects over a wide range of conditions. The improved dose metric can then be used in place of traditional dose metrics (e.g., administered dose) or can be generated as a time-dependent input for a more biologically based response model to simulate the time course of the drug. The physiologic pharmacokinetic model, which accounts for processes of drug distribution, drug binding, metabolism, and drug flow to the body organs, is much more realistic. Disease-related changes in physiologic processes are more readily related to changes in the pharmacokinetics of the drug. Furthermore, organ mass, volumes, and blood perfusion rates are often scalable, based on size, among different individuals and even among different species. This allows a perturbation in one parameter and the prediction of changing physiology on drug distribution and elimination (Sawada et al., 1985; Shargel et al., 2005).

A typical PBPK compartment model can be written based on the total amount of increase in concentration:

$$dC_{oil} = \left(k_{oil}\left(t \right) C_{oil}\left(t \right) + k_{blood}\left(t \right) C_{blood}\left(t \right) + k_h H \right) dt,$$

where $k_{oil}\left(t \right)$ and $k_{blood}\left(t \right)$ have the approximate form of

$$k_i = \beta_i t^{-\alpha_i}, \ \beta_i > 0, \alpha_i > 0, i = oil \text{ or } blood.$$

In general, a compartment model can be viewed as a stochastic network, where the transition probability distribution is a permeability matrix. The Monte Carlo implementation of the PBPK model can be accomplished using OOP.

11.8   Exercises

Exercise 11.1: Describe the objectives of PK analysis and ADME.

Exercise 11.2: What are the differences between traditional PK compartment models and PBPK models?

Exercise 11.3: Establish a diffusion law (equation for the concentration time course), given the two regions have different diffusion coefficients D_1 and D_2. At the steady state, will the concentrations in the two regions be the same?

Exercise 11.4: For an IV dose at a constant infusion rate q, derive the one-compartment model.

Exercise 11.5: Derive the analytical form for the time course of the concentration in the ith compartment for the catenary model (see Figure 11.6).

Exercise 11.6: Determine (analytically or by Monte Carlo) the time course of the concentration in the ith compartment for the model shown in Figure 11.9.

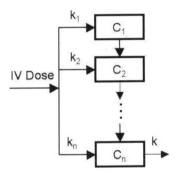

Figure 11.9:   An n-Compartment Model

Exercise 11.7: Given multiple (two or more) IV dose infusions at a constant rate q, derive the one-compartment model and the catenary model with n compartments.

Exercise 11.8: Derive a formulation for AUC and $AUMC$ for a concentration with power function $C(t) = \beta t^{\alpha}$.

Exercise 11.9: Determine the correctness of the following relationship:

$$t^{-\alpha} \propto \sum_{i=1}^{m} k_i^{\alpha+1} t \exp(k_i t), \alpha > 0.$$

Exercise 11.10: What is PBPK simulation and what are the commonly used PK output parameters?

Chapter 12

Pharmacodynamic Simulation

This chapter will cover the following topics:

- Way to Pharmacodynamics
- Enzyme Kinetics
- Pharmacodynamic Models
- Drug–Drug Interactions
- Application of Pharmacodynamic Modeling

12.1 Way to Pharmacodynamics

12.1.1 *Objectives of Pharmacodynamics*

Pharmacodynamics is the study of the relationship between the drug concentration at the site of action and the pharmacological response (biochemical and physiologic effects). According to occupancy theory, originated by Clark (1933; 1937), the drug effect is a function of the following processes: binding of the drug to the receptor, drug-induced activation (inhibition) of the receptor and propagation of this initial receptor activation (inhibition) into the observed pharmacological effect, where the intensity of the pharmacological effect is proportional to the number of receptor sites occupied by the drug. From Chapter 10, we learned that the interaction of a drug molecule with a receptor causes a chain of reactions (events) that could lead to desirable pharmacological effects or undesirable side effects. Therefore, the relationship between pharmacokinetics and pharmacodynamics is a focus of pharmacodynamics. In Chapter 11, we studied the relationship between dose regimen and plasma drug concentration (PK); in this chapter, we study the drug concentration or, more accurately, the time course of the concentration in relation to pharmacological (positive or negative) responses using modeling and simulation. The goal is to use pharmacokinetics to develop dosing regimens that will result in plasma concentrations in the therapeutic window and yield the desired therapeutic or pharmacological response.

In general, a typical PD-PK curve for ideal drugs can be divided into three stages: (1) low-dose level, no biological effect will be seen, (2) moderate dose level, where pharmacological or clinical effects are expected to be seen, but also some infrequent adverse events will be observed, and (3) pharmacological response has no significant changes, but toxicity increases dramatically (Figure 12.1). We should choose a dose regimen such that situations (1) and (3) can be avoided, and situation (2) is targeted.

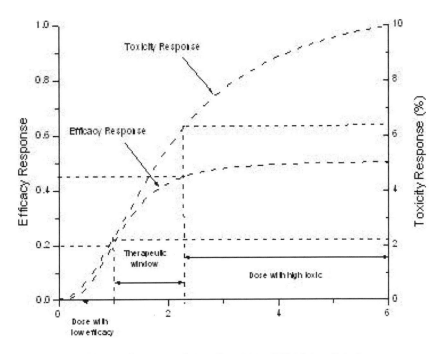

Figure 12.1:   Therapeutic Window

In Chapters 3 and 10, we have discussed the therapeutic index (window), the potency, and the specificity of an NME. In pharmacodynamic study, the response measured is a PD marker, which is different from a response in a clinical endpoint that is ultimately used for regulatory approval of the drug. The PD marker or biomarker can be classified into three categories: classifier, prognostic, and predictive markers.

A classifier biomarker is a marker (e.g., a DNA marker) that usually does not change over the course of a study. A classifier biomarker can be used to select the most appropriate target population or even for personalized treatment. On the other hand, some biomarkers, such as RNA markers, are expected to change over the course of a study. This type of marker can be either a prognostic or a predictive marker.

A prognostic biomarker informs the clinical outcomes, independent of treatment. Biomarkers provide information about the natural course of a disease in persons who have or have not received the treatment under study. Prognostic markers can be used to separate good-prognosis and poor-prognosis patients at the time of diagnosis. If an expression of the marker clearly separates patients with an excellent prognosis from those with a poor prognosis, the marker can be used to aid the decision as to how aggressive the therapy needs to be.

A predictive biomarker informs the treatment effect on the clinical endpoint. Compared to a gold-standard endpoint such as survival, a biomarker can often be measured earlier, more easily, and more frequently. A biomarker is less subject to competing risks and less affected by other treatment modalities. A biomarker could lead to faster decision making (Chang, 2007b).

12.1.2 ADME Review

After it is delivered to the body by a proper dose form (IV, oral, or others), a drug is absorbed into plasma and distributed throughout the body by the systemic circulation. The drug molecules reach the target site (usually a receptor) for desirable drug action as well as undesirable sites, causing side effects or adverse reactions. Drug molecules are distributed to the liver, causing the metabolized, to the kidney for excretion. A substantial portion of the drug may be bound to proteins in the plasma and/or tissues. The circulatory system consists of a series of blood vessels; these include the arteries that carry blood to tissues, and the veins that return the blood back to the heart. An average subject (70 kg) has about 5 L of blood, which is equivalent to 3 L of plasma. About 50% of the blood is in the large veins or venous sinuses. The volume of blood pumped by the heart per minute, the cardiac output, is the product of the stroke volume of the heart and the number of heart beats per minute (69 contractions or heart beats per min). A left ventricular contraction may produce a systolic blood pressure of 120 mm Hg, and moves blood at a linear speed of 300 mm/sec. Fast drug distribution powered by the blood pressure difference is termed perfusion and the slower distribution of drug powered by a concentration difference is termed diffusion.

The interstitial fluid plus the plasma water is termed extracellular water, because these fluids reside outside the cells. Drug molecules may further
diffuse from the interstitial fluid across the cell membrane into the cell cytoplasm. Most small drug molecules permeate capillary membranes easily;
the transportability of drug molecules across a cell membrane depends on
the molecular size and the physicochemical nature of both the drug and the
cell membrane. Cell membranes are composed of protein and a bilayer of
phospholipid, which act as a lipid barrier to drug uptake. Thus, lipid-soluble
drugs generally diffuse across cell membranes more easily than highly polar or water-soluble drugs. If the drug is bound to a plasma protein such
as albumin, the drug-protein complex becomes too large for easy diffusion
across the cell or even capillary membranes.

The typical time courses of plasma concentration distribution following
different routes are presented in Figure 12.2.

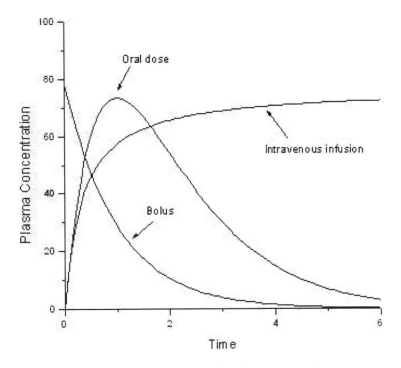

Figure 12.2:   Concentration Curves: Oral, Infusion, and Bolus Doses

A comparison of concentration curves for an oral dose is presented in
Figure 12.3 for single and multiple dose regimens. The troughs and peaks in
the concentration curve for multiple doses at steady state are also presented
in Figure 12.3.

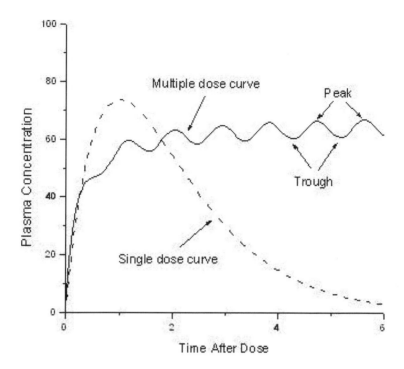

Figure 12.3:   Concentration: Single Oral Dose vs. Multiple Doses

12.1.3   *Intraspecies and Interspecies Scaling*

Interspecies scaling is a method used in toxicokinetics and the extrapolation of therapeutic drug doses in humans from nonclinical animal drug studies. Toxicokinetics is the application of pharmacokinetics to toxicology and pharmacokinetics for interpolation and extrapolation based on anatomic, physiologic, and biochemical similarities (Shargel et al., 2005; Mordenti and Chappell, 1989; Bonate and Howard, 2000; Mahmood, 2000; Hu and Hayton, 2001).

The basic assumption in interspecies scaling is that physiologic variables, such as drug concentration, clearance, heart rate, organ weight, and biochemical processes, are related to the weight or body surface area of the animal species. It is commonly assumed that all mammals use the same energy source (oxygen) and energy transport systems are similar across animal species (Hu and Hayton, 2001). The general allometric equation obtained can be written as (Shargel et al., 2005)

$$\theta = \beta \omega^a, \tag{12.1}$$

where θ is the pharmacokinetic or physiologic property of interest, β is an allometric coefficient, ω is the weight or surface area of the animal species, and constant a is the allometric exponent.

The allometric equation (12.1) can also be derived based on assumptions about the fractal structures of animals. As we discussed earlier, the fractal structure leads to a power law for a geometric or physiologic property. A list of allometric relationships for interspecies parameters is presented in Table 12.1.

Table 12.1: Allometric Relationship for Interspecies Parameters

Physiologic or Pharmacokinetic Property	Allometric Exponent a	Allometric Coefficient b
Basal O_2 consumption (mL/hr)	0.734	3.8
Endogenous N output (g/hr)	0.72	0.000042
O_2 consumption by liver slices (mL/hr)	0.77	3.3
Creatinine clearance (mL/hr)	0.69	8.72
Methotrexate apparent volume (L/kg)	0.92	0.859
Kidney weight (g)	0.85	0.0212
Uvea weight (g)	0.87	0.082
Heart weight (g)	0.98	0.0066
Stomach and intestine weight (g)	0.94	0.112
Blood weight (g)	0.99	0.055
Total volume (mL)	1.0 1	0.0062
Methotrexate half-life (min)	0.23	54.6

Source: Adapted from Ritschel and Banerjee, 1986

12.2   Enzyme Kinetics

12.2.1   *Enzyme Inducer and Inhibitor*

Enzyme induction is the process whereby an (inducible) enzyme is synthesized in response to a specific inducer molecule. The inducer molecule (often a substrate that needs the catalytic activity of the inducible enzyme for its metabolism) combines with a repressor and thereby prevents the blocking of an operator by the repressor that leads to the translation of the gene for the enzyme.

Enzyme inhibitors are molecules that bind to enzymes and decrease their activities. Since blocking an enzyme's activity can kill a pathogen or correct a metabolic imbalance, many drugs are enzyme inhibitors. Inhibitors are also used as herbicides and pesticides. Not all molecules that bind to enzymes are inhibitors; enzyme activators bind to enzymes and increase their enzymatic activities.

The binding of an inhibitor can stop a substrate from entering the enzyme's active site or hinder the enzyme from catalyzing its reaction. Inhibitor binding is either reversible or irreversible. Reversible inhibitors bind noncovalently and different types of inhibition are produced depending on whether these inhibitors bind the enzyme, the enzyme-substrate complex, or both. Inhibitions by most drugs are reversible. In contrast, irreversible inhibitors usually react with the enzyme and change it chemically. These inhibitors modify key amino acid residues needed for enzymatic activity.

Many drug molecules are enzyme inhibitors, so their discovery and improvement is an active area of research in biochemistry and pharmacology. An enzyme inhibitor is often judged by its potency (the concentration needed to inhibit the enzyme) and its specificity (lack of binding to other proteins). A high potency and specificity ensure that a drug will have robust efficacy and few side effects or low toxicity.

Enzyme inhibitors also occur naturally and are involved in the regulation of metabolism. For example, enzymes in a metabolic pathway can be inhibited by downstream products. This type of negative feedback slows flux through a pathway when the products begin to build up and is an important way to maintain homeostasis in a cell. Other cellular enzyme inhibitors are proteins that specifically bind to and inhibit an enzyme target. This can help control enzymes that may be damaging to a cell, such as proteases or nucleases; a well-characterized example is the ribonuclease inhibitor, which binds to ribonucleases in one of the tightest known protein-protein interactions (Shapiro and Vallee, 1991). Natural enzyme inhibitors can also be poisons and are used as defenses against predators or as ways of killing prey (Wikipedia.com).

According to the effect of varying the concentration of the enzyme's substrate on the inhibitor, reversible enzyme inhibitors can be classified as uncompetitive, competitive, and mixed inhibitors.

In uncompetitive inhibition, the inhibitor binds only to the substrate-enzyme complex; it should not be confused with a noncompetitive inhibitor. In competitive inhibition, the substrate and inhibitor compete for the same enzyme's active site because competitive inhibitors are often similar in structure to the real substrate. This type of inhibition can be overcome by sufficiently high concentrations of substrate, i.e., by out-competing the inhibitor. In mixed inhibition, the inhibitor can bind to the enzyme at the same time as the enzyme's substrate. However, the binding of the inhibitor affects the binding of the substrate, and vice versa. This type of inhibition can be reduced, but not overcome, by increasing concentrations of substrate. Omission noncompetitive inhibition is a form of mixed inhibition where the binding of the inhibitor to the enzyme reduces its activity but does not affect the binding of substrate. As a result, the extent of inhibition depends only on the concentration of the inhibitor.

12.2.2 *Occupancy Theory*

The process of biotransformation or metabolism is the enzymatic conversion of a drug to a metabolite. When the drug (substrate) concentration is low relative to the enzyme concentration, there are abundant enzymes to catalyze the reaction, and the rate of metabolism is a first-order process. Saturation of the enzyme occurs when the drug concentration is high, all the enzyme molecules become complex with the drug, and the reaction rate reaches its maximum rate.

Mathematically, the rate process for drug metabolism is described by the Michaelis-Menten equation (see Chapter 11), which assumes that the rate of an enzymatic reaction is dependent on the concentrations of both the enzyme and the drug and that an energetically favored drug-enzyme intermediate is initially formed, followed by the formation of the product and regeneration of the enzyme.

From a previous chapter, we know that

$$\frac{d[ED]}{dt} = k_1[E_0][D] - (k_1[D] - k_2 - k_3)[ED]. \tag{12.2}$$

At equilibrium, both $[ED]$ and $[D]$ are constants and (12.2) can be written as:

$$[ED] = \frac{[E_0][D]}{K_m + [D]} \tag{12.3}$$

where $K_m = (k_2 + k_3)/k_1$ is the so-called Michaelis constant.

Letting $C_d = [D]$, from (12.3) the reaction speed can be obtained:

$$V = \frac{V_{max}C_d}{C_d + K_m}. \tag{12.4}$$

A more illustrative version of the Michaelis-Menten equation is the so-called Lineweaver-Burk equation:

$$\frac{1}{V} = \frac{K_M}{V_{max}C_d} + \frac{1}{V_{max}}. \tag{12.5}$$

When the enzyme is saturated, it reaches its maximum reaction speed $V_{max} = k_3E_0$. We can plot (12.5) in the $x - y$ plan, where $x = 1/C_d$ and

$y = 1/V$. The Lineweaver-Burk equation affords a line with a slope of $K_m/V_{\max}$ and a y-intercept of $1/V_{\max}$. The x-intercept, a theoretical point, since $1/C_d$ can't be negative, is $-1/K_m$.

In the case of competitive enzyme inhibition, the inhibitor and drug substrate compete for the same active center on the enzyme. The drug and the inhibitor may have similar chemical structures. An increase in the drug (substrate) concentration may displace the inhibitor from the enzyme and partially or fully reverse the inhibition. Competitive enzyme inhibition is usually observed by a change in the K_M, but the V_{max} remains the same.

In the case of competitive inhibition, the drug and the inhibitor compete at the same active site; the reaction speed for competitive inhibition is

$$V = \frac{V_{\max}C_d}{C_d + K_M\left\{1 + C_i/k_i\right\}}, \tag{12.6}$$

where C_i is the inhibitor concentration and k_i is the inhibition constant, which is determined experimentally.

The liver is the major site of drug metabolism, and the type of metabolism is based on the reaction involved. Oxidation, reduction, hydrolysis, and conjugation are the most common reactions. The enzymes responsible for oxidation and reduction of drugs (xenobiotics) and certain natural metabolites, such as steroids, are monoxygenase enzymes known as mixed-function oxidases.

The most important enzyme accounting for variation in Phase I metabolism of drugs is the cytochrome P-450 enzyme group, which exists in many forms among individuals because of genetic differences (May, 1994; Tucker, 1994; Parkinson, 1996). There are now at least eight families of cytochrome isozymes known in humans and animals. Cytochrome P-450 I-III (GYP 1-3) is best known for metabolizing clinically useful drugs in humans.

In noncompetitive enzyme inhibition, the inhibitor may inhibit the enzyme by combining at a site on the enzyme that is different from the active site (i.e., an allosteric site). In this case, enzyme inhibition depends only on the inhibitor concentration. In noncompetitive enzyme inhibition, K_m is not altered, but $V_{\max}$ is lower (Shargel et al., 2005).

For a noncompetitive reaction, the reaction speed is given by

$$V = \frac{V_{\max}C_d\left(1 + C_i/k_i\right)}{C_d + K_m}. \tag{12.7}$$

The Michaelis-Menten equation assumes that one drug molecule is catalyzed sequentially by one enzyme at a time. The drug may be eliminated by enzymatic reactions (metabolism) to one or more metabolites, as described above. Protein molecules are quite large compared to drug molecules and may contain more than one type of binding site for the drug.

The receptor occupation theory is not consistent with all kinetic observations. Alternatively, the rate theory states that the pharmacological response is not dependent on drug-receptor complex concentration but rather depends on the rate of association of the drug and the receptor. Each time a drug molecule hits a receptor, a response is produced.

12.2.3   *Feedback Mechanism*

The biomedical literature, particularly that of functional and biochemical pharmacology, is rich with detailed descriptive mechanisms of control and its modification induced by an extensive list of drugs and chemicals. Mathematical analysis of using negative feedback mechanics is discussed by Macheras & Iliadis (2006).

In the feedback model, the ligand or drug is continuously released at rate $R(t)$, and eliminated exponentially with a rate constant k, and there exists a negative feedback control function $F(V)$ that depends on the concentration of occupied receptor $V(t)$ that modulates the release; thus the drug concentration is modeled by

$$\frac{dC(t)}{dt} = -kC(t) + F(V) + R(t). \tag{12.8}$$

This model is based on evidence that the release of neurotransmitters is modulated by the nerve terminal itself as a result of stimulation by the neurotransmitter of a subset of receptors termed "autoreceptors" (Kennakin, 1997). Thus, receptor stimulation not only produces effects but also inhibits or augments release, thereby maintaining a basal level of the ligand. The feedback signal may originate at a site other than the occupied receptor, but it functionally is related to $V(t)$.

12.3   Pharmacodynamic Models

12.3.1   *Pharmacodynamics–Pharmacokinetic Relationship*

Theoretically, pharmacodynamics refers to the relationship between drug concentrations at the site of action (receptor) and pharmacological response, including the biochemical and physiologic effects that influence the interaction of drug with the receptor. Practically, the concentration at the active site is often replaced with the plasma concentration. As we have discussed earlier, the pharmacodynamic response produced by the drug depends on the chemical structure of the drug molecule. The receptors can be classified according to the type of pharmacodynamic response induced. Since most pharmacological responses are due to noncovalent interaction between the drug and the receptor, the nature of the interaction is generally assumed to be reversible.

The plasma protein concentration is dependent on: (1) protein synthesis, (2) protein catabolism, (3) distribution of albumin between intravascular and extravascular space, and (4) excessive elimination of plasma protein, particularly albumin.

A decrease in protein binding and an increase in free drug concentration will allow more drug to cross cell membranes into all tissues and become available to interact at a receptor site to produce a stronger pharmacological effect. Therefore, a drug regimen must be chosen to provide sufficiently high unbound drug concentrations so that an adequate amount of drug reaches the site of drug action (receptor). The onset time is often dependent on the rate of drug uptake and distribution to the receptor site. The intensity of a drug action depends on the total drug concentration of the receptor site and the number of receptors occupied by the drug.

When considering drug safety, how high and how long the free plasma drug level will be sustained are more important to a toxicokineticist and often measured by the AUC for the free drug concentration.

The receptor occupancy concept was extended to show how a drug elicits a pharmacological response as an agonist, or produces an opposing pharmacological response as an antagonist through drug-receptor interactions. Basically, three types of related responses may occur at the receptor: (1) a drug molecule that interacts with the receptor and elicits a maximal pharmacological response is referred to as an agonist; (2) a drug that elicits a partial (below maximal) response is termed a partial agonist; and (3) an agent that elicits no response from the receptor, but inhibits the receptor interaction of a second agent, is termed an antagonist. An antagonist may prevent the action of an agonist by competitive (reversible) or noncompetitive (irreversible) inhibition.

A pharmacological response in drug therapy is often a product of physiologic adaptation to a drug response. As mentioned in Chapter 10, many drugs trigger a pharmacological response through a cascade of enzymatic events highly regulated by the body, whereas clinical measurement of drug response may only occur after many such biologic events. Pharmacodynamic modeling must account for biologic processes involved in eliciting drug induced responses. In general, the onset, intensity, and duration of the pharmacological effect depend on the dose and the pharmacokinetics of the drug. As the dose increases, the drug concentration at the receptor site increases, and the pharmacological response increases until the maximum effect is reached.

12.3.2   *Maximum Effect (E_{max}) Model*

The maximum effect (E_{max}) model is a widely used empirical model that relates pharmacological response to plasma drug concentrations. The E_{max} model describes drug action in terms of the maximum effect (E_{max}) and the drug potency EC_{50}, the drug concentration that produces 50% maximum pharmacological effect.

$$E(t) = kV(t) = E_0 + \frac{E_{max}C(t)}{EC_{50} + C(t)} \qquad (12.9)$$

where $E(t)$ is the pharmacological effect, $C(t)$ is the plasma drug concentration at time t, and E_0 is a constant. Equation (12.9) is a saturable process resembling Michaelis-Menton enzyme kinetics (Figure 12.4). In model (12.9), both E_{max} and EC_{50} can be measured.

To consider the pharmacological response for a wide range of concentrations, the so-called sigmoid model (S-shaped) is often more appropriate. The sigmoid E_{max} model is defined as:

$$E = E_0 + \frac{E_{max}C^{\gamma}}{EC_{50} + C^{\gamma}} \qquad (12.10)$$

where γ is a constant for data fitting. Figure 12.4 is a comparison of E_{max} and sigmoid E_{max} models.

12.3.3   *Logistic Regression*

To model the probability of response, the rate of response, the percent of inhibition, etc., where the dependent variable p ranges from 0 to 1, the logistic model is the most common model:

$$p = \frac{1}{1 + e^{-x}}, \qquad (12.11)$$

$$x = a_0 + a_1 x_1 + \cdots + a_m x_m. \qquad (12.12)$$

Function (12.11) is called a simple perceptron or two-layer artificial neural network in bioinformatics (see next section).

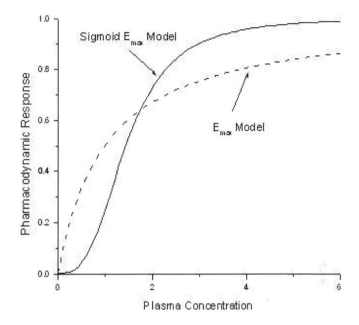

Figure 12.4:   Graphics for $E_{\max}$ and Sigmoid $E_{\max}$ Models

12.3.4   *Artificial Neural Network*

As discussed in Chapter 1, an artificial neural network (ANN) is an artificial intelligence method for system modeling. An ANN mimics the mechanism of the human neural network using adaptive weights between the layers in the network to be able to model very complicated systems. An ANN can be used in supervised learning (classification) and predictions. An ANN can be locally linear (relationship between two adjacent layers), but collectively it shows global nonlinear behaviors.

An ANN is configured for a specific application, such as pattern recognition or data classification, through a learning process. Learning in biological systems involves adjustments to the synaptic connections that exist between neurons; the same is true for ANNs. An ANN features adaptive learning (an ability to learn how to do tasks based on the data given for training or initial experience) and self-organization (creating its own organization or representation of the information it receives at the learning phase).

What we know about how the brain trains itself to process information is very limited. In the human brain, a typical neuron collects signals from others through a host of fine structures called dendrites. The neuron sends out spikes of electrical activity through a long, thin strand known as an axon, which splits into thousands of branches. At the end of each branch, a structure called a synapse converts the activity from the axon into electrical effects that inhibit or excite activity from the axon into electrical effects that inhibit or excite activity in the connected neurons. When a neuron receives excitatory input that is sufficiently large compared with its inhibitory input, it sends a spike of electrical activity down its axon (Figure 12.5). Learning occurs by changing the effectiveness of the synapses so that the influence of one neuron on another changes (Stergiou and Siganos, 2009. www.doc.ic.ac.uk).

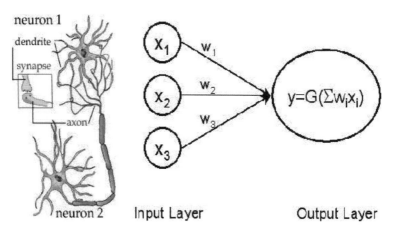

Figure 12.5:   Neural Network and Perceptron in an ANN
(Source: Laerhoven, 2003)

The simplest ANN model is the so-called two-layer one-output perceptron (Figure 12.5). This is simply a linear model with independent variable (input) x_i and dependent variable (output) $y = G\left(\Sigma_i w_i x_i\right)$, where $G\left(\cdot\right)$ is called the link-function and weights w_i between two layers evolute by means of back-propagation or negative feedback using training data sets (sets of inputs x_i and observed responses $\hat{y}$), which is a significant difference from traditional regression methods. Algorithm 12.1 illustrates the perceptron training process.

Algorithm 12.1: ANN Perceptron Training
Objective: train perceptron for prediction.

(1) Choose initial weights $\boldsymbol{w} = \{w_1, .., w_K\}$ and learning rate α.
(2) Input a set of observed $\boldsymbol{x} = \{x_1, ..., x_K\}$ and $\hat{y}$.
(3) Calculate y based on the linear combination of inputs, i.e.,

$$y = G\left(\Sigma_{i=1}^{K} w_i x_i\right).$$ (12.13)

(4) Calculate the derivatives of the square errors $E = \frac{1}{2}(\hat{y} - y)^2$:

$$\frac{\partial E}{\partial w_i} = -(\hat{y} - y)G'x_i. \tag{12.14}$$

(5) Use back-propagation training the system, i.e., update K weights:

$$w_i := w_i + \Delta w_i, \quad i = 1, ..., K. \tag{12.15}$$

$$\Delta w_i = \alpha (\hat{y} - y)G'x_i. \tag{12.16}$$

(6) Go to step 2 with new inputs x and $\hat{y}$.

§

Note that learning rate α is usually choosen such that $0 < \alpha < 1$. The rationale for the constant learning rate is that the amount of weight adjustment is proportional to its effect on the output so that the overall weight adjustment will be minimized. The same data can be used to train the ANN several times. This is very different from traditional regression. In a regression model, coefficients are determined once or the same dataset can only be used once. However, the same dataset should not be used too many times in training the model to avoid overtraining the ANN or overfitting the data.

Multiple-Layer Model
We have discussed a simple two-layer perceptron. However, this simple model barely meets practical requirements. The commonly used ANN model is of multiple-layer perceptrons. Figure 12.6 is an example of a perceptron with a hidden layer where data are not measurable or observable.

The local models (link functions) for the hidden layer and the output layer are:

$$y_k = G_a \left(\Sigma_i a_{ik} x_i \right), \tag{12.17}$$

and

$$z_m = G_b \left(\Sigma_j b_{jm} y_j \right), \tag{12.18}$$

respectively. The squared error loss is expressed as

$$E = \frac{1}{2} \sum_m (\hat{z}_m - z_m)^2, \tag{12.19}$$

where $\hat{z}_m$ and z_m are the observed and model outputs at the mth node, respectively.

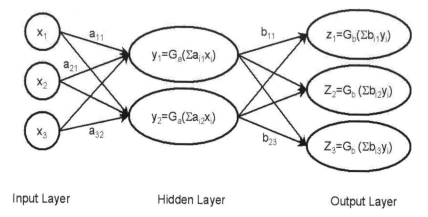

Input Layer   Hidden Layer   Output Layer

Figure 12.6:   A Multilayer Feedforward ANN

The partial derivatives of the squared error are derived as follows.

$$\frac{\partial E}{\partial b_{ik}} = -\sum_m \left[(\hat{z}_m - z_m) \frac{\partial z_m}{\partial b_{ik}} \right] = -\sum_m \left[(\hat{z}_m - z_m) G_b' \sum_j \left[\frac{\partial b_{jm}}{\partial b_{ik}} y_j \right] \right]$$

$$= -\sum_m \left[(\hat{z}_m - z_m) G_b' \sum_j [\delta_{ji}\delta_{mk} y_j] \right] = -\sum_m [(\hat{z}_m - z_m) G_b' \delta_{mk} y_i]$$

$$= -[(\hat{z}_k - z_k) G_b' y_i]$$

$$\frac{\partial E}{\partial a_{ik}} = -\sum_m \left[(\hat{z}_m - z_m) \frac{\partial z_m}{\partial b_{ik}} \right] = -\sum_m \left[(\hat{z}_m - z_m) G_b' \sum_j \left[b_{jm} \frac{\partial y_j}{\partial a_{ik}} \right] \right]$$

$$= -\sum_m \left[(\hat{z}_m - z_m) G_b' \sum_j \left[b_{jm} G_a' \sum_l \frac{\partial a_{lj}}{\partial a_{ik}} x_l \right] \right]$$

$$= -\sum_m \left[(\hat{z}_m - z_m) G_b' \sum_j \left[b_{jm} G_a' \sum_l \delta_{li}\delta_{jk} x_l \right] \right]$$

$$= -\sum_m [(\hat{z}_m - z_m) G_b' [b_{km} G_a' x_i]]$$

where the Kronecker δ_{ik} function is defined as $\delta_{ik} = 1$ if $i = k$; otherwise 0.

Therefore we have:

$$\frac{\partial E}{\partial b_{ik}} = -G_b' \left(\hat{z}_k - z_k \right) y_i \tag{12.20}$$

$$\frac{\partial E}{\partial a_{ik}} = -G_b' G_a' x_i \sum_m \left[\left(\hat{z}_m - z_m \right) b_{km} \right] \tag{12.21}$$

Given these derivatives, a gradient decent update at the $(r+1)^{th}$ iteration can be formed:

$$b_{ik}^{(r+1)} = b_{ik}^{(r)} - \beta^{(r)} \frac{\partial E}{\partial b_{ik}^{(r)}}$$

$$= b_{ik}^{(r)} + \beta^{(r)} G_b' \left(\hat{z}_k - z_k \right) y_i \tag{12.22}$$

$$a_{ik}^{(r+1)} = a_{ik}^{(r)} - \alpha^{(r)} \frac{\partial E}{\partial a_{ik}^{(r)}}$$

$$= a_{ik}^{(r)} + \alpha^{(r)} G_b' G_a' x_i \sum_m \left[\left(\hat{z}_m - z_m \right) b_{km} \right], \tag{12.23}$$

where $\alpha^{(r)}$ is the learning rate at the rth iteration.

Algorithm 11.2 is a back-propagation training algorithm for updating coefficients a_{ik} and b_{ik} in (12.17) and (12.18) for the two-layer ANN in Figure 12.6.

Algorithm 11.2: Back-Propagation Algorithm for an ANN

Objective: back-propagation training for an ANN.
Select initial weights $a_{ik}^{(0)}$ and $b_{ik}^{(0)}$.
Input n (the total number of patients or sets of observations)
For $r := 1$ **To** n
    Input r^{th} data set $\boldsymbol{x}^{(r)}$ and $\hat{\boldsymbol{z}}^{(r)}$, learning rates $\alpha^{(r)}$ and $\beta^{(r)}$
    Calculate z_m using (12.18) and (12.17)
    Update $b_{ik}^{(r)}$ using (12.22)
    Update $a_{ik}^{(r)}$ using (12.23)
Endfor
Return $\left\langle a_{ik}^{(n)}, b_{ik}^{(n)} \right\rangle$
§

To ensure convergence, learning rates $\alpha^{(r)}$ and $\beta^{(r)}$ should satisfy the conditions of stochastic approximation (Robbins and Monro, 1951): $\alpha^{(r)} \to 0, \sum_r \alpha^{(r)} = \infty$, and $\sum_r \alpha^{(r)} \alpha^{(r)} < \infty$ (for example $\alpha^{(r)} = 1/r^\theta, \theta > 1/2$). Similar convergence conditions are required for $\beta^{(r)}$.

ANN Link-Functions

The behavior of an ANN depends on the weights and the link-function. Commonly used link-functions are given below.

Step-function (threshold):

$$G\left(x\right) = \begin{cases} 1, & \text{if } x \geq c \\ 0, & \text{otherwise} \end{cases}; G'\left(x\right) = \delta\left(x - c\right) \tag{12.24}$$

where c is a constant and $\delta\left(x - c\right)$ is the Dirac-δ general function defined as

$$\int_{\Omega_\varepsilon} \delta\left(x\right) dx = \begin{cases} 1 & \text{if } x \in \Omega_\varepsilon \\ 0, & \text{otherwise} \end{cases} \tag{12.25}$$

with Ω_ε being an arbitrary small subspace. From (12.25) we can see that the general function has the property: $\delta\left(x\right) = 0$ if $x \neq 0$ and $\delta\left(x\right) = \infty$ if $x = 0$, which is different from the conventional function definition.

Logit (sigmoid) function:

$$G\left(x\right) = \frac{1}{1 + \exp\left(-x\right)}; \ G'\left(x\right) = \frac{-\exp\left(-x\right)}{\left[1 + \exp\left(-x\right)\right]^2}. \tag{12.26}$$

A generalized logit function is given by

$$G\left(x\right) = \frac{1}{1 + \exp\left(-f\left(x\right)\right)}; \ G'\left(x\right) = G\left(x\right)\left(1 - G\left(x\right)\right)\frac{df\left(x\right)}{dx}, \tag{12.27}$$

where $f\left(\cdot\right)$ is a real function.

Absolute function:

$$G\left(x\right) = |x|; \ G'\left(x\right) = \frac{x}{|x|}. \tag{12.28}$$

Softmax function:

$$G\left(x\right) = \frac{\exp\left(x_i\right)}{\sum_i \exp\left(x_i\right)}. \tag{12.29}$$

Hyperbolic tangent (Tanh) function:

$$G\left(x\right) = \frac{e^{-x} - e^x}{e^{-x} + e^x}. \tag{12.30}$$

Gaussian:

$$G\left(x\right) = \exp\left(-\frac{x^2}{2\pi}\right); \ G'\left(x\right) = -\frac{x}{\pi}\exp\left(-\frac{x^2}{2\pi}\right). \tag{12.31}$$

There are many possible ANNs for pharmacodynamic analysis. Figure 12.7 presents an ANN with four layers: input, PK compartment, receptor, and pharmacological output layers.

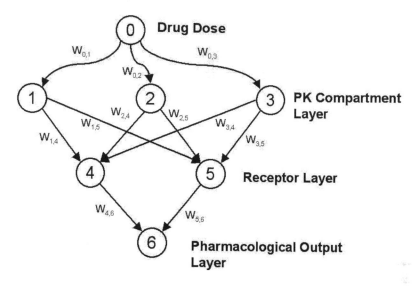

Figure 12.7:   Artificial Neural Network for PD

The layer structure such as the one in an ANN is very common in our lives. The nodes in each layer perform a similar role but differ in magnitude or efficiency (weights differ). Once some nodes fail, other nodes in the same layer will take more "responsibilities" or weights to accomplish the mission. There are plenty of examples that several units in a system have the same functionality but differ in efficiency or time (it seems that redundant = robust). For example, many people can accomplish the same task but their speed and the quality of the outcome differ. There are many cells that carry out similar functions or several biological pathways for causing the same disease. For this reason, we can consider them as nodes in the same layer and use a linear combination for the outcome.

In a regression method, the less significant parameters are removed from the final model to avoid overfitting. In an ANN, no parameters are removed from the model, but the weights are adjusted gradually based on observed (training) data using algorithms such as the back-propagation method.

ANNs for Abstract Drug Design

ANNs have been used for so-called abstract drug design (Abraham, Grosan, and Tigan, 2007), in which three learning algorithms, namely, an evolutionary artificial neural network, a Takagi-Sugeno neuro-fuzzy system, and an artificial neural network are combined. The ensemble combination is optimized by a particle swarm optimization algorithm. The experimental data were obtained from the Laboratory of Pharmaceutical Techniques of the Faculty of Pharmacy in Cluj-Napoca, Romania. Additional data were generated using the bootstrap method.

Hypothesis Test for an ANN

A hypothesis test for a parameter (e.g., treatment) can be performed using a bootstrap method. In this method, we draw a random sample of the original sample size from the data with replacement. For each sample, we train the ANN the same way as with the original data. Then the distribution of the outcomes/output from the ANN can provide a way to calculate the confidence interval (see Chapter 13).

12.3.5 *Genetic Programming for Pharmacodynamics*

In an ANN, the network topology is predetermined and weights are adjusted based on training data. In contrast, GP (see Chapters 1 and 13 for more information) aims to create the topology and numerical parameters (called sizing) for the network simultaneously based on observed data. Is it possible? Koza and colleagues (Koza et al., 2005) have proved that it can be done using a metabolic network involving four chemical reactions that takes glycerol and fatty acid as input, uses ATP as a cofactor, and produces diacyl-glycerol as its final product. In their model, the topology of a network of chemical reactions comprises:

(1) The total number of reactions in the network,
(2) The number of substrate(s) consumed by each reaction,
(3) The number of product(s) produced by each reaction,
(4) The pathways supplying the substrate(s),
(5) The pathways dispersing each reaction's product(s), and
(6) An indication of which enzyme (if any) acts as a catalyst for a particular reaction.

These chemical and enzymic reactions are represented by a program tree that contains:

(1) Internal nodes representing chemical reaction functions,
(2) Internal nodes representing selector functions that select the reaction's first versus the reaction's second product (if any),
(3) External points (leaves) representing substances that are consumed by a reaction,
(4) External points (leaves) representing substances that are produced by a reaction,

(5) External points representing enzymes that catalyze a reaction, and

(6) External points representing numerical constants (reaction rates).

Koza and colleagues conclude that there are numerous opportunities to incorporate and exploit preexisting knowledge about chemistry and biology in the application of PG. Genetic programming could be used to generate diverse alternatives to naturally occurring pathways (Mendes and Kell, 1998; Mittenthal et al., 1998). Conceivably, realizable alternative metabolisms might emerge from such evolutionary runs in GP.

12.4 Drug–Drug Interaction

12.4.1 *Drug–Drug Interaction Mechanisms*

Drug–drug interactions are possible whenever a person takes two or more medications concurrently. Recent advances in the area of cytochrome P-450 drug metabolizing enzymes have made a dramatic impact on drug interaction studies. The drug affected by the interaction is called the "object drug," and the drug causing the interaction is called the "precipitant drug." The drugs' interactions can be categorized into pharmacokinetic and pharmacodynamic interactions. Pharmacokinetic drug interactions refer to one drug affecting the ADME of another, whereas pharmacodynamic drug interactions imply the two drugs have synergistic, additive, or antagonistic pharmacological effects.

12.4.2 *Pharmacokinetic Drug Interactions*

Drugs that act as binding agents can impair the bioavailability of other drugs. This will result in a reduction in the therapeutic effect of the object drug. The effects of drugs that have pH dependent absorption will be affected by drugs that increase stomach pH. Some drugs (prodrugs) require activation by enzymes in the body before they can produce their effects. Inhibition of the metabolism of these prodrugs may reduce the amount of active drug formed and decrease or eliminate the therapeutic effect. Other drugs (enzyme inducers) are capable of increasing the activity of drug metabolizing enzymes, resulting in a decrease in the effect of certain other drugs. Some drugs are converted to toxic metabolites by drug metabolizing enzymes and some can alter the renal route of elimination.

12.4.3   *Pharmacodynamic Drug Interactions*

Pharmacodynamic interactions can occur when two or more drugs have mechanisms of action that result in the same physiological outcome. Most drugs are metabolized to inactive or less active metabolites by enzymes in the liver and intestine. Inhibition of this metabolism can increase the effect of the object drug and increase the chance of drug toxicity.

Pharmacodynamic interactions can be characterized into: (1) synergistic when the effect of two drugs is greater than the sum of their individual effects, (2) antagonistic when the effect of two drugs is less than the sum of their individual effects, (3) additive when the effect of two drugs is merely the sum of the effects of each, and (4) sequence dependent when the order in which two drugs is given governs their effects.

Synergistic Interactions

In oncology, synergistic effects can result in increased cytotoxic activity and translate into an improved clinical response. For example, leucovorin increases the activity of 5-FU in the treatment of colorectal cancer by stabilizing the complex of 5-FU and thymidylate synthase (TS). However, synergistic interactions can also increase adverse effects. Although leucovorin is commonly used as a modulator to increase the anti-tumor effectiveness of 5-FU, its use can also increase 5-FU toxicity (Scripture and Figg, 2006).

Additive Pharmacodynamic Effects

When two or more drugs with similar pharmacodynamic effects are given, the additive effects may result in the sum of the individual responses and toxicities. Examples given by Hansten and Horn (2003) include combinations of drugs that prolong the QTc interval resulting in ventricular arrhythmias, and combining drugs with hyperkalemic effects resulting in hyperkalemia.

Antagonistic Pharmacodynamic Effects

Drugs with opposing pharmacodynamic effects may reduce the response to one or both drugs (Hansten and Horn, 2003). For example, drugs that tend to increase blood pressure (such as nonsteroidal anti-inflammatory drugs) may inhibit the antihypertensive effect of drugs such as ACE inhibitors. Another example would be inhibition of the response to benzodiazepines by the concurrent use of theophylline.

As pointed out by Hansten and Horn (2003), although dramatic advances have been made in the study of drug interaction mechanisms over the past few decades, there is still much to learn. Thus, many of the mechanism concepts useful today will be refined in the future, yielding a picture closer to the truth. It also should be kept in mind that for some drug–drug interactions more than one mechanism may be occurring simultaneously.

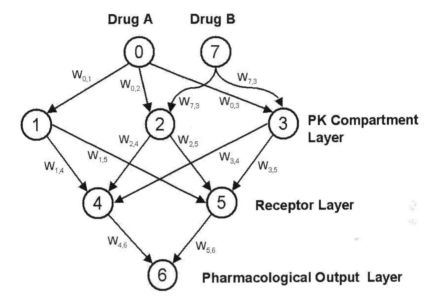

Figure 12.8:   Artificial Neural Network for Drug–Drug Interaction

ANNs provide nice features to model and simulate drug–drug interactions. Figure 12.8 provides such an artificial neural network. Although there are only two drug nodes and one output node in this example, one can add as many drug nodes and output nodes as necessary to the network.

The algorithm for the drug–drug interaction network is essentially the same as Algorithm 11.2. After the initial weights are chosen, the patient (or animal) data are collected. The weights are updated using the back-propagation method whenever data for a new patient becomes available. When the ANN is adequately trained, it can be used for predictions.

12.5   Application of Pharmacodynamic Modeling

Case Study 12.1: Prostate Cancer Trial

The prostate is a gland found only in men. There are several types of cells in the prostate, but nearly all prostate cancers start in the gland cells. Many cases of prostate cancer aren't detected until the cancer has spread beyond the prostate. For most men, prostate cancer is first detected during a routine screening such as a prostate-specific antigen (PSA) test.

The investigative therapy XYZ combines the chemotherapeutic maytansinoid drug DM1. This Phase Ib dose-escalation trial for men with metastatic androgen-independent prostate cancer was designed to determine (1) the therapy's dose-limiting toxicity (DLT) and maximum tolerated dose (MTD) and (2) the therapy's response rate. At the interim analysis, the efficacy response based on the PD marker, meaning PSA reduction 50% from baseline, showed promising results. However, there was a concern regarding the moderately high rate of neuropathy ($\geq$ grade 2). Therefore, the question was raised: can we modify the dose regimen to improve the safety profile without jeopardizing efficacy? Theoretically we can if the mechanism for efficacy and safety is different (e.g., if efficacy is largely controlled by AUC and safety is substantially contributed to $C_{\max}$). The following PD modeling and simulations were conducted. The ultimate goal of this simulation was to identify an optimal dose regimen that would provide a satisfactory safety and efficacy profile for the drug.

Univariate logistic regressions for neuropathy and PSA reduction were first performed, followed by a multivariate logistic regression using a stepwise-elimination method. The final model only includes the factors that are both clinically and statistically significant. Twelve potential risk factors causing neuropathy were considered and grouped into three categories: (1) baseline characteristics, (2) PK parameters, i.e., mechanics of action (controlled by AUC or C_{max} or both), (3) dose regimen including dose intensity and frequency/interval for an optimal dose regimen. The univariate safety modeling results are presented in Table 12.2 and the univariate PD modeling results are presented in Table 12.3.

Ideally, effects of AUC and $C_{\max}$ on neuropathy and PSA are different. To confirm that, the predictive model was considered, based on which an optimal regimen was expected to be found. Multivariate analyses were performed and the main conclusions are: All baseline variables were not significant; $C_{\max}$ of xyz-DM1 complex was a good predictor for safety and efficacy. The multivariate analysis indicated that PSA reduction is basically characterized by plasma concentration $C_{\max}$ of xyz-DM1 and neuropathy occurrence is characterized by $C_{\max}$ and AUC.

Table 12.2: Univariate Analysis for Neuropathy ($\geq$Grade 2)

Risk Factor (unit)	Odds Ratio	P-value
Dose to onset of neuropathy (100 mg/m^2)	1.02	0.790
Dose to maximum grade (100 mg/m^2)	1.13	0.074
Scheduled dose (10 mg/m^2) in cycle 1	1.09	0.007
Dose intensity (10 mg/(m^2.wk)) in cycle 1	1.33	0.001
Dose interval (wk) in cycle 1	0.81	0.394
Prior neuropathy (Y/N)	0.46	0.364
Taxanes (Y/N)	0.62	0.482
Diabetes (Y/N)	0.95	0.958
xyz-DM1 C$_{max}$ (25 μg/mL) in cycle 1	4.57	0.003
Free DM1 C$_{max}$ (0.05 mg/mL) in cycle 1	1.36	0.007
xyz –DM1 AUC (1000 μg/mL·h) in cycle 1	1.23	0.004
Free DM1 AUC (mg/mL·h) in cycle 1	1.19	0.009

Table 12.3: Univariate Analysis for PSA Decline ($\geq$50%)

Factor (unit)	Odds Ratio	P-value
Dose to onset of neuropathy (100 mg/m^2)	1.23	0.039
Dose to maximum grade (100 mg/m^2)	1.16	0.089
Scheduled dose (10 mg/m^2) in cycle 1	1.08	0.088
Dose intensity (10 mg/(m^2·wk)) in cycle 1	1.10	0.333
Dose interval (wk) in cycle 1	1.06	0.887
Prior neuropathy (Y/N)	0.93	0.947
Taxanes (Y/N)	0.41	0.438
Diabetes (Y/N)	1.71	0.656
xyz-DM1 C$_{max}$ (25 μg/mL) in cycle 1	2.15	0.145
Free DM1 C$_{max}$ (0.05 mg/mL) in cycle 1	1.08	0.459
xyz-DM1 AUC (1000 μg/mL·h) in cycle 1	1.13	0.146
Free DM1 AUC (mg/mL·h) in cycle 1	1.05	0.499

The predicted probability of neuropathy ($\geq$grade 2) turns out to be

$$Pr = [1 + \exp(1.706 - 0.0107D + 0.563D_I)] - 1,$$

where D is dose and D_I is dose interval.

The predicted probability of PSA decline ($\geq$50%) is given by:

$$Pr = [1 + \exp(3.985 - 0.00743D)] - 1.$$

Based on this predictive model, the conclusion was that the dose regimen with 300 mg/m^2 every 4 weeks is a good choice, and will have a probability of efficacy (50% decline in PSA) of 18% and a probability of toxicity (grade 2 neuropathy) of 40%. These simulation results triggered a protocol amendment for the new treatment with 300 mg/m^2 every 4 weeks.

12.6   Summary

Theoretically, pharmacodynamics refers to the relationship between drug concentrations at the site of action (receptor) and pharmacological response, including the biochemical and physiologic effects that influence the interaction of drug with the receptor. Practically, the concentration at an active site in the relationship is often replaced with the plasma concentration because the former is difficult to measure.

According to occupancy theory, the drug effect is a function of the following processes: binding of the drug to the receptor, drug-induced activation (inhibition) of the receptor, and propagation of this initial receptor activation (inhibition) into the observed pharmacological effect, where the intensity of the pharmacological effect is proportional to the number of receptor sites occupied by the drug. The receptor occupancy concept shows how a drug elicits a pharmacological response as an agonist, or produces an opposing pharmacological response as an antagonist through drug-receptor interactions.

The pharmacological response in drug therapy is often a product of physiologic adaptation to a drug response. Many drugs trigger the pharmacological response through a cascade of enzymatic events highly regulated by the body, whereas clinical measurement of a drug response may only occur after many such biologic events. Pharmacodynamic modeling must account for biologic processes involved in eliciting drug induced responses. In general, the onset, intensity, and duration of the pharmacological effect depend on the dose and the pharmacokinetics of the drug. As the dose increases, the drug concentration at the receptor site increases, and the pharmacological response increases until the maximum effect is reached.

Understanding different types of enzymes is important in drug development. Enzyme induction is the process whereby an enzyme is synthesized in response to a specific inducer molecule. The inducer molecule combines with a repressor and thereby prevents the blocking of an operator by the repressor that leads to the translation of the gene for the enzyme. In contrast, enzyme inhibitors are molecules that bind to enzymes and decrease their activities.

Enzyme inhibitors can be classified as uncompetitive, competitive, and mixed inhibitors. In uncompetitive inhibition, the inhibitor binds only to the substrate-enzyme complex. In competitive inhibition, the substrate and inhibitor compete for the same enzyme's active site because competitive inhibitors are often similar in structure to the real substrate. This type of inhibition can be overcome by sufficiently high concentrations of substrate, i.e., by out-competing the inhibitor. In mixed inhibition, the inhibitor can bind to the enzyme at the same time as the enzyme's substrate. However, the binding of the inhibitor affects the binding of the substrate, and vice versa. This type of inhibition can be reduced, but not overcome, by increasing concentrations of substrate.

The liver is the major site of drug metabolism, and the type of metabolism is based on the reaction involved. Oxidation, reduction, hydrolysis, and conjugation are the most common reactions. The enzymes responsible for oxidation and reduction of drugs (xenobiotics) and certain natural metabolites, such as steroids, are monoxygenase enzymes known as mixed-function oxidases.

Pharmacodynamic interactions can occur when two or more drugs have mechanisms of action that result in the same physiological outcome. Most drugs are metabolized to inactive or less active metabolites by enzymes in the liver and intestine. Inhibition of this metabolism can increase the effect of the object drug and increase the chance of drug toxicity.

Pharmacodynamic interactions can be characterized into: (1) synergistic when the effect of two drugs is greater than the sum of their individual effects, (2) antagonistic when the effect of two drugs is less than the sum of their individual effects, (3) additive when the effect of two drugs is merely the sum of the effects of each, and (4) sequence dependent when the order in which two drugs is given governs their effects.

The maximum effect model is a widely used empirical model that relates pharmacological response to plasma drug concentrations. The model describes drug action in terms of maximum effect and drug potency.

An artificial neural network (ANN) mimics the mechanism of the human neural network using adaptive weights between the layers in the network to model very complicated systems. An ANN consists of layers of nodes, each of which, though it may have different abilities, carries the same task, and hence can be linearly weighted. The effects of those nodes collectively contribute the output to the next layer through a link function. A distinction between a conventional regression approach and an ANN is that the same data can be used to train the ANN more than once, whereas in a regression model, coefficients are determined once, i.e., the same data set can only be used once.

Unlike ANNs, where the network topology is predetermined and weights are adjusted based on training data, genetic programming (GP) aims to create the topology and numerical parameters for the network simultaneously based on observed data such as in the case of a metabolic network involving chemical reactions studied by Koza and colleagues (Koza et al., 2005).

12.7 Exercises

Exercise 12.1: What are the purposes of pharmacodynamic studies and how can simulation help?

Exercise 12.2: What factors will affect the plasma protein concentration?

Exercise 12.3: Describe enzyme inducers and inhibitors.

Exercise 12.4: How does the plasma concentration differ between single dose and multiple dose regimens?

Exercise 12.5: What are the bases for interspecies scaling?

Exercise 12.6: What is a two-layer perceptron?

Exercise 12.7: If there is more than one type of binding site and the drug binds independently on each binding site with its own association constant, derive the Michaelis-Menten equation for the rate of the reaction for the formulation of the product (metabolic) or the forward rate of decomposition of the ED intermediate.

Exercise 12.8: Devise an algorithm (corresponding to Algorithm 12.1) using p-order error $E = |y_k - \hat{y}_k|^p$ and link function $G(x) = 1/(1 + \exp(-x))$.

Exercise 12.9: Use cross-entropy (deviance) $E = -\sum \hat{z}_m \ln z_m$ to derive the back-propagation algorithms for the ANN in Figure 12.6.

Exercise 12.10: Study the multiple sites and multiple molecules Michaelis-Menten equation using the occupation theory for enzyme dynamics.

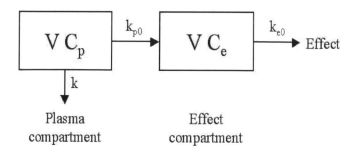

Figure 12.9:   Effect Compartment Model

Exercise 12.11: The maximum pharmacological response produced by a drug may be observed some time after the plasma drug concentration reaches its peak, i.e., there is a delayed pharmacological response. To account for the pharmacodynamics of delayed drug response, an effect compartment model can be used in addition to the PK compartment (Figure

12.9). This effect compartment is a hypothetical pharmacodynamic compartment that links to the plasma compartment containing the drug. The drug substance transfers from the plasma compartment to the effect compartment. Only a free drug will diffuse into the effect compartment, and the transfer rate constants are usually first order. The pharmacological response is determined from the rate constant. Study this model.

Exercise 12.12: Derive the back-propagation algorithm for a four-layer ANN (Figure 12.10) and train the ANN using random data generated from some distribution.

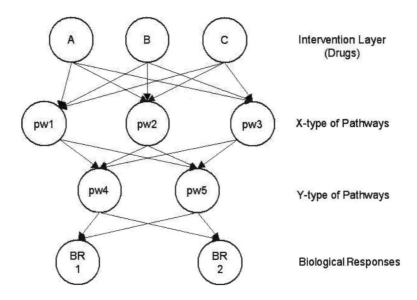

Figure 12.10:   An ANN for Biological Pathways Modeling

Chapter 13

Monte Carlo for Inference and Beyond

This chapter will cover the following topics:

- Sorting Algorithm
- Resampling Methods
- Genetic Programming

13.1 Sorting Algorithm

13.1.1 *Quicksorting Algorithms*

Sorting is one of the most common tasks in Monte Carlo computing. Two very important sorting algorithms are Quicksort by Hoare (Hoare, 1960) and Heapsort by Press et al. (2007). Quicksort is the fastest known general sorting algorithm. In this section, we are going to discuss several useful sorting algorithms.

The Quicksort algorithm was proposed by Tony Hoare in 1962 (Hoare, 1962). It is a simple and fast sorting technique. The basic idea behind the algorithm is to partition the array C into two subarrays: C_{small}, containing all elements from C that are smaller than m, and C_{large}, containing all elements larger than m, where m is selected from C (e.g., the first element). This partitioning can be done in linear time, and by following a divide-and-conquer strategy. Quicksort recursively sorts each subarray in the same way (Jones and Pevzner, 2004). The sorted list returned is the concatenation of the sorted C_{small}, element m, and the sorted C_{large}.

Algorithm 13.1: Quicksorting
Objective: Return sorted array of C using Quicksort.
Function Quicksort(C)
$\qquad m := C_1$

  Determine the set of elements C_{small} smaller than m
  Determine the set of elements C_{large} larger than m
  Quicksort(C_{small})
  Quicksort(C_{large})
  Concatenate C_{small}, m, and C_{large} into C_{sorted}
Return C_{sorted}.
§

  The implementation of Quicksort using the object-oriented language C^{++} is available (e.g., Press et al., 2007).

  The efficiency of Quicksort depends on the value of m. If m divides C into C_{small} and C_{large} with even size, then it leads to $O(n \ln n)$ running time. However, if we choose m in such a way that it splits C unevenly, the running time could be up to $O(n^2)$. However, if we choose m uniformly at random, there is at least a 50% chance that it will be a good splitter. This observation motivates the following randomized algorithm (Algorithm 13.2) with the expected running time $O(n \ln n)$ (Jones and Pevzner, 2004):

Algorithm 13.2: Randomized Quicksort
Objective: Return sorted array using Randomized Quicksort.
Function RandomizedQuicksort(C)
  Randomly choose element m uniformly from C
  Determine the set of elements C_{small} smaller than m
  Determine the set of elements C_{large} larger than m
  RandomizedQuicksort(C_{small})
  RandomizedQuicksort(C_{large})
  Concatenate C_{small}, m, and C_{large} into C_{sorted}
Return C_{sorted}.
§

  Heapsort is an "in-place" sort, requiring no auxiliary storage. It is lower than Quicksort by a constant factor, but it is so beautiful that people sometimes use it anyway, just for the sheer joy of it (see Press et al., 2007).

13.1.2   *Indexing and Ranking*

Indexing is a central part of any search engine such as Google and Yahoo. It is also important for any other larger database search. For a data file with multiple fields (variables) with N records, the sorting task is usually accomplished by means of the so-called index table. In such an index table I_j, $j = 0, 1, ..., N - 1$, the smallest K_i has $i = I_0$, the second smallest has

$i = I_1$, and so on up to the largest K_i with $i = I_{N-1}$. In other words, the array

$$K_{I_j}, \ j = 0, 1, ...N - 1$$

is in sorted order when indexed by j.

Using various index tables created and sorted, we can sort the data file without actually moving the records from their original order. The algorithm for constructing an index table is straightforward, as outlined in Algorithm 13.3.

Algorithm 13.3: Index Table
Objective: Create an index table.

(1) Initialize the index array C with integers 0 to $N - 1$.
(2) Perform the Quicksorting algorithm for C, moving the elements around as if one were sorting the keys.
(3) The integer that initially numbered the smallest key thus ends up in the number one position, and so on.

§

The implementation of Algorithm 13.3 using C^{++} is available (see Press et al., 2007).

Another type of sorting task is ranking or selecting the kth largest element, as is often required in statistical analyses. A commonly used algorithm for this task with a large dataset is single-pass selection, where we have a stream of input values, each of which we get to see only once. At any time after N input values, we can report the kth smallest value. The fastest general method for the selection, allowing rearrangement, is partitioning, exactly as for the Quicksort algorithm. See Press et al. (2007) for implementation with C^{++}.

13.2 Resampling Methods

13.2.1 *Bootstrap: The Plug-in Principle*

Bootstrapping is a resampling method which estimates the distribution of an estimator by sampling with replacement from the original sample. Bootstrapping is useful when the analytical form of distribution is not available or is unknown. Bootstrapping is often used for deriving robust estimates of standard errors and confidence intervals of a population parameter like a mean, median, proportion, odds ratio, correlation coefficient, or regression coefficient. It can also be used for constructing a hypothesis test.

Suppose $x_1, x_2, ..., x_n$ is i.i.d. from probability distribution F. The empirical distribution function $\hat{F}$ is defined to be the discrete distribution that puts $1/n$ on each value x_i $(i = 1, ..., n)$, i.e.,

$$\hat{\Pr}\{A\} = \frac{\#\{x_i \in A\}}{n}. \tag{13.1}$$

The Plug-in Principle

The plug-in principle is a simple method of estimating parameters from samples. The plug-in estimate of a parameter $\theta = t(F)$ is defined to be (Efron and Tibshirami, 1994; Chernick, 2007)

$$\hat{\theta} = t\left(\hat{F}\right). \tag{13.2}$$

In other words, we estimate the function $\theta = t(F)$ of the probability distribution F by the same function of the empirical distribution $\hat{F}$, $\hat{\theta} = t\left(\hat{F}\right)$.

Algorithm 13.4 is an algorithm for the plug-in principle.

Algorithm 13.4: Bootstrapping Distribution of Estimator
Objective: Return bootstrapping distribution of estimator $\theta(x_1, ..., x_n)$.
Input observations $\{x_1, ..., x_n\}$ and nRuns.
For $i := 1$ **To** nRuns
    For $j := 1$ **To** n
        Draw k from the equal distribution $U_c(n)$
        $y_j^{(i)} := x_k$
    Endfor
    $\hat{\theta}_i := \theta\left(y_1^{(i)}, y_2^{(i)} ..., y_m^{(i)}\right)$
Endfor
Sort $\left\{\hat{\theta}_1, \hat{\theta}_2, ..., \hat{\theta}_{\text{nRuns}}\right\}$
Return $\left\{\hat{\theta}_1, \hat{\theta}_2, ..., \hat{\theta}_{\text{nRuns}}\right\}$
§

Having obtained the sorted $\left\{\hat{\theta}_1, \hat{\theta}_2, ..., \hat{\theta}_{\text{nRuns}}\right\}$, its median, quantiles, mean, standard error, and confidence interval can be easily calculated.

Resampling Methods in Clinical Trials

Confidence intervals (CI), hypothesis test, and p-value calculations are common statistical analyses in clinical trials. The following is a clinical trial example with two parallel groups and sample size n per group. Assume the total number of responses observed is m and the observed proportions in groups 1 and 2 are $\hat{p}_1$ and $\hat{p}_2$, respectively. In Algorithm 13.5, the goal is to calculate the confidence interval for the difference between the response rates p_1 and p_2. The main step in the bootstrap approach is to sort the bootstrap values for $T_k = p_2 - p_1$ ($k = 1, 2, ...$). With these sorted values T_k, the confidence interval (CI) and the p-value can be obtained. Because the CI and p-value are calculated based on the assumption of the null hypothesis condition, meaning there is no treatment effect, the response data can be pooled, and the treatment code can be scrambled. In Algorithm 13.5, the pooled data are represented by $\{x_1, x_2, ..., x_{2n}\}$, for each simulation run, the treatment code is randomly assigned for each observation x_i, and the response rate is calculated for each group p_1 and p_2, from which the test statistic $T_k := p_2 - p_1$ is calculated. These T_ks then are sorted for calculating the confidence interval for the rate difference. The histogram of T_k is the empirical distribution of the test statistic T_k under the null hypothesis; by comparing this distribution with the observed value $\hat{T} = \hat{p}_2 - \hat{p}_1$, the p-value can be calculated.

Algorithm 13.5: Bootstrapping CI for Rate Difference
Objective: Return a bootstrap $100(1 - \alpha)\%$ CI for $\hat{p}_2 - \hat{p}_1$
Input n, m, $\hat{p}_1$, $\hat{p}_2$, and binary responses $\{x_1, x_2, ..., x_{2n}\}$.
For $k := 1$ **To** nRuns
    $p_1 := 0$
    $p_2 := 0$
    For $i := 1$ **To** $2n$
        Generate a random sample u from $U_c(n)$
        If $u = 1$ **Then** $p_1 := p_1 + x_i/n$
        If $u = 2$ **Then** $p_2 := p_2 + x_i/n$
    Endfor
    $T_k := p_2 - p_1$
Endfor
Sort $\{T_1, T_2, ..., T_{\text{nRuns}}\}$ in ascending order
CI$:= \{T_{\lfloor \alpha \cdot \text{nRuns} \rfloor}, T_{\lceil (1-\alpha) \cdot \text{nRuns} \rceil}\}$
Return CI and $\{T_1, T_2, ..., T_{\text{nRuns}}\}$
§

The general steps in the bootstrap method can be described as follows:

(1) Substitute the empirical (sample) distribution for the population distribution.
(2) Repeat the experiment procedure using the sample distribution instead of the population distribution.

(3) Use the estimator (or test statistic) to calculate the estimate for the parameter for each sample.
(4) Sort the values of the parameter estimate.
(5) The rest of the calculations are dependent on a particular question but usually are a trivial task.

The stagewise-ordering p-value is a measure of the statistical strength of the evidence in an adaptive trial (see Chapter 6). Algorithm 13.6 can be used to calculate this p-value using a bootstrap method.

Algorithm 13.6: Bootstrap for the Stagewise-Ordering p-value
Objective: Bootstrap for the stagewise-ordering p-value in an adaptive trial. The method is useful when the distribution of test statistics under H_o is not fully determined.

(1) Repeat the experiment procedure using the sample distribution instead of the population distribution.
(2) For the kth stage stagewise-ordering p-value, collect all samples that pass the $(k-1)^{th}$ stage and calculate their corresponding test statistic.
(3) Sort the test statistics by their values.
(4) Stagewise p-value p_i is the proportion of the observed statistical values larger than the single value observed from actual trial $\hat{t}_i$.
(5) The stagewise ordering p-value is $p_{adj} = \sum_{i=1}^{k-1} \pi_i + p_i$.
§

13.2.2 *Asymptotic Theory of Bootstrap*

Let $X_1, ..., X_n$ be i.i.d. from distribution F and $\Re_n = \Re_n(X_1, ..., X_n, F)$ be a random variable. We are interested in estimating the sampling distribution R_n, i.e.,

$$H_{n,F} = P\{\Re_n \le x|F\}. \tag{13.3}$$

Because F is not always available, we approximate F by its empirical distribution F_n based on $X_1, ...,$ and X_n in (13.3), i.e.,

$$H_{n,F_n} = P^*\{\Re_n(X_1^*, ..., X_n^*, F_n) \le x|F_n\}, \tag{13.4}$$

where $X_1^*, ..., X_n^*$ are i.i.d. from F_n.

Efron's Plug-In Principle suggests using bootstrap estimation (13.4) to approximate $H_{n,F}$ in (13.3).

In general, we use notations $T_n = T_n (X_1, ..., X_n)$ for an estimator of parameter θ and $T_n^* = T_n (X_1^*, ..., X_n^*)$ for the corresponding bootstrap estimator. If $\Re_n = T_n - \theta$ and

$$H_{n,F} = P\{T_n - \theta \le x | F\}, \tag{13.5}$$

then the bootstrap estimator of $H_{n,F}$ can be written as

$$H_{n,F_n} = P\{T_n^* - T_n \le x | F_n\}. \tag{13.6}$$

Example 13.1: For constructing a confidence interval of unknown parameter θ related to F, we use $\Re_n = T_n - \theta$ or the studentized version $(T_n - \theta)/S_n$, where T_n is an estimator of θ and S_n is a estimator of the standard deviation of T_n.

In the following, we present some important theoretical results, where the measure ρ_m $(m = 1, 2., ..., \infty)$ is the Mallows distance (Shao and Tu, 1995).

Theorem 13.1 *Let $X_1, ..., X_n$ be i.i.d. random variables from F and $T_n = \sum_{j=1}^m a_j F_n^{-1}(p_j)$. Suppose that F is differentiable at each $F^{-1}(p_j)$ and $f(F^{-1}(p_j)) > 0$ where $f = \frac{dF}{dt}$. Then, the bootstrap estimator $H_{n,F_n} = P\{\sqrt{n}(T_n^* - T_n) \le x\}$ for $H_{n,F} = P\{\sqrt{n}(T_n - \theta) \le x\}$ is strongly consistent, i.e., $\rho_\infty(H_{n,F_n}, H_{n,F}) \to_{a.s.} 0$ as $n \to \infty$.*

Theorem 13.2 *Suppose that $E\|X_1\|^2 < \infty$, $T_n = g(\bar{X}_n)$, and g is continuously differentiable at $\theta = E(X_1)$ with $\nabla g(\mu) \ne 0$. Then the bootstrap estimator H_{n,F_n} defined by (13.6) is strongly consistent for $H_{n,F}$ in (13.5), i.e., $\rho_\infty(H_{n,F_n}, H_{n,F}) \to_{a.s.} 0$ as $n \to \infty$.*

Standardized Mean

Bickel and Freedman (1980) and Singh (1981), among others, studied the accuracy of

$$H_{n,F_n}(x) = P^*\{\sqrt{n}(\bar{X}_n^* - \bar{X}_n) \le x\}, \tag{13.7}$$

the bootstrap estimator of

$$H_n(x) = P\{\sqrt{n}(\bar{X}_n - \mu) \le x\} \tag{13.8}$$

and the accuracy of $\tilde{H}_{n,F_n}(x) = H_{n,F_n}(\hat{\sigma}x)$ as an estimator of $\tilde{H}_{n,F}(x) = H_{n,F_n}(\sigma x)$, the distribution of the standardized sample mean $\sqrt{n}(\bar{X}_n - \mu)/\sigma$. Some of the key results are summarized in the following theorems:

Theorem 13.3 *Let $X_1, ..., X_n$ be i.i.d. random variables.*

(i) If $E\left(X_1^4\right) < \infty$, then

$$\lim_{n\to\infty} \sup \frac{\sqrt{n}\rho_\infty \left(H_{n,F_n}, H_{n,F}\right)}{\sqrt{\ln(\ln n)}} = \frac{\sqrt{var(X_1 - \mu)^2}}{2\sigma^2\sqrt{\pi e}} \quad a.s. \tag{13.9}$$

(ii) If $E|X_1|^3 < \infty$ and F is lattice in the sense that there are a constant c and h such that $P\{X_1 = c + kh, k = 0, 1, 2, ...\} = 1$, then

$$\lim_{n\to\infty} \sup \sqrt{n}\rho_\infty \left(\tilde{H}_{n,F_n}(x), \tilde{H}_{n,F}(x)\right) = \frac{h}{\sqrt{2\pi\sigma}} \quad a.s. \tag{13.10}$$

(iii) If $E|X_1|^3 < \infty$ and F is nonlattice, then

$$\lim_{n\to\infty} \sqrt{n}\rho_\infty \left(\tilde{H}_{n,F_n}(x), \tilde{H}_{n,F}(x)\right) \to_{a.s.} 0. \tag{13.11}$$

See, e.g., Shao and Tu (1995, p. 92–93) for proofs of the theorem.

Studentized Statistics

Let $\{Y_{j1}, ...Y_{jn_j}\}$ be i.i.d. samples taken from G_j, $j = 1, 2, ..., k$. The corresponding bootstrap sample is denoted by $\left\{Y_{j1}^*, ...Y_{jn_j}^*\right\}$. Denote the jth sample mean $\bar{Y}_j = \frac{1}{n_j}\sum_{i=1}^{n_j} Y_{ji}$ with variance $\hat{\sigma}_j^2 = var\left(\bar{Y}_j\right)$ and the corresponding bootstrap sample mean $\bar{Y}_j^* = \frac{1}{n_j}\sum_{i=1}^{n_j} Y_{ji}^*$ with variance $\hat{\sigma}_j^{*2} = var\left(\bar{Y}_j^*\right)$. Then the student t-statistic

$$t_{kn} = \frac{\sum_{j=1}^k l_j\bar{Y}_j - \theta}{\sqrt{\sum_{j=1}^k \frac{1}{n_j}l_j^2\hat{\sigma}_j^2}} \tag{13.12}$$

can be approximated by the corresponding bootstrap t-statistic

$$t_{kn}^* = \frac{\sum_{j=1}^k l_j\bar{Y}_j^* - \theta}{\sqrt{\sum_{j=1}^k \frac{1}{n_j}l_j^2\hat{\sigma}_j^{*2}}}, \tag{13.13}$$

where $\theta = EY_j$ and l_j $(j = 1, ..., k)$ are predetermined constants.

Theorem 13.4 *(Babu and Singh, 1983) Let $n = \sum_{j=1}^k n_j$, where $n_j \neq 0$ $(j = 1, ..., k)$. Suppose that G_j is continuous and has a finite 6th moment for $\forall j \in \{1, ..., k\}$. Then*

$$\lim_{n\to\infty} \sqrt{n} \sup |P_*\{t_{kn}^* \leq x\} - P\{t_{kn} \leq x\}| \to_{a.s} 0. \tag{13.14}$$

An estimator is usually said to be k^{th} order accurate if its convergence rate is $O(n^{-k/2})$. It is expected that the convergence rate of the bootstrap estimator of the distribution of a standardized or studentized statistic is $O(n^{-1/2})$ or $O(n^{-1})$.

13.2.3 Bayesian Bootstrap

We use a missing data problem to show the application of Bayesian bootstrapping in practice. Missing data are common in clinical trials and data analyses (Gilks, Richardson, and Spiegelhalter 1998). Practically missing data usually refer to to any data points that were intended to be collected but were not obtained. Philosophically, any unobserved variable at any timepoint can be considered as missing or there are no missing data at all. In the most general and abstract form, the "missing data" can refer to any augmented component of the probabilistic system under consideration and the inclusion of this component often results in a simpler structure and easier computation (Liu, 2003).

A Bayesian missing data problem can be formulated as follows (Liu, 2003, p. 19–21): Suppose the "complete-data" model $f(x, \theta)$ has a known analytical posterior distribution form, where θ is a parameter vector and x can partition into the observed part x_{obs} and the missing part x_{mis}, i.e., $x = (x_{obs}, x_{mis})$. The joint posterior distribution of x_{mis} and θ is (see Section 5.4.2)

$$\varphi(\theta, x_{mis}) \propto f(x_{mis}, x_{obs}|\theta) \pi(\theta), \qquad (13.15)$$

and the marginal posterior of θ is given by

$$\pi(\theta|x_{obs}) = \varphi(\theta) = \int \varphi(\theta, x_{mis}) \, dx_{mis}. \qquad (13.16)$$

If we can draw Monte Carlo samples $\left(\theta^{(1)}, x_{mis}^{(1)}\right), ..., \left(\theta^{(m)}, x_{mis}^{(m)}\right)$ from $\varphi(\theta, x_{mis})$, then the "empirical distribution" characterized by the histogram based on $\theta^{(1)}, ..., \theta^{(m)}$ can serve as an approximation to $\pi(\theta|x_{obs})$. Furthermore, for a function $h(\theta)$, we have

$$E\{h(\theta|x_{obs})\} \simeq \frac{1}{m}\left[h(\theta^1) + ... + h\left(\theta^{(m)}\right)\right]. \qquad (13.17)$$

In the case that there is no analytical form available, we can easily obtain the marginal distributions $p\left(x_{mis}|\theta^{(t)}, x_{obs}\right)$ and $p\left(\theta|x_{mis}^{(t+1)}, x_{obs}\right)$ from the joint distribution $\varphi(\theta, x_{mis})$. With the two marginal distributions, we can use the following iterative algorithm to obtain the posterior distribution of θ.

Algorithm 13.7 Posterior With Missing Data
Objective: Return the posterior of parameter θ
$i := 0$
rejection := **True**

While rejection := **True**:

Draw $x_{mis}^{(t+1)}$ from $p\left(x_{mis}|\theta^{(t)}, x_{obs}\right)$

Draw $\theta^{(t+1)}$ from $p\left(\theta|x_{mis}^{(t+1)}, x_{obs}\right)$

$i := i+1$

If stop criterion met **Then** rejection := **False**

Endwhile

Return $\left\{\theta^{(i+1)}\right\}$

§

13.2.4 Jackknife

Jackknifing is a resampling method used to estimate the bias and standard error for an estimator. The basic idea behind jackknifing lies in systematically recomputing the statistic estimate based on subsets of observations, which are obtained from the original set of the observations but leaving one observation out at a time.

Suppose we have a sample $x = (x_1, x_2, ...x_n)$ and an estimator $\hat{\theta}(x)$. We wish to estimate the bias and standard error of $\hat{\theta}$. The kth jackknife sample is

$$x^{(k)} = (x_1, .., k_{k-1}, x_{k+1}, ...x_n) \tag{13.18}$$

where $k = 1, 2, ..., n$. In other words, $x^{(k)}$ is obtained from the original sample x by removing the kth observation. The corresponding k^{th} jackknife replication of $\hat{\theta}$ is given by $\hat{\theta}\left(x^{(k)}\right)$.

The jackknife estimate of bias is defined as

$$\Delta\hat{\theta} = (n-1)\left(\frac{1}{n}\sum_{k=1}^{n}\hat{\theta}^{(k)}\right) \tag{13.19}$$

and the jackknife estimate of standard error is defined as

$$\hat{S}_e = \sqrt{\frac{n-1}{n}\sum_{k=1}^{n}\left(\hat{\theta}^{(k)} - \frac{1}{n}\sum_{k=1}^{n}\hat{\theta}^{(k)}\right)^2}. \tag{13.20}$$

Similar to the jackknife, in the cross-validation of a predictive model, different subsets of the observations, by leaving out a single (or multiple) observation at a time, are used for building the model and validation. Another method, K-fold cross-validation, splits the data into K subsets; each is held out in turn as the validation set.

13.2.5 Permutation Tests

A permutation test (also called a randomization test, re-randomization test, or an exact test) is a type of statistical significance test in which a reference distribution is obtained by calculating all possible values of the test statistic under rearrangements of the treatment labels on the observed data points. The rationale behind the label rearrangement is that we intend to obtain the distribution of the test statistic under the null hypothesis, i.e., no treatment effect or no effect of label rearrangement. This label rearrangement should be consistent with randomization (e.g., 1:1 or 1:2 for a trial with two independent groups). An important assumption behind a permutation test is that the observations are exchangeable under the null hypothesis. This implies that tests of difference in location require equal variance.

The theory has evolved from the works of R.A. Fisher (Fisher, 1953) and E.J.G. Pitman (Pitman, 1937, 1938) and more recently by Good (2005) and Metha, Patel, and Senchaudhuri (1988). For binary responses with two treatment groups, the p-value for testing no difference in response between groups, conditioning the total number of responses, can be calculated exactly.

Let m_i be the number of responses in the ith group with sample size n_i $(i = 1, 2)$. Under the null hypothesis of the same response rate $p_1 = p_2$ in the two groups and a fixed total number of responses $m = m_1 + m_2$, m_1 follows a hypergeometric distribution with parameters (m, n_1, n_2), i.e.,

$$P(m_1 = i | m, n_1, n_2) = \frac{\binom{n_1}{i}\binom{n_2}{m-i}}{\binom{n_1+n_2}{m}}. \tag{13.21}$$

From (13.21), the p-value p, defined as the probability of having equal to or more than m_1 responses, can be calculated as

$$p = \sum_{i=m_1}^{m} \frac{\binom{n_1}{i}\binom{n_2}{m-i}}{\binom{n_1+n_2}{m}}. \tag{13.22}$$

For a continuous response or complex experiment design, the general steps for a permutation test are (1) selecting a test statistic, (2) calculating the observed test statistic for the original treatment label, (3) rearranging (permuting) the labels and computing the corresponding test statistic, repeating for all possible permutations.

The key step in this process is to generate all possible permutations. In the permutation algorithm below (Algorithm 13.8), the idea is to swap only two elements in the target array such that a unique combination is produced (Fuchs, 2008). This algorithm is faster than recursion algorithms.

Algorithm 13.8: Quick Permutation

Objective: Generate all permutations for array $A = (a_0, a_1, ..., a_{N-1})$.

For $i := 0$ **To** $N - 1$

    $p_i = 0$

Endfor

$i := 1$

While $i < N$:

    If $p_i < i$ **Then**

        If i is odd **Then**

            $j := p_i$

        Else

            $j := 0$

        Endif

        swap(a_j, a_i)

        $p_i := p_i + 1$

        Display the array

        $i := 1$

    Else

        $p_i := 0$

        $i := i + 1$

    Endif

Endwhile

§

Sometimes, permutation may not be necessary, meaning there are more efficient algorithms than permutation to solve the problem. Let's illustrate the permutation test for two parallel groups with observed continuous responses $(x_1, x_2, ..., x_n)$. Without loss of generality, suppose the first n_1 observations are for group 1 and the rest for group 2. We calculate the test statistic $T_{obs} = \frac{1}{n_2} \sum_{i=n_1+1}^{n_1+n_2} x_i - \frac{1}{n_1} \sum_{i=1}^{n_1} x_i$ (or another statistic we defined). Next, during permutation we always label the first n_1 observations as treatment 1 and the rest as treatment 2. However, to exhaustively list all the possible permeations and calculate the test statistic for each permutation can be computationally intensive for a large sample size. We can use the following algorithm to greatly reduce the computing time: (1) select $\binom{n_1+n_2}{n_1}$ possible combinations of n_1 observations from $(x_1, x_2, ..., x_n)$. (2) For each such combination j, calculate the test statistic T_j. (3) Compute the frequency for such a test statistic T_j, which is equal to $n_1! n_2!$. In this approach, a combination algorithm is required (Exercise 13.11).

13.3   Genetic Programming

13.3.1   *Genetics and Inheritance*

DNA and Genes

Base pairs are the low-level alphabet of DNA instructions, encoding instructions for the creation of a particular amino acid. The base pairs of two nucleic acid bases then chemically bond to each other, forming a 3D double helix ladder of base pairs. There are only four different bases that appear in DNA, i.e., adenine (A), guanine (G), cytosine (C), and thymine (T). The rules for base pairings are simply A pairs with T; G pairs with C. Thus, any one of the following four base pair configurations comprises a single piece of information in the DNA molecule: $A \sim T$, $T \sim A$, $G \sim C$, $C \sim G$.

A chromosome is an organized structure of DNA and protein in cells. It is a single piece of coiled DNA containing many genes, regulatory elements, and other nucleotide sequences. Chromosomes also contain DNA-bound proteins, which serve to package the DNA and control its functions.

A codon is a template for the production of a particular amino acid or a sequence termination codon. There are 64 different codons or different ways to order four different bases in three different locations. But there are only twenty amino acids for which DNA codes. This is because there are often several different codons that produce the same amino acid — redundancy often implies robustness—in case some of them failed.

Producing amino acids is not the end product of DNA instructions. Instead, DNA acts on the rest of the world by providing the information necessary to manufacture polypeptides, proteins, and nontranslated RNA (tRNA and rRNA) molecules, each of which carries out various tasks in the development of the organism. Proteins are complex organic molecules that are made up of many amino acids. Polypeptides are protein fragments.

Reproduction and Inheritance

The exchange of genetic material in sexual reproduction take places through recombination. The DNA from both parents is recombined to produce an entirely new DNA molecule for the child.

Mendelian inheritance (Mendel, 1865 and 1866) is a set of primary tenets relating to the transmission of hereditary characteristics from parent organisms to their children. Mendel's findings allowed other scientists to predict the expression of traits on the basis of mathematical probabilities. Mendelism became the core of classical genetics after it was integrated with the chromosome theory of inheritance by Thomas Hunt Morgan in 1915.

Mendel discovered that in crossing white flower and purple flower plants, the offspring were not a mix of the two. Instead, the offspring had a ratio of 1:3 between the purples and whites.

This can be explained as follows. An individual possesses two alleles (alternative forms for the same gene) for each trait; one allele is given by the female parent and the other by the male parent. They are passed on when an individual matures and produces gametes: egg and sperm. When gametes form, the paired alleles separate randomly so that each gamete receives a copy of one of the two alleles. The presence of an allele doesn't promise that the trait will be expressed in the individual that possesses it. In heterozygous individuals the only allele that is expressed is the dominant. The recessive allele is present but its expression (appearance or phenotype) is hidden. For Mendel's experiment, genes can be paired in four ways: AA, Aa, aA, aa with equal probability. The capital A represents the dominant factor and lowercase a represents the recessive. In heterozygous pairs (Aa or aA), only gene A is expressed, i.e., the same as the homozygous pairs, AA. The only pair with different expression is the homozygous pair aa. In other words, the ratio of offspring with the two colors is 1:3.

Mendel's findings were summarized in two laws: the law of segregation and the law of independent assortment.

Law of Segregation (The "First Law"): When any individual produces gametes, the copies of a gene separate, so that each gamete receives only one copy. A gamete will receive one allele or the other.

Law of Independent Assortment (The "Second Law"): Alleles of different genes assort independently of one another during gamete formation.

Of the 46 chromosomes in a normal diploid human cell, half are maternally derived and half are paternally derived. This occurs as sexual reproduction involves the fusion of two haploid gametes (the egg and sperm) to produce a new organism having the full complement of chromosomes. In independent assortment the chromosomes that end up in a newly formed gamete are randomly sorted from all possible combinations of maternal and paternal chromosomes. For human gametes, with 23 pairs of chromosomes, the number of possibilities is 2^{23} or 8,388,608 possible combinations with equal probability.

13.3.2 *Natural Selection*

Natural Selection

> ... if variations useful to any organic being do occur, assuredly individuals thus characterized will have the best chance of being preserved in the struggle for life; and from the strong principle of inheritance they will tend to produce offspring similarly character-ized. This principle of preservation, I have called, for the sake of brevity, Natural Selection. – C. Darwin, 1859

Darwin implied here the four essential conditions for the occurrence of evolution by natural selection:

(1) Reproduction of individuals in the population
(2) Heredity in reproduction
(3) Variation that affects the individual, survival
(4) Finite resources causing competition

Those factors result in natural selection that changes the characteristics of the population with an increasing fitness over time. However, in my view, the fourth one is not a necessary condition, but its existence will speed up the evolution process.

The term "fitness" has undergone a semantic shift in its migration from population biology to evolutionary computation. In population biology, fit-ness generally refers to the actual rate at which an individual type ends up being sampled in contributing to the next generation (Altenberg, 1995). In contrast, an evolutionary computation such as genetic programming (GP), fitness is often an artificial function and the probability of selecting a par-ent to produce offspring is a monotonic function of the fitness, thus forcing more offspring for parents with high fitness.

Ontogeny

Ontogeny is the development of the organism from fertilization to matu-rity. Ontogeny is the link between the genotype (DNA), the phenotype (the organism's body and behavior), and the environment in which the organ-ism's development takes place. The organism's DNA mediates the growth and development of the organism from birth to death. Natural selection acts on the phenotype (not on the genotype) because the phenotype (the body) is necessary for biological reproduction. In other words, the organism (the phenotype) must survive to reproduce.

Mutation

Entropy-driven variation, such as mutation, is the principal source of variability in evolution. A mutation is a randomly derived change to the nucleotide sequence of the genetic material of an organism. There are small-scale and large-scale mutations. For GP, we are not interested in large-scale mutations because of the high risk of a fatal consequence. Small-scale mutations include three types of mutations: point mutations, insertions, and deletions.

Point mutations, often caused by chemicals or malfunction of DNA replication, exchange a single nucleotide for another. These changes are classified as transitions or transversions. Most common is the transition that exchanges a purine for a purine ($A \leftrightarrow G$) or a pyrimidine for a pyrimidine, ($C \leftrightarrow T$). In GP, point mutation is most commonly used. Insertions add one or more extra nucleotides into the DNA. They are usually caused by transposable elements, or errors during replication of repeating elements. Deletions remove one or more nucleotides from the DNA. Like insertions, these mutations can alter the reading frame of the gene. They are generally irreversible. Insertions and deletions, called frameshift mutations, often have drastic consequences on the functioning of the gene.

13.3.3   *Genetic Algorithm and Price's Theorem*

Genetic Algorithm

A genetic algorithm (GA) represents a school of directed search algorithms based on the mechanics of biological evolution developed in the 1970s. A genetic algorithm iterates three steps: selection, random mating, and production of offspring to constitute the population in the next generation. The core of GA is the transmission probability of certain characteristics from a generation to the next. Mathematically, the canonical genetic algorithm can be defined as follows (Slatkin, 1970, Altenberg, 1995).

Definition 13.1   *Canonical Genetic Algorithm.* The dynamic system representing the "canonical" genetic algorithm is in the form of transmission probability:

$$p_{i+1}(x) = \sum_{y,z \in S_i} T(x \leftarrow y, z) \frac{\omega(y)\,\omega(z)}{\bar{\omega}^2} p_i(y)\, p_i(z), \qquad (13.23)$$

where $p_{i+1}(x)$ is the frequencies of chromosome in the $(i+1)^{th}$ generation, S_i is the search space of n chromosomal types in the ith generation, and $T(x \leftarrow y, z)$, the transmission function, is the probability that the offspring genotype is produced by parental genotypes and as a result of the action of genetic operators on the representation, with $T\left(x \leftarrow y, z\right) = T\left(x \leftarrow z, y\right)$, and $\Sigma_x T\left(x \leftarrow y, z\right) = 1$ for all $y, z \in S_i$ and $\omega\left(\cdot\right)$ is the *fitness of chromosome* with the average fitness of the population $\bar{\omega} = \Sigma_{g \in S_i} \omega\left(g\right) p\left(g\right)$.

For mutation, only a single parent is chosen, hence

$$p_{i+1}\left(x\right) = \sum_{y \in S_i} T\left(x \leftarrow y\right) \frac{\omega\left(y\right)}{\bar{\omega}} p_i\left(y\right). \tag{13.24}$$

Practically we are more interested in macroscopic properties than the transmission probability, i.e., the change in the population average of a measurement function that measures how the population is evolving:

$$\bar{C}_i = \sum_{x \in S_i} C\left(x\right) p_i\left(x\right) \tag{13.25}$$

$$\bar{C}_{i+1} = \sum_{x \in S_{i+1}} C\left(x\right) p_{i+1}\left(x\right), \tag{13.26}$$

where $C\left(x\right)$ represents some property of genotype x.

Price (1970) developed a theorem that partitions the effect of selection on a population in terms of covariances between fitness and the property of interest $C\left(x\right)$ (e.g., allele frequencies) and effects due to transmission.

Theorem 13.5 *(Covariance and Selection, Price, 1970). For any parental pair $\{y, z\}$ with certain genotypes in population S_i, let $\tilde{C}\left(y, z\right)$ represent the expected value of C among their offspring with population S_{i+1}, i.e.,*

$$\tilde{C}\left(y, z\right) = \sum_{x \in S_{i+1}} C\left(x\right) T\left(x \leftarrow y, z\right). \tag{13.27}$$

Then the population average of the function in the $(i+1)^{th}$ generation is given by

$$\bar{C}_{i+1} = \bar{C}_i + cov\left(\tilde{C}\left(y, z\right), \omega\left(y\right) \omega\left(z\right) / \bar{\omega}^2\right), \tag{13.28}$$

where

$$\bar{C}_i = \sum_{y, z \in S_i} \tilde{C}\left(y, z\right) p_i\left(y\right) p_i\left(z\right) \tag{13.29}$$

is the average offspring value in a population reproducing without selection based fitness, and

$$cov\left(\tilde{C}\left(y, z\right), \omega\left(y\right) \omega\left(z\right) / \bar{\omega}^2\right) = \sum_{y, z \in S_i} \frac{\omega\left(y\right) \omega\left(z\right)}{\bar{\omega}^2} p_i\left(y\right) p_i\left(z\right) - \bar{C}_i \tag{13.30}$$

is the population covariance between the parental fitness values and the measured values of their offspring.

Proof.   *One must assume that for functions (13.23) and (13.24), the expectation always exists. Substitution of (13.23), (13.27), and (13.30) into (13.25) directly produces (13.28).*   □

Price's theorem shows that the covariance between parental fitness and offspring traits is the means by which selection directs the evolution of the population. Price's theorem is often expressed in terms of frequency changes ΔQ from one generation to the next. For reproduction by mutation only,

$$\Delta Q = \frac{cov\,(C\,(y)\,,\omega\,(y))}{\bar{\omega}}, \tag{13.31}$$

where $C\,(y)$ = frequency of the gene y, $\omega\,(y)$ = fitness or number of offspring produced by parents with gene y; $\bar{\omega}$ = mean number of children produced.

The probability of an individual being selected by a tournament is determined by its fitness rank r within the population of size M ($r = 1$ for the worst and $r = M$ for the best) and the tournament size T by the formula (Blick and Thiele, 1995; Langdon, 1996):

$$\Delta Q = \frac{T}{\bar{z}}cov\left(\left(\frac{r}{M}\right)^{T-1},q\right). \tag{13.32}$$

Keep in mind that there are no assumptions about chromosomal structure in Price's theorem; thus it holds for a single gene or for any linear combination of genes at any number of loci, and for any sort of dominance or epistasis, for sexual or asexual reproduction, for random or nonrandom mating, for diloid, haploid, or polyploid species, and even for imaginary species with more than two sexes (Price, 1970).

Price's theorem has been applied in kin selection (Grafen, 1985; Taylor, 1988), group selection (Wade, 1985), and the evolution of mating systems (Uyenoyama, 1988).

13.3.4   *Concept of Genetic Programming*

Genetic programming was developed from the genetic algorithm. We have discussed the concept of GP with a simple example in Chapter 1. Genetic programming, inspired by biological evolution, is an evolutionary computation technique that automatically solves problems without requiring the user to know or specify the form or structure of the solution in advance. The simplest case is that GP generates different functions automatically by recombining different but predetermined function elements to fit the target function as closely as possible.

To study GP conceptually and theoretically, it is not convenient to use actual GP directly; rather, an appropriate representation of GP is required. Commonly used representations are Syntax Tree (Figure 13.1) and GP Schema. Syntax tree is very intuitive, but GP schema is helpful for theoretical study. Different schemata have been proposed with very limited theoretical results. GP representation requires unambiguity, i.e., a GP representation has to lead to a unique (mathematical) model or program. With an appropriate representation, we can develop algorithms for implementing it into particular program languages.

GP generates new programs by means of so-called genetic operators, e.g., crossover, mutation, and cloning. Crossover is a way to produce offspring. Crossover is to take (copy) a subtree from each of the parents and combine them into a new tree (offspring or child) (Figure 13.1). Mutation is to replace some nodes or subtree with some random symbols in the func-

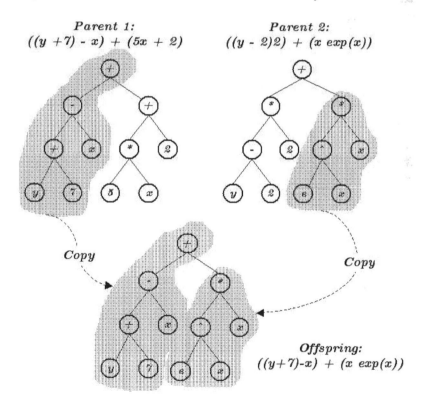

Figure 13.1: Crossover Operation in Genetic Programming

tion, subtree, or terminal set. The most commonly used mutation is a point mutation. Unlike crossover, which requires two parents, a point mutation only requires a single parent. Cloning is to make a copy of a parent program such that the chance of selecting this type of program to generate offspring increases. Thus we don't need to actually make a copy, but to change the count for this program.

The fitness measure is used to determine the survival time of an individual syntax tree or program and the probability of being selected to generate offspring during program evolution.

13.3.5 *Adaptive Genetic Programming*

Representation

We use a string to represent the program. The starting point of a GP string is the root of the tree, gradually going to the leaves. In order to perform effectively homologous genetic operations (crossover and mutation), we need to determine the "similarity" between strings or substrings. An exchange of two similar substrings is a crossover-like operation, whereas the replacement of a substring with a very different substring is a mutation-like operation. As mentioned previously, crossover involves two individuals (parents), but mutation can only involve one parent.

Let's limit our discussion on math operators for the moment. For programming purposes, it is convenient to write "+," "−," "×," "÷," and "^" in function form as "sum," "dif," "prd," "quo," and "pow," respectively. We now can see that the GP tree is nothing but nested functions. For example, the GP tree in Figure 13.2 is equivalent to the string of nested functions:

$$sum\left(dif\left(sum\left(\sin\left(y\right),7\right),x\right),prd\left(\exp\left(quo\left(x,5\right)\right),2\right)\right). \qquad (13.33)$$

Crossover and Mutation

Conventionally, homologous genetic transfers mean two parents crossover at the same GP location, which is equivalent to counting the number of functions or left parentheses from the left-hand side of the string. Both homologous reproduction (crossover) and nonhomologous reproduction (mutation) are necessary; the former should be used more often than the latter to avoid chaos or fatal consequences for the entire population. Examples of similarity determination (homologously) are presented in Table 13.1.

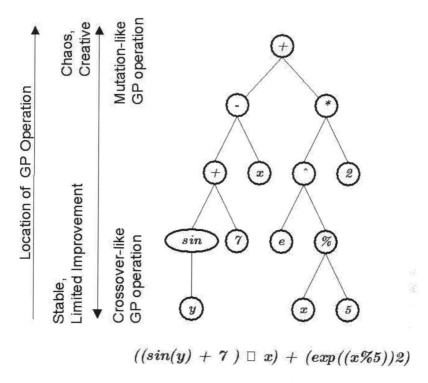

$$((sin(y) + 7) \Box x) + (exp((x\%5))2)$$

Figure 13.2:   Characteristics of GP Operations at Different Locations

Table 13.1: Definitions of Similarity Between Primitive Sets

Symbol 1	Symbol 2	Degree of symbolic (functional) similarity
+	-	0.8
*	%	0.5
^	*, %	0.6
sin	cos	0.9
x	y	0.1
exp	sin, cos	0.2
And	Or	
Not		
If-Then-Else		
Loop		
∀ anything	⊔ nothing	−1

Note: Default similarity between any two units is zero if not defined.

The overall similarity of a symbol can be defined as

Overall similarity = functional similarity × location similarity

The genetic operations can be performed probabilistically based on the similarity after a parent(s) is selected for generating an offspring. However, the current homologous reproduction methods available are based on the same location only.

In GP, we can assume each individual (tree) has a limited survival time, i.e., it will die after k generations, where k can be inversely proportional to its fitness function.

13.3.6   *GP Algorithm*

Typical GP preparation steps include determinations of function set, terminal set, population initialization, reproduction, fitness function, survival time and population control, and termination. These steps are outlined as follows:

1. Function Set
The function set F can be mathematical functions or other actions/operations such as moves of an object. The function may return a value, a variable, or a string of a program.

$$F = \{+, -, \times, \div, \exp, AND, OR, NOT, ...\}. \tag{13.34}$$

The input arguments can be any element (even a GP tree) legal for the function.

2. Terminal Set
A terminal set typically consists of input constants (pre-specified, randomly generated as part of the tree creation process, or created by mutation), variables, and functions with no arguments. In general, terminal sets are function specific.

The terminal and function sets compose the primitive set. It is ideal to select the primitive set that is sufficient to express a solution to the problem. Unfortunately, sufficiency can't be guaranteed in most practical settings. An example of a sufficient primitive set is $\{AND, OR, NOT, x_1, x_2, ..., x_n\}$. An example of an insufficient set is $\{+, -, *, /, x, 0, 1, 2\}$, which is unable to represent transcendental functions such as $exp(x)$ — $exp(x)$ can't be expressed as a rational function (basically, a ratio of polynomials), so it cannot be represented exactly by any finite combination of $\{+, -, *, /, x, 0, 1, 2\}$.

3. Population Initialization

A commonly used method to create the initial population randomly is the so-called ramped half-and-half with a depth range of 2 to 6. The initial tree sizes will depend upon the number of functions, the number of terminals, and the arities of the functions.

Random generation of the initial population can be based on a randomization list, a list of primitives with their associated probability of being selected. Population initialization can be adaptive using, e.g., Lachin's randomization model, the Urn model, or the biased-coin model. The probability of selecting symbols in a function set or terminal set can be reduced as the number of selected symbols in that set increases.

4. Reproduction

The main form of GP reproduction is crossover and only a small portion is generated by means of mutation. This is because mutation often results in an interruption of the normal function (deadly) of an individual. It is suggested that about 90% of children be created by subtree crossover and 10% by mutation.

Crossover is to copy some parts from each of the parents and combine them into a new individual or program. It is important to be homologous in crossover. Homology usually refers to location similarity, but can also be additionally functionally similar, as discussed earlier.

The probability of selecting a parent for crossover can be based on its fitness (an individual with high fitness will have a high probability of being selected) and the probability of selecting its spouse can be based on similarity between the two individuals.

After parents are selected, the probability of selecting the crossover point can be based on the uniform distribution (or equal probability) for all nodes except the root node or based on the location of the node. For example, smaller probabilities will associate the nodes near the root of the tree so the similarity between parents and child is most likely kept.

Although a mutation can be any meaningful substring (token) replacement by a random generated token, it's usually a replacement of a subtree by a randomly generated subtree. The probability of a mutation location will also be based on the location of the mutation point in a similar way as for crossover.

5. Fitness Function

Fitness can be measured in different ways, e.g., in terms of the amount of error between the output and the desired output, the amount of time (fuel, money, etc.) required to bring a system to a desired target state, the accuracy of the program in recognizing patterns or classifying objects, the payoff that a game-playing program produces, or the compliance of a structure with user-specified design criteria (Poli, Langdon, and McPhee, 2008).

The following probability of selection can be used in our GP implementation:

$$\Pr(parent = i) = \frac{fitness_i}{\sum_j fitness_j}. \tag{13.35}$$

Because the structures being evolved in GP are computer programs, fitness evaluation normally requires executing all the programs in the population, typically multiple times. While one can compile the GP programs that make up the population, the overhead of building a compiler is usually substantial, so it is much more common to use an interpreter to evaluate the evolved programs (Poli, Langdon, and McPhee, 2008). Ruby, JavaScript, PHP, and VB scripts are examples of scripts languages that do not require precompiling the programs.

6. Survival Time and Population Control

To avoid the population getting too large and exceeding computer memory, we can set up a survival time for individuals. Survival time can be measured by number of generations and is proportional to individual fitness. Another simple way to control the population size is to keep only the top n best fit individuals. When a new offspring comes to the world, its fitness is calculated and compared to the fitness of the nth individual: if the new fitness is small, the offspring will be removed; otherwise the $(n+1)^{th}$ best fit individual will be removed and the new offspring will be kept. Meanwhile, the new n^{th} best fit individual is recalculated and marked. The survival time consideration implies that GP allows for different generations living at the same time, which is different from conventional GP.

7. Termination

Termination criteria may include a maximum number of generations to run as well as a problem-specific success predication or the achievement of target fitness. After termination, the single best fit individual is the solution for the problem.

A five hundred or larger population size is preferable to the population size in each generation, but that is usually limited by computer power. Typically, the number of generations is $10 \sim 50$. It is observed that the most productive search is usually performed in those early generations, but there are those who suggest using many runs with much smaller populations instead.

GP runtime can be estimated by the product of the number of runs, the number of generations, the size of the population, the average size of the programs, and the number of fitness cases.

In GP, we should avoid the so-called bloat. Starting in the early 1990s, researchers began to notice that, in addition to progressively increasing their mean and best fitness, the average size (number of nodes) of the programs in a population after a certain number of generations often started growing at a rapid pace. This type of increase in program size was typically not accompanied by any meaningful increase in fitness. This phenomenon, called bloat, has been a mystery for over a decade.

From a statistical point of view, a large program has a large probability of fitting well or a high fitness value (it can be overfitting statistically). Over time there are more and more large programs than small programs. If the selecting probability for parents is proportional to the fitness rank, the program size could exponentially increase. However, if the selecting probability is proportional to the difference in fitness (13.36), not the ranks, the bloat, should be largely avoided. There are many other ways to avoid bloat such as using a fitness function with an over size penalty.

Algorithm 13.9: Generic Programming for Symbolic Regression

For implementation of GP (symbolic regression) with Javascript (as mentioned earlier, a scripts language is preferred) you just need an internet browser. It can be imbedded in an html page.

(1) Preparations:

   (a) Implementing function set, sum(a,b):=a+b; dif(a,b)=a-b; prd(a,b): =a·b, quo(a,b):=a/max(0.00001,b); pow(a,b):=a^b; sin(x); cos(x); log(x).

   (b) Functions:

      i. Target function
      ii. Subtree generator
      iii. Crossover
      iv. Mutation
      v. Fitness

   (c) Terminal set: $x \in [0.1, 5], e, \pi$, constant range from 0.01 to 100.

(2) Generate an initial population

(3) Determine genetic operation location

   (a) The kth level from the root = the kth "(" from the left of the program string.

(b) The ith node at the kth level = the ith ")" from the left after the kth "(" from the left.

(4) Calculate the fitness for each individual based on squared error.
(5) Offspring generation

   (a) Randomly select genetic operator
   (b) Randomly select one or two parents based on mutation or crossover with the probability of selection:

$$\Pr\left(parent = i\right) = \frac{fitness_i}{\sum_j fitness_j}.$$

(6) Termination
    If the best fitness reaches the target, terminate the execution.
    §

GP for symbolic regression, Algorithm 13.9, is implemented in Javascript in the appendix and at www.statisticians.org. You can double-click the file to run the program. Another interesting implementation example, TinyGP, is available in Poli, Langdon, and McPhee (2008) and on the web.

13.3.7   *GP Schema Theory*

A schema, in psychology and cognitive science, is a mental structure that represents some aspect of the world. In GP, schemata are similarity templates representing entire groups of chromosomes (Langdon and Poli, 2002). The schema theorem is the study of statistical properties of schema dynamics or propagation from generation to generation under the effects of selection. Because of the complexity of the topic and lack of theoretical development, the usefulness of schemata is questioned (see, e.g., Altenberg, 1995). In the following, we will present the major results in GP schema theory; the practical usefulness of the theorems is to be further explored.

   A schema is represented as a set of a program subtree (S-expression) with a certain pattern. For example, $H = [(+2\ x), (-\ x\ y)]$ represents all subprograms that include at least one occurrence of the expression $(+2\ x)$ and at least one occurrence of $(-\ x\ y)$.

   In GP, various processes contribute to the overall production and loss of individuals matching a schema H. The probability of schema transmission for schema H at generation i is dependent on characteristics of individual selection and genetic operations (crossover, cloning, and mutation).

If the genetic operations are mutually independent and generate mutually exclusive schema, then the chance of each child matching H will be the same, so the total $n(H, i+1)$ will be binomially distributed, with mean $\mu = N\alpha$ and variance $\sigma^2 = N\alpha(1-\alpha)$ for a population of size N, where α is a shorthand notation of $\alpha(H, i)$. Using Chebyshev's inequality, $\Pr\{|X - \mu| < k\sigma\} \geq 1 - 1/k^2$, we can obtain the following theorem.

Theorem 13.6 *For any given constant $k > 0$,*

$$\Pr\left\{n(H, i+1) > N\alpha - k\sqrt{N\alpha(1-\alpha)}\right\} \geq 1 - 1/k^2. \qquad (13.36)$$

There are microscopic and macroscopic schema theorems. Microscopic schema theorems concern in detail each member of the population rather than an average. Macroscopic schema theorems use the concept of hyperschema as defined in Definition 13.2.

Definition 13.2 *GP Hyperschema.* A GP hyperschema is a rooted tree composed of initial nodes from the set $F \cup \{=\}$ and leaves from $T \cup \{=, \#\}$, where F and T denote the function set and terminal set, respectively; the operator $=$ is a "don't care" symbol which stands for exactly one node, and the operator $\#$ stands for any valid subtree.

Theorem 13.7 *(Microscopic Exact GP Schema theorem). Let p_{xo} be the fraction of children created by crossover between two parents in population S, $N_C(g_1, g_2)$ be the number of nodes in the tree fragment representing the common region Ω between program g_1 and program g_2, $I(g_1, g_2)$ be the set of indices of the crossover points in Ω, $U(H, j)$ be the hyperschema obtained by replacing the subtree below crossover point j with a $\#$ node, and $L(H, j)$ be the hyperschema obtained by replacing all the nodes on the path between crossover point j and the root node with $=$ nodes, and all the subtrees connected to those nodes with $\#$ nodes. Then the total transmission probability for a fixed-size-and-shape GP schema H under one-point crossover and no mutation is given by*

$$\alpha(H, i) = (1 - p_{xo})p(H, i) + p_{xo} \sum_{h_1, h_2 \in S} \frac{p(g_1, i)p(g_2, i)}{N_C(g_1, g_2)} \cdot$$

$$\sum_{j \in C(h_1, h_2)} \delta(g_1 \in L(H, j))\delta(g_2 \in U(H, j)),$$

where h_1 and h_2 are two parental programs and indicator function $\delta(x) = 1$ if $x = true$; otherwise, $\delta(x) = 0$.

See Langdon and Poli (2002) for the proof of this theorem. We now consider the global properties of the population and introduce macroscopic schema theorems.

Theorem 13.8   *(GP Schema Theorem with One-Point Crossover). The total transmission probability for a fixed-size-and-shape GP schema H under one-point crossover and no mutation is*

$$\alpha(H, i) = (1 - p_{xo}) \, p(H, i) + p_{xo} \sum_j \sum_k \frac{1}{N_C(g_j, g_k)} \cdot$$

$$\sum_{m \in C(G_j, G_k)} p(L(H, m) \cap g_j, i) \, p(U(H, m) \cap g_k, i),$$

where the sets $L(H, m) \cap g_j$ and $U(H, m) \cap g_k$ are either fixed-size-and-shape schema or the empty set ϕ.

For GP with standard crossover the macroscopic schema theorem is also available (Langdon and Poli, 2002). Before we state the theorem, we have to introduce some concepts/definitions.

Definition 13.3   A variable arity V_A hyperschema is a rooted tree composed of internal nodes from the set $F \cup \{=, \#\}$ and leaves from $T \cup \{=, \#\}$.

Definition 13.4   The function $L(H, i, j)$ returns the variable arity hyperschema obtained by (1) rooting at coordinate j in an empty reference system the subschema of the schema H below crossover point i, (2) labeling all the nodes on the path between node j and the root node with $\#$ function nodes, and (3) labeling the arguments of those nodes which are to the left of such a path with $\#$ terminal nodes.

Definition 13.5   The function $U(H, i)$ returns the V_A hyperschema obtained by replacing the subtree below crossover point i with a $\#$ node.

Theorem 13.9   *(GP Schema Theorem with Standard Crossover). The total transmission probability for a fixed-size-and-shape GP schema H under standard crossover with uniform selection of a crossover point is*

$$\alpha(H, i) = (1 - p_{xo}) \, p(H, i) + p_{xo} \sum_{k, l} \frac{1}{N(G_k) \, N(G_l)} \cdot$$

$$\sum_{m \in H \cap G_k} \sum_{j \in G_l} p(U(H, m) \cap G_k, i) \, p(L(H, m, j) \cap G_l, i),$$

where the first two summations are over all the possible program shapes (i.e., all the fixed-size-and-shape schemata including only the $=$ symbol) G_1, G_2, ..., and $N(G)$ is the number of nodes in the schema G.

13.4 Summary

Sorting is one of the most common tasks in Monte Carlo computing. Quicksort is the fastest known general sorting algorithm.

Bootstrapping is a resampling method which estimates the distribution of an estimator by sampling with replacement from the original sample. Bootstrapping is useful when the analytical form of distribution is not available or is unknown. Bootstrapping is often used for deriving robust estimates of standard errors and confidence intervals of a population parameter like a mean, median, proportion, odds ratio, correlation coefficient, or regression coefficient. It can also be used for a hypothesis test.

The plug-in principle is a simple method of estimating parameters from samples. The plug-in estimate of a parameter $\theta = t(F)$ is defined to be

$$\hat{\theta} = t\left(\hat{F}\right). \tag{13.2}$$

In other words, we estimate the function $\theta = t(F)$ of the probability distribution F by the same function of the empirical distribution $\hat{F}$, $\hat{\theta} = t\left(\hat{F}\right)$.

Jackknifing is another resampling method used to estimate the bias and standard error for an estimator. The basic idea behind jackknifing lies in systematically recomputing the statistic estimate based on subsets of observations, which are obtained from the original set of observations but leaving one observation out at a time.

A permutation test is a type of statistical significance test in which a reference distribution is obtained by calculating all possible values of the test statistic under rearrangements of the treatment labels on the observed data points. The rationale behind the label rearrangement is that we intend to obtain the distribution of the test statistic under the null hypothesis and that the observations are exchangeable under the null hypothesis. This implies that tests of difference in location require equal variance. Also, this label rearrangement should be consistent with randomization in the experiment.

Genetic algorithms (GA) represent a school of directed search algorithms based on the mechanics of biological evolution. A genetic algorithm iterates three steps: selection, random mating, and production of offspring to constitute the population in the next generation. The core of GA is the transmission probability of certain characteristics from one generation to the next.

Genetic programming, inspired by biological evolution, is an evolutionary computation technique that automatically solves problems without requiring the user to know or specify the form or structure of the solution in advance.

Typical GP preparation steps are determinations of function set, terminal set, population initialization, reproduction, fitness function, survival time and population control, and termination.

13.5   Exercises

Exercise 13.1: Algorithm 13.6 is a proposed bootstrap algorithm for a stagewise-ordering p-value in an adaptive trial. Discuss the validity of the algorithm.

Exercise 13.2: Algorithm 13.5 provides a way of calculating the p-value and the CI calculations and the determination of the rejection boundary using bootstrapping. Can you develop a bootstrap algorithm for power and sample size calculations?

Exercise 13.3: In Algorithm 13.5, the test statistic is the rate difference $T = p_2 - p_1$. Can you use other test statistics such as $T = (p_2 - p_1)/Se$, where $Se = p_1 (1 - p_1)/n + p_2 (1 - p_2)/n$, and compare the two different methods?

Exercise 13.4: Modify Algorithm 13.5 for an unbalanced two-group design with sample size n_1 and n_2, respectively. Study how the sample size ratio n_2/n_1 affects the results (e.g., bias).

Exercise 13.5: Study the effect of sample size $m < n$ in Algorithm 13.5.

Exercise 13.6: We have discussed the asymptotic properties of bootstrapping. Perform Monte Carlo to study the properties of bootstrapping for a small sample size.

Exercise 13.7: Assuming $\hat{\theta} = \bar{x}$, show that the jackknife estimate standard error is equal to the unbiased estimate (13.20).

Exercise 13.8: Develop a bootstrapping algorithm for a confidence interval of a logrank test statistic for testing the survival difference between two groups.

Exercise 13.9: A controversy about the resampling approach is: if the resampling method is OK, then we can multiply any test statistic T by an independent random variable X with unit expectation to form a new test statistic and use the same rejection region without inflating α under repeated experiments, because

$$\Pr(TX > C_\alpha) = \Pr(T > C_\alpha) E(X) = \Pr(T > C_\alpha).$$

Debate this argument.

Exercise 13.10: Develop an algorithm for the p-value calculation using permutation tests for difference the between $\mu_{\max} - \mu_1$ in a clinical trial with three groups, where $\mu_{\max} = max(\mu_2, \mu_3)$. State how to obtain the 95% CI for the difference and compare it to a bootstrap method.

Exercise 13.11: Develop an algorithm for generating all $\binom{n}{m}$ possible combinations for array A=$\{a_1, a_2, ..., a_n\}$.

Exercise 13.12: Use Monte Carlo to obtain $cov(M, q)$ and ΔQ in Equation (13.32).

Exercise 13.13: Develop GP (to be placed in a robot) for finding a coin of $1/2''$ in diameter that is randomly placed in a 10 x $10'$ room.

Exercise 13.14: Describe how to implement operators *if* and *loop* in genetic programming. (Hint: implement a condition function taking two inputs and returning an output.)

Appendix A

JavaScript Programs

To illustrate the implementation of the algorithms presented in this book, three examples are used from an easy to moderate to difficult level. The JavaScript language is chosen because it is easy, even for those with very limited coding experience, and no specific software is required beyond an internet browser. All three programs were tested using MS Internet Explorer 6.0.

A.1 Pi Simulation

The following JavaScript code embedded in html is an implementation of Algorithm 1.1. You can save this file as "Pi.htm." To run the simulation, just double-click the file and you will see the simulation result. You can also use other values for the parameter nRuns and see how the result changes.

```
<html> <body>
<script type="text/javascript">
var nRuns = 100000;
var m=0;
for (iRun=1; iRun<nRuns; iRun++) {
    var x = Math.random();
    var y = Math.random();
    var d = Math.pow((x-0.5),2) + Math.pow((y-0.5),2);
    if(d<0.25) m = m + 1;
}
Pi = 4*m/nRuns;
document.write("Pi = " + Pi);
</script>
</body> </html>
```

A.2   Adaptive Trial Simulation

The following JavaScript code embedded in html is an implementation of Algorithm 6.5 for adaptive design. Algorithm 2.11 has also been implemented as it is necessary for the adaptive trial simulation. You can save this file as "AdaptiveDesign.htm." To run the simulation, just double-click the file and you will see the simulation result.

```
<html> <body>
<script type="text/javascript">
// Ref: Algorithm 6.5, but on z-scale and without futility stopping.
document.write("Adaptive Trial Simulation: " + " <br />"+" <br />");
    var z = new Array(), nc = new Array();
    zc = [0, 2.963, 1.969]; // OF-like boundary
    ns = [0, 66, 66]; // ns[0] will not be used.
    var N = 2;
    var delta = 1.0;
    var sigma = 2.5;
    var nRuns = 10000;
    nc[0] = 0;
    for (var k=1;k<=N; k++) nc[k]=nc[k-1]+ns[k];
var power = 0;
var power2 =0;
for (iRun=1; iRun<=nRuns; iRun++) {
    for (var i=1; i<=N; i++) {
    z[i]= delta*Math.sqrt(ns[i]/2)/sigma+ normRan();
    }
    for (var k=1;k<=N; k++) {
        var Tk = 0;
        for (i=1; i<=k; i++) Tk = Tk +Math.sqrt(ns[i]/nc[k])*z[i];
        if (Tk >= zc[k]) {
            power = power +1/nRuns;
            break;
        }
    }
}
document.write("Power for the trial design is" + power);
function normRan() {
    // return random number from N(0,1 ) Ref: Algorithm 2.11.
    var rejection = 1;
    while (rejection == 1) {
```

```
        var u1 = 2*Math.random()-1;
        var u2 = 2*Math.random()-1;
        var r2 = u1*u1 + u2*u2;
        if (r2<1) {
            var x1 = u1*Math.sqrt(-2*Math.log(r2)/r2);
            return x1; // just need one.
            rejection = 0;
        }
    }
}
</script>
</body> </html>
```

A.3   Genetic Programming

The following JavaScript code embedded in html is an implementation of Algorithm 13.9. You can save this file as "GP.htm." To run the simulation, just double-click the file and you will see the simulation result.

```
<html> <body>
<script type="text/javascript">
//Global variables:
var genSize =3, popSize=30, treeDepth=3, mcRatio=0.1, carryoverSize=3;
// 1) Function set;
var funSet=["sum(xx,yy)", "dif(xx,yy)", "pro(xx,yy)", "quo(xx,yy)", "min(xx,yy)",
"max(xx,yy)", "rod(xx)", "pow(xx,yy)", "abs(xx)", "sin(xx)", "cos(xx)", "log(xx)",
"tan(xx)", "atn(xx)", "neg(xx)"];
nFuns=3;
// 2) Terminal set;
var termSet=["x", 0.5, 1, 3, "pie()", "exp(1)", "rnd()", "2+5*rnd()"];
mTerms=2;
// 3) Population Initialization;
var parents = new Array();
var parentFitness = new Array();
var children = new Array();
var childFitness = new Array();
var cFits = new Array();
// 4) Target function;
var targetFun="sin(x)";
var xMin=1;
```

```
var xMax=2;
var nPoints=50;
document.write("Teeny Genetic Program Input Parameters: " + "<br/>");
document.write("Target Function: " + targetFun + " with the evaluation range of (" +
xMin + ", " + xMax +") and " + nPoints + " evaluation points."+"<br />");
document.write("Function set: ");
for (i=0; i<nFuns; i++) document.write(funSet[i]+" ");
document.write("<br />"+"Terminal set: ");
for (i=0; i<mTerms; i++) document.write(termSet[i]+" ");
document.write("<br />"+"Generation size= "+ genSize + ", population size = " +
popSize + ", initial tree depth = " + treeDepth + ", mutation proportion = " + mcRatio
+", carryover size = " + carryoverSize);
document.write("<br />");
// 5) Population initialization;
for (k=0; k<popSize; k++) {
    myfunTree=new funTree(funSet, nFuns, termSet, mTerms, treeDepth);
    parents[k]=myfunTree.tree;
}
fitness(parents, targetFun, popSize, xMin, xMax, nPoints, parentFitness);
shellSort(parentFitness, parents);
cFit(parentFitness,cFits);
for (childId =0; childId<popSize; childId++) {
    var repdut= reproduction(childId, mcRatio, cFits, parents, children, funSet, nFuns,
termSet, mTerms);
}
fitness(children, targetFun, popSize, xMin, xMax, nPoints, childFitness);
for (id =0; id<min(5,popSize); id++) {
    if (id==min(5,popSize)-1) document.write("<br/>");
}
// 6.1) Reproduction/ evolution;
document.write("Teeny Genetic Program Outcomes: " + "<br/>");
for (mm=1; mm<=genSize; mm++) {
    survivor(children, childFitness, popSize, carryoverSize, parents, parentFitness);
    for (childId =0; childId<popSize; childId++) {
    var repdut= reproduction(childId, mcRatio, cFits, parents, children, funSet, nFuns,
termSet, mTerms);
    }
    fitness(children, targetFun, popSize, xMin, xMax, nPoints, childFitness);
    document.write("Best of individual in generation " + mm + " is " + parents[0]);
    document.write(" with a fitness of " + parentFitness[0] +"<br />");
}
```

```
// 6.2) add termination criterion;
document.write("Best of individual in all generation is " + parents[0]);
document.write(" with a fitness of " + parentFitness[0] +"<br />");
//function set include function names with 3 letters and <3 parameters only.
function sum(a,b){return a+b;}
function dif(a,b){return a-b;}
function pro(a,b){return a*b;}
function quo(a,b){return a/b;}
function rod(a){return Math.round(a);}
function rnd(){return Math.random()};
function sin(x){return Math.sin(x);}
function cos(x){return Math.cos(x);}
function log(x){return Math.log(x);}
function pow(x,a){return Math.pow(x,a);}
function abs(x){return Math.abs(x);}
function tan(x){return Math.tan(x);}
function exp(x){return Math.exp(x);}
function min(x){return Math.min(x);}
function max(x){return Math.max(x);}
function pie(){return Math.PI;}
function atn(x){return Math.atan(x);}
function neg(x){return -x;}
function ran(n){return rod(Math.random()*n+0.5);} //random integer 1 to n;
function shellSort(myA,myB) {
    // Sorts the array a[0..n-1] into ascending numerical order by Shell sort method.
    // and array b is moved simultaneously.
    // The sorting speed is in the order of N^1.25, at least for N<60000.
    // Source: Numerical computation therapies by xxx.
    var j, v, u, inc;
    n=myA.length;
    inc=1; // Determine the starting increment.;
    while (inc <= n) inc *=3, inc++;
    while (inc > 1) {                        // Loop over the partial sorts.
        inc =rod(inc/3);                     //original coed is intN(inc/3);
        for (var k=inc+1; k<= n; k++) {      // Outer loop of straight insertion.
            v=myA[k-1];
            u=myB[k-1];
            j=k;
            while (myA[j-inc-1] > v) {       // Inner loop of straight insertion.
                myA[j-1]=myA[j-inc-1];
                myB[j-1]=myB[j-inc-1];
```

```
                j -= inc;
                if (j <= inc ) break;
            }
            myA[j-1]=v;
            myB[j-1]=u;
        }
    }
}
function getCounts(myTree, me) {
// return the total counts of me.
 var index0=myTree.indexOf(me);
 if (index0 <0) return 0;
 m=1;
 while (index0>0) {
    index0=myTree.indexOf(me,index0+1);
    if (index0>0) m=m+1;
 }
 return m;
}
function nthMe(myStr, me, n) {
// return the position of nth occurrence of str.;
 var index0=myStr.indexOf(me);
 if (index0 <0) return 0;
 m=1;
 while (m<n) {
 index0=myStr.indexOf(me,index0+1);
 m=m+1;
 }
 return index0;
}
function funTree(funSet, nFuns, termSet, mTerms, treeDepth){
 // generate a function string or tree;
 //funSet should have only 1 parameter (xx) or 2 parameters (xx, yy).
 var funcTree=funSet[ran(nFuns)-1];
 for (i=1; i<treeDepth; i++) {
    funcTree=funcTree.replace("xx", funSet[ran(nFuns)-1]);
    funcTree=funcTree.replace("yy", funSet[ran(nFuns)-1]);
    }
 while (funcTree.indexOf("xx")>0) {
    funcTree=funcTree.replace("xx", termSet[ran(mTerms)-1]);
    funcTree=funcTree.replace("yy", termSet[ran(mTerms)-1]);
```

```
        }
    while (funcTree.indexOf("rnd()")>0) funcTree=funcTree.replace("rnd()", rnd());
    this.tree=funcTree;
    this.treeDepth=treeDepth;
}
function treeSplitor(myStr,index0) {
// split string into 3 strings: root+funBranch+Branchs.
    index1=index0;
    index2=index0;
    while (index2<=index1 && index2>0) {
    index1=myStr.indexOf(")",index1+1);
    index2=myStr.indexOf("(",index2+1);
    }
    if (index1<0) index1=myStr.length-1;
    this.root=myStr.substring(0,index0-3);
    this.funBranch=myStr.substring(index0-3,index1+1);
    this.branchs=myStr.substring(index1+1);
    return 1;
}
function parentId(cFits, popSize) {
    fitVar = rnd();
    for (var i=0; i<popSize; i++) {
        if (fitVar <= cFits[i]) return i;
    }
    return popSize;
}
function gPoint(myTree) {
// uniformly select any function, return the position of (.
        var nG=ran(getCounts(myTree, "(")-1)+1; // make sure >1.
        return nthMe(myTree, "(", nG);
}
function fitness(gpFuns, targetFun, popSize, xMin, xMax, nPoints, fits) {
// fitness = abs(gpFun-targetFun)) => small value of fitness = better.
    dx = (xMax-xMin)/nPoints;
    for (k=0; k<popSize; k++) {
        fits[k] = 0;
        for (var j=1; j<nPoints; j++) {
            var x = xMin+ j*dx;
            fits[k]=fits[k]+abs(eval(gpFuns[k] + "-" + targetFun))/nPoints;
        }
    }
```

```
        }
    function reproduction(childId, mcRatio, cFits, parents, children, funSet, nFuns, termSet,
mTerms) {
            var opVar=rnd();
        if (opVar<mcRatio) { // Mutation.
        var parent=parents[parentId(cFits, popSize)];
        var mPoint=gPoint(parent); // mutation point;
        var parentSplitor= new treeSplitor(parent,mPoint);
        var subtreeDepth = rod(0.6*getCounts(parentSplitor.funBranch, "(")); // approximate
        var myfunTree= new funTree(funSet, nFuns, termSet, mTerms, subtreeDepth);
        children[childId]=parentSplitor.root + myfunTree.tree + parentSplitor.branchs;
        }
            else { // Crossover.
        var mom=parents[parentId(cFits, popSize)];
        var dad=parents[parentId(cFits, popSize)];
        var mPoint=gPoint(mom); // genetic operation point;
        var dPoint=gPoint(dad); // genetic operation point;
        var momSplitor= new treeSplitor(mom,mPoint);
        var dadSplitor= new treeSplitor(dad,dPoint);
        children[childId]=momSplitor.root + dadSplitor.funBranch + momSplitor.branchs;
            }
    }
    function cFit(fitness,cFits) {
    // cumulative probability;
    this.cFits[0]=fitness[0];
    for (k=1; k<popSize; k++) this.cFits[k]=this.cFits[k-1]+fitness[k];
    for (k=0; k<popSize; k++) this.cFits[k]=this.cFits[k]/cFits[popSize-1];
    }
    function survivor(children, childFitness, popSize, carryoverSize, parents, parentFitness) {
    sSize=popSize-carryoverSize;
    shellSort(childFitness, children);
    for (k=0; k<sSize; k++) {
            kc=k+carryoverSize;
            parents[kc]=children[k];
            parentFitness[kc]=childFitness[k];
    }
        shellSort(parentFitness, parents);
    }
    </script>
    </body> </html>
```

K-Stage Adaptive Design Stopping Boundaries

B.1 Stopping Boundaries with MSP

Derivations of stopping boundaries using MSP are given below:

$\pi_1 = \alpha_1.$

$\pi_2 = \frac{1}{2}\left(\alpha_2 - \alpha_1\right)^2.$

$\pi_3 = \int_{\alpha_1}^{\alpha_3} \int_{\max(0,\alpha_2-p_1)}^{\alpha_3} \int_0^{\max(0,\alpha_3-p_2-p_1)} dp_3 dp_2 dp_1$

$= \int_{\alpha_2}^{\alpha_3} \int_0^{\alpha_3-p_1} (\alpha_3-p_1-p_2) dp_2 dp_1 + \int_{\alpha_1}^{\alpha_2} \int_{\alpha_2-p_1}^{\alpha_3-p_1} (\alpha_3-p_1-p_2) dp_2 dp_1$

$= \alpha_1\alpha_2\alpha_3 + \frac{1}{3}\alpha_2^3 + \frac{1}{6}\alpha_3^3 - \frac{1}{2}\alpha_1\alpha_2^2 - \frac{1}{2}\alpha_1\alpha_3^2 - \frac{1}{2}\alpha_2^2\alpha_3.$

$\pi_4 = \int_{\alpha_1}^{\alpha_4} \int_{\max(0,\alpha_2-p_1)}^{\alpha_4} \int_{\max(0,\alpha_3-p_2-p_1)}^{\alpha_4} \int_0^{\max(0,\alpha_4-p_3-p_2-p_1)} dp_4 dp_3 dp_2 dp_1$

$= \int_{\alpha_1}^{\alpha_2} \int_{\max(0,\alpha_2-p_1)}^{\alpha_4} \int_{\max(0,\alpha_3-p_1-p_2)}^{\alpha_4} \max\left(0, \alpha_4-p_1-p_2-p_3\right) dp_3 dp_2 dp_1$

$+ \int_{\alpha_2}^{\alpha_4} \int_0^{\alpha_4} \int_{\max(0,\alpha_3-p_1-p_2)}^{\alpha_4} \max\left(0, \alpha_4-p_1-p_2-p_3\right) dp_3 dp_2 dp_1$

$= \int_{\alpha_1}^{\alpha_2} \int_{\alpha_2-p_1}^{\alpha_4} \int_{\alpha_3-p_1-p_2}^{\alpha_4-p_1-p_2} (\alpha_4-p_1-p_2-p_3) dp_3 dp_2 dp_1$

$+ \int_{\alpha_1}^{\alpha_2} \int_{\alpha_3-p_1}^{\alpha_4} \int_0^{\max(0,\alpha_4-p_1-p_2)} (\alpha_4-p_1-p_2-p_3) dp_3 dp_2 dp_1$

$+ \int_{\alpha_2}^{\alpha_4} \int_0^{\max(0,\alpha_3-p_1)} \int_{\alpha_3-p_1-p_2}^{\alpha_4-p_1-p_2} (\alpha_4-p_1-p_2-p_3) dp_3 dp_2 dp_1$

$+ \int_{\alpha_2}^{\alpha_4} \int_{\max(0,\alpha_3-p_1)}^{\alpha_4} \int_0^{\max(0,\alpha_4-p_1-p_2)} (\alpha_4-p_1-p_2-p_3) dp_3 dp_2 dp_1$

$= \int_{\alpha_1}^{\alpha_2} \int_{\alpha_2-p_1}^{\alpha_3-p_1} \int_{\alpha_3-p_1-p_2}^{\alpha_4-p_1-p_2} (\alpha_4-p_1-p_2-p_3) dp_3 dp_2 dp_1$

$+ \int_{\alpha_1}^{\alpha_2} \int_{\alpha_3-p_1}^{\alpha_4-p_1} \int_0^{\alpha_4-p_1-p_2} (\alpha_4-p_1-p_2-p_3) dp_3 dp_2 dp_1$

$+ \int_{\alpha_2}^{\alpha_3} \int_0^{\alpha_3-p_1} \int_{\alpha_3-p_1-p_2}^{\alpha_4-p_1-p_2} (\alpha_4-p_1-p_2-p_3) dp_3 dp_2 dp_1$

$+ \int_{\alpha_2}^{\alpha_4} \int_{\max(0,\alpha_3-p_1)}^{\alpha_4-p_1} \int_0^{\alpha_4-p_1-p_2} (\alpha_4-p_1-p_2-p_3) dp_3 dp_2 dp_1$

$+ \frac{1}{2}\alpha_1\alpha_2\alpha_3^2 + \frac{1}{2}\alpha_1\alpha_2\alpha_4^2 + \frac{1}{2}\alpha_1\alpha_3^2\alpha_4 + \frac{1}{2}\alpha_2^2\alpha_3\alpha_4 - \frac{1}{4}\alpha_2^2\alpha_3^2 - \frac{1}{4}\alpha_2^2\alpha_4^2$

$= \int_{\alpha_1}^{\alpha_2} \int_{\alpha_2-p_1}^{\alpha_3-p_1} \int_{\alpha_3-p_1-p_2}^{\alpha_4-p_1-p_2} (\alpha_4-p_1-p_2-p_3) dp_3 dp_2 dp_1$

$+ \int_{\alpha_1}^{\alpha_2} \int_{\alpha_3-p_1}^{\alpha_4-p_1} \int_0^{\alpha_4-p_1-p_2} (\alpha_4-p_1-p_2-p_3) dp_3 dp_2 dp_1$

$+ \int_{\alpha_2}^{\alpha_3} \int_0^{\alpha_3-p_1} \int_{\alpha_3-p_1-p_2}^{\alpha_4-p_1-p_2} (\alpha_4-p_1-p_2-p_3) dp_3 dp_2 dp_1$

$+ \int_{\alpha_2}^{\alpha_3} \int_{\alpha_3-p_1}^{\alpha_4-p_1} \int_0^{\alpha_4-p_1-p_2} (\alpha_4-p_1-p_2-p_3) dp_3 dp_2 dp_1$

$+ \int_{\alpha_3}^{\alpha_4} \int_0^{\alpha_4-p_1} \int_0^{\alpha_4-p_1-p_2} (\alpha_4-p_1-p_2-p_3) dp_3 dp_2 dp_1$

$$= \tfrac{1}{8}\alpha_3^4 - \alpha_1\alpha_2\alpha_3\alpha_4 + \tfrac{1}{24}\alpha_4^4 - \tfrac{1}{3}\alpha_1\alpha_3^3 - \tfrac{1}{6}\alpha_1\alpha_4^3 - \tfrac{1}{6}\alpha_3^3\alpha_4 + \tfrac{1}{2}\alpha_1\alpha_2\alpha_3^2$$
$$+ \tfrac{1}{2}\alpha_1\alpha_2\alpha_4^2 + \tfrac{1}{2}\alpha_1\alpha_3^2\alpha_4 + \tfrac{1}{2}\alpha_2^2\alpha_3\alpha_4 - \tfrac{1}{4}\alpha_2^2\alpha_3^2 - \tfrac{1}{4}\alpha_2^2\alpha_4^2.$$

$$\pi_5 = \int_{\alpha_1}^{\alpha_5} \int_{\max(0,\alpha_2-p_1)}^{\alpha_5} \int_{\max(0,\alpha_3-p_2-p_1)}^{\alpha_5} \int_{\max(0,\alpha_4-\sum_{i=1}^{3}p_i)}^{\alpha_5}$$
$$\max\left(0, \alpha_5 - \sum_{i=1}^{4} p_i\right) dp_4 dp_3 dp_2 dp_1$$
$$= \int_{\alpha_1}^{\alpha_5} \int_{\max(0,\alpha_2-p_1)}^{\alpha_5} \int_{\max(0,\alpha_3-p_2-p_1)}^{\alpha_5} \int_{\max(0,\alpha_4-\sum_{i=1}^{3}p_i)}^{\alpha_5-\sum_{i=1}^{3}p_i}$$
$$\left(\alpha_5 - \sum_{i=1}^{4} p_i\right) dp_4 dp_3 dp_2 dp_1$$
$$= \int_{\alpha_1}^{\alpha_2} \int_{\alpha_2-p_1}^{\alpha_5} \int_{\max(0,\alpha_3-p_2-p_1)}^{\alpha_5} \int_{\max(0,\alpha_4-p_3-p_2-p_1)}^{\alpha_5-p_3-p_2-p_1} f_5 dp_4 dp_3 dp_2 dp_1$$
$$+ \int_{\alpha_2}^{\alpha_5} \int_{0}^{\alpha_5} \int_{\max(0,\alpha_3-p_2-p_1)}^{\alpha_5} \int_{\max(0,\alpha_4-p_3-p_2-p_1)}^{\alpha_5-p_3-p_2-p_1} f_5 dp_4 dp_3 dp_2 dp_1$$
$$= \left[\int_{\alpha_1}^{\alpha_2} \int_{\alpha_2-p_1}^{\alpha_3-p_1} \int_{\alpha_3-p_2-p_1}^{\alpha_5} \int_{\max(0,\alpha_4-p_3-p_2-p_1)}^{\alpha_5-p_3-p_2-p_1} f_5 dp_4 dp_3 dp_2 dp_1\right.$$
$$\left.+ \int_{\alpha_1}^{\alpha_2} \int_{\alpha_3-p_1}^{\alpha_5} \int_{0}^{\alpha_5} \int_{\max(0,\alpha_4-p_3-p_2-p_1)}^{\alpha_5-p_3-p_2-p_1} f_5 dp_4 dp_3 dp_2 dp_1\right]$$
$$+ \left[\int_{\alpha_2}^{\alpha_5} \int_{0}^{\alpha_3-p_1} \int_{\alpha_3-p_2-p_1}^{\alpha_5} \int_{\max(0,\alpha_4-p_3-p_2-p_1)}^{\alpha_5-p_3-p_2-p_1} f_5 dp_4 dp_3 dp_2 dp_1\right.$$
$$\left.+ \int_{\alpha_2}^{\alpha_5} \int_{\alpha_3-p_1}^{\alpha_5} \int_{0}^{\alpha_5} \int_{\max(0,\alpha_4-p_3-p_2-p_1)}^{\alpha_5-p_3-p_2-p_1} f_5 dp_4 dp_3 dp_2 dp_1\right]$$
$$= \left[\int_{\alpha_1}^{\alpha_2} \int_{\alpha_2-p_1}^{\alpha_3-p_1} \int_{\alpha_3-p_2-p_1}^{\alpha_4-p_2-p_1} \int_{\alpha_4-p_3-p_2-p_1}^{\alpha_5-p_3-p_2-p_1} f_5 dp_4 dp_3 dp_2 dp_1\right.$$
$$\left.+ \int_{\alpha_1}^{\alpha_2} \int_{\alpha_2-p_1}^{\alpha_3-p_1} \int_{\alpha_4-p_2-p_1}^{\alpha_5} \int_{0}^{\alpha_5-p_3-p_2-p_1} f_5 dp_4 dp_3 dp_2 dp_1\right]$$
$$+ \left[\int_{\alpha_1}^{\alpha_2} \int_{\alpha_3-p_1}^{\alpha_5} \int_{0}^{\alpha_4-p_2-p_1} \int_{\alpha_4-p_3-p_2-p_1}^{\alpha_5-p_3-p_2-p_1} f_5 dp_4 dp_3 dp_2 dp_1\right.$$
$$\left.+ \int_{\alpha_1}^{\alpha_2} \int_{\alpha_3-p_1}^{\alpha_5} \int_{\alpha_4-p_2-p_1}^{\alpha_5} \int_{0}^{\alpha_5-p_3-p_2-p_1} f_5 dp_4 dp_3 dp_2 dp_1\right]$$
$$+ \left[\int_{\alpha_2}^{\alpha_5} \int_{0}^{\alpha_3-p_1} \int_{\alpha_3-p_2-p_1}^{\alpha_4-p_2-p_1} \int_{\alpha_4-p_3-p_2-p_1}^{\alpha_5-p_3-p_2-p_1} f_5 dp_4 dp_3 dp_2 dp_1\right.$$
$$\left.+ \int_{\alpha_2}^{\alpha_5} \int_{0}^{\alpha_3-p_1} \int_{\alpha_4}^{\alpha_5} \int_{0}^{\alpha_5-p_3-p_2-p_1} f_5 dp_4 dp_3 dp_2 dp_1\right]$$
$$+ \left[\int_{\alpha_2}^{\alpha_5} \int_{\alpha_3-p_1}^{\alpha_5} \int_{0}^{\alpha_4-p_2-p_1} \int_{\alpha_4-p_3-p_2-p_1}^{\alpha_5-p_3-p_2-p_1} f_5 dp_4 dp_3 dp_2 dp_1\right.$$
$$\left.+ \int_{\alpha_2}^{\alpha_5} \int_{\alpha_3-p_1}^{\alpha_5} \int_{\alpha_4-p_2-p_1}^{\alpha_5} \int_{0}^{\alpha_5-p_3-p_2-p_1} f_5 dp_4 dp_3 dp_2 dp_1\right].$$

To further eliminate the negative upper limits in the integrations, let $\pi_5 = \pi_{51} + \pi_{52}$, where

$$\pi_{51} = \left[\int_{\alpha_1}^{\alpha_2} \int_{\alpha_2-p_1}^{\alpha_3-p_1} \int_{\alpha_3-p_2-p_1}^{\alpha_4-p_2-p_1} \int_{\alpha_4-p_3-p_2-p_1}^{\alpha_5-p_3-p_2-p_1} f_5 dp_4 dp_3 dp_2 dp_1\right.$$
$$\left.+ \int_{\alpha_1}^{\alpha_2} \int_{\alpha_2-p_1}^{\alpha_3-p_1} \int_{\alpha_4-p_2-p_1}^{\alpha_5-p_2-p_1} \int_{0}^{\alpha_5-p_3-p_2-p_1} f_5 dp_4 dp_3 dp_2 dp_1\right]$$
$$+ \left[\int_{\alpha_1}^{\alpha_2} \int_{\alpha_3-p_1}^{\alpha_4-p_1} \int_{0}^{\alpha_4-p_2-p_1} \int_{\alpha_4-p_3-p_2-p_1}^{\alpha_5-p_3-p_2-p_1} f_5 dp_4 dp_3 dp_2 dp_1\right.$$
$$+ \int_{\alpha_1}^{\alpha_2} \int_{\alpha_3-p_1}^{\alpha_4-p_1} \int_{\alpha_4-p_2-p_1}^{\alpha_5-p_2-p_1} \int_{0}^{\alpha_5-p_3-p_2-p_1} f_5 dp_4 dp_3 dp_2 dp_1$$
$$\left.+ \int_{\alpha_1}^{\alpha_2} \int_{\alpha_4-p_1}^{\alpha_5} \int_{0}^{\alpha_5-p_2-p_1} \int_{0}^{\alpha_5-p_3-p_2-p_1} f_5 dp_4 dp_3 dp_2 dp_1\right]$$
$$+ \left[\int_{\alpha_2}^{\alpha_3} \int_{0}^{\alpha_3-p_1} \int_{\alpha_3-p_2-p_1}^{\alpha_4-p_2-p_1} \int_{\alpha_4-p_3-p_2-p_1}^{\alpha_5-p_3-p_2-p_1} f_5 dp_4 dp_3 dp_2 dp_1\right.$$
$$\left.+ \int_{\alpha_2}^{\alpha_3} \int_{0}^{\alpha_3-p_1} \int_{\alpha_4-p_2-p_1}^{\alpha_5-p_2-p_1} \int_{0}^{\alpha_5-p_3-p_2-p_1} f_5 dp_4 dp_3 dp_2 dp_1\right]$$

and

$$\pi_{52} = \left[\int_{\alpha_2}^{\alpha_3} \int_{\alpha_3-p_1}^{\alpha_5} \int_{0}^{\alpha_4-p_2-p_1} \int_{\alpha_4-p_3-p_2-p_1}^{\alpha_5-p_3-p_2-p_1} f_5 dp_4 dp_3 dp_2 dp_1\right.$$
$$+ \int_{\alpha_3}^{\alpha_5} \int_{0}^{\alpha_5} \int_{0}^{\alpha_4-p_2-p_1} \int_{\alpha_4-p_3-p_2-p_1}^{\alpha_5-p_3-p_2-p_1} f_5 dp_4 dp_3 dp_2 dp_1$$
$$\left.+ \int_{\alpha_2}^{\alpha_3} \int_{\alpha_3-p_1}^{\alpha_5} \int_{\alpha_4-p_2-p_1}^{\alpha_5} \int_{0}^{\alpha_5-p_3-p_2-p_1} f_5 dp_4 dp_3 dp_2 dp_1\right.$$

$$+ \int_{\alpha_3}^{\alpha_5} \int_0^{\alpha_5} \int_{\alpha_4-p_2-p_1}^{\alpha_5} \int_0^{\alpha_5-p_3-p_2-p_1} f_5 dp_4 dp_3 dp_2 dp_1]$$
$$= [\int_{\alpha_2}^{\alpha_3} \int_{\alpha_3-p_1}^{\alpha_4-p_1} \int_0^{\alpha_4-p_2-p_1} \int_{\alpha_4-p_3-p_2-p_1}^{\alpha_5-p_3-p_2-p_1} (\alpha_5-p_4-p_3-p_2-p_1)dp_4 \cdots dp_1$$
$$+ \int_{\alpha_3}^{\alpha_4} \int_0^{\alpha_4-p_1} \int_0^{\alpha_4-p_2-p_1} \int_{\alpha_4-p_3-p_2-p_1}^{\alpha_5-p_3-p_2-p_1} (\alpha_5-p_4-p_3-p_2-p_1)dp_4 \cdots dp_1$$
$$+ \int_{\alpha_2}^{\alpha_3} \int_{\alpha_3-p_1}^{\alpha_4-p_1} \int_{\alpha_4-p_2-p_1}^{\alpha_5-p_2-p_1} \int_0^{\alpha_5-p_3-p_2-p_1} (\alpha_5-p_4-p_3-p_2-p_1)dp_4 \cdots dp_1$$
$$+ \int_{\alpha_2}^{\alpha_3} \int_{\alpha_4-p_1}^{\alpha_5-p_1} \int_0^{\alpha_5-p_2-p_1} \int_0^{\alpha_5-p_3-p_2-p_1} (\alpha_5-p_4-p_3-p_2-p_1)dp_4 \cdots dp_1$$
$$+ \int_{\alpha_3}^{\alpha_4} \int_0^{\alpha_4-p_1} \int_{\alpha_4-p_2-p_1}^{\alpha_5-p_2-p_1} \int_0^{\alpha_5-p_3-p_2-p_1} (\alpha_5-p_4-p_3-p_2-p_1)dp_4 \cdots dp_1$$
$$+ \int_{\alpha_3}^{\alpha_4} \int_{\alpha_4-p_1}^{\alpha_5-p_1} \int_0^{\alpha_5-p_2-p_1} \int_0^{\alpha_5-p_3-p_2-p_1} (\alpha_5-p_4-p_3-p_2-p_1)dp_4 \cdots dp_1$$
$$+ \int_{\alpha_4}^{\alpha_5} \int_0^{\alpha_5-p_1} \int_0^{\alpha_5-p_2-p_1} \int_0^{\alpha_5-p_3-p_2-p_1} (\alpha_5-p_4-p_3-p_2-p_1)dp_4 \cdots dp_1.$$

Finally we obtain

$$\pi_5 = \alpha_1\alpha_2\alpha_3\alpha_4\alpha_5 + \frac{1}{30}\alpha_4^5 + \frac{1}{120}\alpha_5^5 - \frac{1}{8}\alpha_1\alpha_4^4 - \frac{1}{24}\alpha_1\alpha_5^4 - \frac{1}{24}\alpha_4^4\alpha_5$$
$$+ \frac{1}{3}\alpha_1\alpha_2\alpha_4^3 + \frac{1}{6}\alpha_1\alpha_2\alpha_5^3 + \frac{1}{6}\alpha_1\alpha_4^3\alpha_5 + \frac{1}{6}\alpha_3^3\alpha_4\alpha_5 - \frac{1}{2}\alpha_1\alpha_2\alpha_3\alpha_4^2 - \frac{1}{2}\alpha_1\alpha_2\alpha_3\alpha_5^2$$
$$- \frac{1}{2}\alpha_1\alpha_2\alpha_4^2\alpha_5 - \frac{1}{2}\alpha_1\alpha_3^2\alpha_4\alpha_5 - \frac{1}{2}\alpha_2^2\alpha_3\alpha_4\alpha_5 - \frac{1}{6}\alpha_2^2\alpha_4^3 - \frac{1}{12}\alpha_2^2\alpha_5^3 - \frac{1}{12}\alpha_3^3\alpha_4^2$$
$$- \frac{1}{12}\alpha_3^3\alpha_5^2 + \frac{1}{4}\alpha_1\alpha_3^2\alpha_4^2 + \frac{1}{4}\alpha_1\alpha_3^2\alpha_5^2 + \frac{1}{4}\alpha_2^2\alpha_3\alpha_4^2 + \frac{1}{4}\alpha_2^2\alpha_3\alpha_5^2 + \frac{1}{4}\alpha_2^2\alpha_4^2\alpha_5.$$

B.2 Stopping Boundaries with MPP

Derivations of stopping boundary using Fisher's combination (MPP):

$\pi_1 = \alpha_1$.

$\pi_2 = \alpha_2 \ln \frac{1}{\alpha_1}$.

$\pi_3 = \int_{\alpha_1}^1 \int_{\alpha_2/p_1}^1 \int_0^{\alpha_3/(p_1p_2)} dp_3 dp_2 dp_1 = \int_{\alpha_1}^1 \int_{\alpha_2/p_1}^1 \frac{\alpha_3}{p_1 p_2} dp_2 dp_1$

$= \int_{\alpha_1}^1 \frac{\alpha_3}{p_1} (\ln p_1 - \ln \alpha_2) dp_1 = \alpha_3 \left[\frac{1}{2}\ln^2 p_1 - \ln \alpha_2 \ln p_1 \right]_{\alpha_1}^1$

$= \alpha_3 \left(\ln \alpha_2 \ln \alpha_1 - \frac{1}{2}\ln^2 \alpha_1 \right).$

$\pi_4 = \int_{\alpha_1}^1 \int_{\alpha_2/p_1}^1 \int_{\alpha_3/(p_1p_2)}^1 \int_0^{\alpha_4/(p_1p_2p_3)} dp_4 dp_3 dp_2 dp_1$

$= \int_{\alpha_1}^1 \int_{\alpha_2/p_1}^1 \int_{\alpha_3/(p_1p_2)}^1 \frac{\alpha_4}{p_1 p_2 p_3} dp_3 dp_2 dp_1$

$= \int_{\alpha_1}^1 \int_{\alpha_2/p_1}^1 \frac{\alpha_4}{p_1 p_2} (\ln p_1 + \ln p_2 - \ln \alpha_3) dp_2 dp_1$

$= \int_{\alpha_1}^1 \frac{\alpha_4}{p_1} \left[\ln p_1 \ln p_2 + \frac{1}{2}\ln^2 p_2 - \ln \alpha_3 \ln p_2 \right]_{\alpha_2/p_1}^1 dp_1$

$= \int_{\alpha_1}^1 \alpha_4 \left[\ln p_1 (\ln p_1 - \ln \alpha_2) + \frac{1}{2}(\ln p_1 - \ln \alpha_2)^2 - \ln \alpha_3 (\ln p_1 - \ln \alpha_2) \right] d\ln p_1$

$= \int_{\ln \alpha_1}^0 \alpha_4 \left[x(x - \ln \alpha_2) + \frac{1}{2}(x - \ln \alpha_2)^2 - \ln \alpha_3 (x - \ln \alpha_2) \right] dx$

$= \int_{\ln \alpha_1}^0 \alpha_4 \left[\frac{3}{2}x^2 - x(2\ln \alpha_2 + \ln \alpha_3) + \ln \alpha_2 \ln \alpha_3 + \frac{1}{2}\ln^2 \alpha_2 \right] dx$

$= \alpha_4 \left[\frac{1}{2}x^3 - \frac{x^2}{2}(2\ln \alpha_2 + \ln \alpha_3) + x\ln \alpha_2 \ln \alpha_3 + \frac{x}{2}\ln^2 \alpha_2 \right]_{\ln \alpha_1}^0$

$= \alpha_4 \left((\ln \alpha_1 - \ln \alpha_3 - \ln \alpha_2) \ln \alpha_2 + \frac{1}{2}(\ln \alpha_3 - \ln \alpha_1) \ln \alpha_1 \right) \ln \alpha_1.$

$$\pi_5 = \int_{\alpha_1}^1 \int_{\alpha_2/p_1}^1 \int_{\alpha_3/(p_1 p_2)}^1 \int_{\alpha_4/(p_1 p_2 p_3)}^1 \frac{\alpha_5}{p_1 p_2 p_3 p_4} dp_4 dp_3 dp_2 dp_1$$

$$= \int_{\alpha_1}^1 \int_{\alpha_2/p_1}^1 \int_{\alpha_3/(p_1 p_2)}^1 \frac{\alpha_5}{p_1 p_2 p_3} \left(\ln p_1 + \ln p_2 + \ln p_3 - \ln \alpha_4 \right) dp_3 dp_2 dp_1$$

$$= \int_{\alpha_1}^1 \int_{\alpha_2/p_1}^1 \frac{\alpha_5}{p_1 p_2} \left(\ln p_1 \ln p_3 + \ln p_2 \ln p_3 + \tfrac{1}{2} \ln^2 p_3 - \ln \alpha_4 \ln p_3 \right)_{\alpha_3/(p_1 p_2)}^1 dp_2 dp_1$$

$$= \int_{\alpha_1}^1 \int_{\alpha_2/p_1}^1 \frac{\alpha_5}{p_1 p_2} \left((\ln p_1 + \ln p_2 - \ln \alpha_4) \ln p_3 + \tfrac{1}{2} \ln^2 p_3 \right)_{\alpha_3/(p_1 p_2)}^1 dp_2 dp_1$$

$$= \int_{\alpha_1}^1 \int_{\alpha_2/p_1}^1 \frac{\alpha_5 (\ln p_1 + \ln p_2 - \ln \alpha_5)}{p_1 p_2}$$
$$\left((\ln p_1 + \ln p_2 - \ln \alpha_4) + \tfrac{1}{2} (\ln p_1 + \ln p_2 - \ln \alpha_5) \right) dp_2 dp_1$$

$$= \int_{\alpha_1}^1 \int_{\ln(\alpha_2/p_1)}^0 \frac{\alpha_5 (\ln p_1 + x - \ln \alpha_5)}{p_1}$$
$$\left((\ln p_1 + x - \ln \alpha_4) + \tfrac{1}{2} (\ln p_1 + x - \ln \alpha_5) \right) dx dp_1$$

$$= \int_{\alpha_1}^1 \frac{\alpha_5}{p_1} \left(\tfrac{3}{2} \ln^2 p_1 + \tfrac{1}{2} \ln^2 \alpha_5 - \ln p_1 \ln \alpha_4 - 2 \ln p_1 \ln \alpha_5 + \ln \alpha_4 \ln \alpha_5 \right)$$
$$(\ln p_1 - \ln \alpha_2) dp_1 + \int_{\alpha_1}^1 \frac{\alpha_5}{p_1} (3 \ln p_1 - \ln \alpha_4 - 2 \ln \alpha_5) \tfrac{1}{2} (\ln p_1 - \ln \alpha_2)^2 dp_1$$

$$+ \int_{\alpha_1}^1 \tfrac{1}{2} \frac{\alpha_5}{p_1} (\ln p_1 - \ln \alpha_2)^3 dp_1$$

$$= -\alpha_5 [(-\tfrac{1}{2} \ln^3 \alpha_2 + \tfrac{1}{2} (\ln^2 \alpha_2) (-\ln \alpha_4 - 2 \ln \alpha_5)$$
$$- (\ln \alpha_2) (\ln \alpha_4 \ln \alpha_5 + \tfrac{1}{2} \ln^2 \alpha_5)) \ln \alpha_1$$
$$+ \tfrac{1}{2} (\ln \alpha_4 \ln \alpha_5 + 3 \ln^2 \alpha_2 + \tfrac{1}{2} \ln^2 \alpha_5 - 2 (\ln \alpha_2) (-\ln \alpha_4 - 2 \ln \alpha_5)) \ln^2 \alpha_1$$
$$+ \tfrac{1}{3} (-6 \ln \alpha_2 - \tfrac{3}{2} \ln \alpha_4 - 3 \ln \alpha_5) \ln^3 \alpha_1 + \tfrac{7}{8} \ln^4 \alpha_1].$$

References

Abdo, A. and Salim, N. (2008). *Molecular Similarity Searching Using Inference Network*. University of Technology Malaysia. www.UTM.my.

Abraham, A., Grosan, C., and Tigan, S. (2007). Ensemble of hybrid neural network learning approaches for designing pharmaceutical drugs. *Neural Computing & Applications*. Volume 16, Number 3 / May, 2007.

Abrahamsson, B., et al. (1998). Drug absorption from nifedipine hydrophilic matrix extended release (ed) tablet—Comparison with an osmotic pump tablet and effect of food. *J. Controlled Release* (Netherlands), 52:301-310.

Agarwal, R. (2008). Collaborating for innovation. http://www.business.uiuc.edu /agarwalr/. Feb. 20, 2008.

Altenberg, L. (1995). The Schema Theorem and Price's Theorem. In *Foundations of Genetic Algorithms 3*, ed. Darrell Whitley and Michael Vose. Morgan Kaufmann, San Francisco, pp. 23-49.

An, G. (2004). In-silico experiments of existing and hypothetical cytokine-directed clinical trials using agent based modeling. *Critical Care Medicine* 32(10):2050-2060.

Artzner, R, Delbaen, R, Bber, M. and Heath, D. (1999). Coherent measures of risk. *Mathematical Finance* 9:203-228.

Association of Medical Publications (2001). *ROI Analysis of Pharmaceutical Promotion* (RAPP): *An Independent Study by Scott A. Neslin*. Available from http://www.rappstudy.org.

Association of Medical Publications (2002). www.vioworks.com/clients/amp. September 18, 2002.

Ausk, B.J, Gross, T.S. and Srinivasan, S. (2005). An agent based model for real-time signaling induced in osteocytic networks by mechanical stimuli. *Journal of Biomechanics*.

Avitabile, D. (2006). Product Management Today, December 2006. www. thefreelibrary.com.

Babu, G.J. and Singh, K. (1983). Inference on means using the bootstrap. *Ann. Statist.*, 11:999-1003.

Baldi, P. and Hirschberg, D.S. (2009). An intersection inequality sharper than the Tanimoto triangle inequality for efficiently searching large databases. *J. Chem. Inf. Model.* (to be published).

Banzhaf, W., et al. (1998). Genetic Programming — An Introduction. Morgan

Kaufmann Publishers. San Francisco, CA, USA.

Barfield, C.E. and Groom bridge, M.A. (1998). Parallel Trade in the Pharmaceutical Industry: Implications for Innovation, Consumer Welfare, and Health Policy. Fordham Intellectual Property, *Media & Entertainment Law Journal*, Vol. 10 (1999), pp. 185-265.

Barfield, C.E. and Groombridge, M.A. (1998). The economic case for copyright and owner control over parallel imports. *Journal of World Intellectual Property*, Vol. 1, pp. 903-939.

Bass, F.M. (1969). A new-product growth model for consumer durables. *Management Science*, 15(5):215-227.

Bather, J. (2000). Decision Theory, *an Introduction to Dynamic Programming and Sequential Decisions*. John Wiley & Sons. Baffins Lane, Chichester, West Sussex, England.

Bauer, P. and Kohne K. (1994). Evaluation of experiments with adaptive interim analyses. *Biometrics*, 50:1029-1041.

Bauer, P. and Rohmel, J. (1995). An adaptive method for establishing a dose-response relationship. *Statist. Med.*, 14:1595-1607.

Beard, D.A. and Bassingthwaighte, J.B. (1998). Power-law kinetics of tracer washout from physiological systems. *Ann Biomed Eng.*, 26(5):775-9.

Bellman, R. (1957a). A Markovian decision process. *Journal of Mathematics and Mechanics* 6.

Bellman, R. (1957b). *Dynamic Programming*. Princeton University Press, Princeton, NJ.

Berlekamp, E.R., Conway, J.H., and Guy, R.K. (1982). *Winning Ways for Your Mathematical Plays*, Academic Press, London.

Bernard, S. (2002). The drug drought. *Pharmaceutical Executive*, Nov 1, 2002.

Berndt, E. R., Bui, L.T., Lucking-Rciley, D.H., and Urban, G.L. (1997). The Roles of Marketing, Product Quality, and Price Competition in the Growth and Composition of the U.S. Antiulcer Drug Industry. In Timothy F. Bresnahan and Robert J. Gordon (Eds.), *The Economics of New Goods* (pp. 277-322). The University of Chicago Press, Chicago, IL.

Berndt, E.R., Pindyck, R., and Azoulay, P. (1999). Network Effects and Diffusion in Pharmaceutical Markets: Antiuncer Drugs. NBER Working Paper, number 7024.

Berndt, E.R, Pindyck, R.S., and Azoulay P. (2003). Consumption externalities and diffusion in pharmaceutical markets: antiulcer drug. *Journal of Industry Economics*, 0022-1821.Vol. LI, No. 2.

Bertsekas, D. (1995). *Dynamic Programming and Optimal Control*. Volume 2, Athena Scientific, MA.

Bickel, P.J. and Freedman, D.A. (1980). On Edgeworth expansions for bootstrap, *Ann. Statist.*, 9:1196-1217.

Biining, H. K, Lettmann, T., and Mayr, E. W. (1988). *Projections of Vector Addition System Reachability Sets Are Semilinear*. March 1988 Report No. STAN-CS-88- 1199. Department of Computer Science, Stanford University, Stanford, California.

Bonate, P.L. and Howard, D. Prospective allometic scaling: Does the emperor have clothes? *J. Clin. Pharmacol.* 40:665-670, 2000.

Booth, B. and Zemmel, R. (2004). Prospects for productivity, *Nature Reviews*

Drug Discovery, Vol 3, May 2004.

Borwein, J., Bailey, D., and Girgensohn, R. (2004). *Experimentation in Mathematics: Computational Paths to Discovery*. AK Peters, New York.

Breusch, T.S (1978). Testing for autocorrelation in dynamic linear models. *Australian Economic Papers*, 17:334-355.

Briggs, G. G., Freeman, R. K., and Yaffe, S. J., Eds. (2005). *Drugs in Pregnancy and Lactation*, 7th ed.,Williams & Wilkins, Philadelphia, pp. xxi-xxvi.

Butler, T.C. (1972). The distribution of drugs. In LaDu, B.N., Mandel, H.G., Way, E.L. (Eds), *Fundamentals of Drug Metabolism and Disposition*. Williams &Wilkins, Baltimore.

Byrom, B. (2002). Using IVRS in clinical trial management. *Applied Clinical Trials*, October 2002, 36-42.

Cambridge Pharma Consultancy. (2004). Pricing and Reimbursement Review 2003. Cambridge, UK: IMS Health-Management Consulting.

Chambers, J.M., Mallows, C.L. and Stuck, B.W. (1976). A method for simulating stable random variables. *Journal of the American Statistical Association* 71:340-344.

Chandon, P. (2004). Innovative marketing strategies after patent expiry: The case of GSK's antibiotic Clamoxyl in France. *International Journal of Medical Marketing*. Henry Stewart Publications. 1469-7025 Vol. 4, 1 65-73.

Chang, M. (2007a). Adaptive design method based on sum of p-values. *Statistics in Medicine*, 26:2772–2784.

Chang, M. (2007b). *Adaptive Design Theory and Implementation Using SAS and R*. Chapman & Hall/CRC, Taylor & Francis, Boca Raton, FL.

Chang, M. (2008). Classical and Adaptive Designs using ExpDesign Studio. John-Wiley and Sons, Inc., New York.

Chaouiya, C., Remy E., and Thieffry, D. (2008). Petri net modelling of biological regulatory networks. *Journal of Discrete Algorithms*, Volume 6, Issue 2, pages 165-177.

Chard, J.S. and Mellor, C.J. (1989). Intellectual property rights and parallel imports. *World Economy*, Vol. 12, pp. 69-83.

Chen M. and Hofestädt, R. (2003). Quantitative Petri net model of gene regulated metabolic networks in the cell. In *Silico Biology* 3:0029.

Chernick, M.R. (2007). *Bootstrap Methods* (2nd ed.): *A Guide for Practitioners and Researchers*. John Wiley and Sons, Inc.

Chesbrough, H.W. (2007). Why companies should have open business models. *MIT Sloan Management Review* 48(2).

Chib, S. (1993). Bayes regression with autoregressive errors: A Gibbs sampling approach. *Journal of Econometrics*, 58(3):275-294.

Chien, C. (2003). Cheap drugs at what price to innovation: Does the compulsory licensing of pharmaceuticals hurt innovation? *Berkeley Technology Law Journal*, 18, Summer 2003.

Chintagunta, P. K. and Desiraju, R. (2002). Strategic pricing and detailing behavior in international markets. Forthcoming, *Marketing Science*.

Chow, S.C. and Chang, M. (2006). *Adaptive Design Methods in Clinical Trials*. Chapman & Hall/CRC, Boca Raton, FL.

Clark, A. (1933). *Applied Pharmacology* (5th ed.) Churchill, London.

Clark, A. (1937). *General Pharmacology*, Vol. 4 of Handbook of Experimental

Pharmacology Series, Springer-Verlag, Berlin.

Coleman, J., Katz, E., and Menzel, H. (1966). *Medical Innovation: A Diffusion Study*. Indianapolis, IN, Bobbs-Merrill.

Cope, D. (1993). Virtual music. *Electronic Musician*, 9/5:80-5.

Cope, D. (2001). *Virtual Music, Computer Synthesis of Music Style*. MIT Press.

Cui, L., Hung, H.M.J., and Wang, S.J. (1999). Modification of sample-size in group sequential trials. *Biometrics*, 55:853-857.

Danzon, P.M. (1997). *Pharmaceutical Price Regulation*. Washington, DC: American Enterprise Institute Press.

Danzon, P.M. (1998). The economics of parallel trade. *PharmacoEconomics*, Vol. 13, pp. 293-304.

Danzon, P.M. and Towse, A. (2003). Differential pricing for pharmaceuticals: reconciling access, Research and Development and patents. *International Journal of Health Care Finance and Economics*, Vol. 3, pp. 183-205.

Dearden, R., Friedman, N., and Russell, S. (1998). *Bayesian Q-learning*. American Association for Artificial Intelligence (www.aaai.org).

Decisionview. (2009). Automating Clinical Trial Enrollment. www.decisionviewsoftware.com.

Dekimpe, M.G., Parker, P.M. and Sarvary, M. (2000a). Multimarket and Global Diffusion. In Mahajan, V., Muller, E. and Wind, Y. (Eds). *New-Product Diffusion Models* (pp. 49-73). Kluwer Academic Publishers, Boston, MA.

Dekimpe, M.G., Parker, P.M., and Sarvary, M. (2000b). Global diffusion of technological innovations: A coupled-hazard approach. *Journal of Marketing Research*, XXXVII (February), 47-59.

Desiraju, R., Nair, H., and Chintagunta, P. (2004). *Diffusion of New Pharmaceutical Drugs in Developing and Developed Nations*. Research Paper No. 1950. Research Paper series, Stanford School of Business.

d'Inverno, M. and Prophet, J. (2005). Multidisciplinary investigation into adult stem cell behaviour. Lecture Notes Computer Science 3737:49-64.

Domino, M.E., Frank, O.Q, and Rosenheck R. (2003). The diffusion of new antipsychotic medications and formulary policy. *Schizophrenia Bulletin*, Vol. 29, No. 1.

Donohue, J.M., Cevasco, M., and Rosenthal, M.B. (2007). A decade of direct-to-consumer advertising of prescription drugs. *N. Engl. J. Med.* 357;7 www.nejm.org, August 16, 2007.

Dowlman, N. (2001). Intelligent medication management—Using IVR to optimise the drug supply process. *Pharmaceutical Manufacturing and Packaging Sourcer*, (Summer) 24–28.

Dresher M. (1961). *Games of Strategy: Theory and Applications*. Prentice-Hall, Inc., Englewood Cliffs, NJ.

Durbin, J. (1970). Testing for serial correlation in least-squares regression when some of the regressors are lagged dependent variables. *Econometrica*, 38 (3):410-421.

Earll, M. (2006). A guide to log P and pKa measurements and their use. http://www.raell.demon.co.uk.

Ebisch, R. (2005). Prescription for change. *Teradata Magazine*, March 2005.

Eldridge, M., et al. (1997) Empirical scoring functions: I. The development of a fast empirical scoring function to estimate the binding affinity of ligands in receptor complexes. *Journal of Computer-Aided Molecular Design*, 11:425-45.

Emonet, T., et al. (2005) AgentCell: A digital single-cell assay for bacterial chemotaxis. *Bioinformatics* 21:2714-2721

Ewing, T.J., et al. (2001). DOCK 4.0: Search strategies for automated molecular docking of flexible molecule databases. *Journal of Computer-Aided Molecular Design.* 15:411-28.

Fabio, A., et al. (2008). Trends in the globalization of clinical trials. *Natural.* Vol.7:13.

Farkas, Julius (Gyula) (1902). Über die Theorie der Einfachen Ungleichungen, *Journal für die Reine und Angewandte Mathematik* 124:1-27.

FDA (1988). Guideline for Format and Content of the Clinical and Statistical Sections of New Drug Applications. U.S. Food and Drug Administration, Rockville, MD.

FDA (2006). Guidance for Clinical Trial Sponsors: Establishment and Operation of Clinical Trial Data Monitoring Committees.

FDA Approval Study. (2008). BioMedTracker, Sagient Research Systems.

FDA (2008). Orange Book. www.fda.gov/cder/ob/default.

Feig, M., et al. (2004). Performance comparison of generalized born and Poisson methods in the calculation of electrostatic solvation energies for protein structures. *Journal of Computational Chemistry* 25(2):265-84.

Ferguson, T.S. (1996). *A Course in Large Sample Theory: Texts in Statistical Science.* Chapman & Hall/CRC, London, UK.

Fisher, J. C. and Pry, R. H. (1971). A simple substitution model of technological change. *Technological Forecasting and Social Change*, 3 (March), 75-88.

Fisher, M.R., Roecker, E.B., and DeMets, D.L. (2001). The role of an independent statistical analysis center in the industry-modified National Institutes of Health model. *Drug Information Journal*, Vol. 35, pp. 115-129.

Fisher, R. A. (1953). *The Design of Experiment*, Hafner, New York.

Fishman, G. (2000). *Monte Carlo, Concepts, Algorithms and Applications.* Springer, NC.

Frank, S. A. and M. Slatkin. (1990). The distribution of allelic effects under mutation and selection. *Genetical Research*, Cambridge 55:111-117.

Fuchs, P. P. (2008). Permutation algorithm. www.geocities.com/permute_it.

Ganslandt, M. and Maskus, K.E. (2004). The price impact of parallel imports in pharmaceuticals: Evidence from the European Union. *Journal of Health Economics*, Vol. 23, pp. 1035-1057.

Gardner, M. (1988). *Combinatorial Card Problems, in Time Travel and Other Mathematical Bewilderments.* W. H. Freeman, New York.

Gelfand A.E. and Smith A.F.M. (1990). Sampling based approaches to calculating marginal densities. *Journal of the American Statistical Association*, 85:398-409.

Geman, S. and Geman, D. (1984). Stochastic relaxation, Gibbs distribution, and the Bayesian restoration of imagines. *IEEE Transactions on Pattern Analysis and Machine Intelligence*, PAMI-6, 721.

Gentle J. E. (2005). *Elements of Computational Statistics.* Springer, VA.

Gentle J. E. (2005). *Random number generation and Monte Carlo Methods* (2nd ed). Springer, VA.

Gentle, J.E. and Härdle W. (2004). *Handbook of Computational Statistics* (1st ed), Y. Mori (Eds). Springer Verlag, Heidelberg, Germany.

Geweke, G., Gowrisankaran, G., and Town, R.T. (2003). Bayesian inference for hospital quality in a selection model. *Econometrika*, Econometric Society, vol. 7(4):1215-1238.

Gibbs Sampling, Version 3.0. Cambridge, MA: Cambridge Medical Research Council Biostatistics Unit.

Godfrey, L. G. (1978). Testing against General Autoregressive and Moving Average Error Models

Gonul, F., Carter, F., Petrova, E., and Srinivasan, K. (2001). Promotion of prescription drugs and its impact on physicians' choice behavior. *Journal of Marketing*, 65(3):79-90.

Good, P.I. (2005). *Permutation, Parametric and Bootstrap Tests of Hypotheses* (3rd ed), Springer.

Gosavi, A. (2003). *Simulation-based Optimization: Parametric Optimization Techniques and Reinforcement Learning.* Springer (Kluwer), Boston, MA.

Grafen, A. (1985). A geometric view of relatedness. *Oxford Surveys in Evolutionary Biology* 2:28-89.

Grossman, G. and Lai, E. (2004). International protection of intellectual property. *American Economic Review*, vol. 94, n. 5, 1635-1653.

Grossman, G. and Lai, E. (2008). Parallel imports and price controls. RAND *Journal of Economics*, 2008, vol. 39, issue 2, pp. 378-402.

Hahn, M., Park, S., Krishnamurthi, L., and Zoltners, A. (1994). Analysis of new-product diffusion using a four-segment trial-repeat model. Marketing Science, 13(3):224-247.

HAI (2000). Drug Pricing and Access to Essential Medicines. Statement by Health Action International (HAI) - Europe for the DG Trade and Civil Society Health Issue Group Meeting (June 2000). http://trade.ec.europa.eu/doclib/docs/2005/april/tradoc_122213.pdf.

Hamilton, S. and Ho, K.F. (2004). Efficient drug supply algorithms for stratified clinical trials by focusing on patient coverage—not just site supplies—this dynamic approach significantly reduces drug waste. *Applied Clinical Trials*, Feb 1, 2004.

Hansten, P. and Horn, J. (2003) *Drug–Drug Interaction Mechanisms.* H&H Publications, http://www.hanstenandhorn.com.

Hausman, J., Leonard, G., and Zona, D. (1994). Competitive analysis with differentiated products. *Annales D'Economie et de Statistique*, 34 (April/June): 159-180.

Hausman, J. and Taylor, W. (1981). Panel data and unobservable individual effects. *Econometrica*, 49(6):1377-1398.

Heerkens, G. (2001). *Project Management* (The Briefcase Book Series). McGraw-Hill.

Heiner, M., et al. (2004). Model validation of biological pathways using Petri nets — demonstrated for apoptosis. *Biosystems*, 75:15-28.

Hinchliffe, A. (2008). *Molecular Modeling for Beginners* (2nd ed). John Wiley & Sons, UK.

Hixson, A. and Crowell. J. (1931). Dependence of reaction velocity upon surface and agitation. I. Theoretical considerations. *Industrial and Engineering*

Chemistry Research, Vol. 51, pp. 923-931.

Hoare, C.A.R. (1962). Quicksort. *Computer Journal.* 5:10-15.

Hofestadt. R. (1994). A Petri net application of metabolic processes. *Journal of System Analysis, Modeling and Simulation*, 16:113-122.

Höltje, H., Sippl, W., et al. (2008). *Molecular Modeling: Basic Principles and Applications* (3rd ed). Wiley-VCH.

Hong, S.H. et al. (2005). Product-line extensions and pricing strategies of brand-name drugs facing patent expiration. *Journal of Managed Care Pharmacy JMCP* November/December 2005, Vol. 11, No. 9. www.amcp.org.

Howard, R.A. *Dynamic Programming and Markov Processes*, The MIT Press, Cambridge, MA.

Hu, M., et al. (2007). The Innovation Gap in *Pharmaceutical Drug Discovery & New Models for Research and Development Success.* www.kellogg.northwestern.edu/academic/biotech/faculty/articles/ NewRDModel.pdf. Access date: 3/2/2009.

Hu, T.M. and Hayton, W.L. (2001). Allometric scaling of xenobiotic clearance: Uncertainty versus universality. *AAPS PharmSci* 3(4), article 29, www.pharmsci.org.

Huang, S. and Zou, X. (2006). An iterative knowledge-based scoring function to predict protein-ligand interactions: I. Derivation of interaction potentials. *Journal of Computational Chemistry*, Published online 18 September 2006 in Wiley InterScience.

Huttin, C. (1995). Comparative Prices and Reimbursement Systems for Regulating Pharmaceutical Expenditures in the European Community. Report to the European Union (October 1995), updated for some countries.

Huttin, C. (1999). Drug Price Divergence In Europe: Regulatory Aspects. *Health Affairs*, May / June 1999. The People-to-People Health Foundation, Inc.

IMS Health Report (2008). *Geographic Variation in Prescription Utilization.* Express Scripts, Inc.

Ingram, R. E. and Scher, C. (1998). Depression. *Encyclopedia of Mental Health*, Volume 1, 723-732.

Joao M., et al. (2002). *Fuzzy Decision Making in Modeling and Control.* World Scientific Publishing Company.

Johnston, J. and Dinardo, J. (1997). *Econometric Methods* (section 6.5, pp. 176-188). McGraw-Hill.

Jones, N. C. and Pevzner, P.A. (2004). *An Introduction to Bioinformatics Algorithms* (1st ed). The MIT Press, Cambridge, MA.

Kamakura, W. and Kossar, B. (1998). *A Factor-Analytic Split Hazard Model for Database Marketing.* University of Iowa, Iowa.

Kanavos, P. and Costa-Font, J. (2005). Pharmaceutical parallel trade in Europe: Stakeholder and competition effects. *Economic Policy*, Vol. 44, pp. 751-798.

Kennakin, T. (1997). *Pharmacological Analysis of Drug-receptor Interaction*, Lippincott-Raven, New York.

Kerzner, H. (2003). *Project Management: A Systems Approach to Planning, Scheduling, and Controlling* (8th ed.).

Kier, L.B., et al. (1996). A cellular automata model of enzyme kinetics. *J. Mol. Graph.* 14:227-231.

Kier, L.B., et al. (1996). A cellular automata model of micelle formation. *Pharm.*

Res 13:1419-1422

Kier, L.B., et al. (1997). A cellular automata model of diffusion in aqueous systems. *J. Pharm. Sci.* 86:774-778.

Kirchmair, J., et al. (2006). Comparative performance assessment of the conformational model generators omega and catalyst: a large-scale survey on the retrieval of protein-bound ligand conformations. *Journal of Chemical Information and Modeling*, 46:1848-61.

Klastorin, T. (2003). *Project Management: Tools and Trade-offs* (3rd ed). Wiley.

Koch I. and Heiner, M. (2008). Petri Net. In Junker B.H. (Eds). *Analysis of Biological Networks*. John-Wiley & Sons, Hoboken, NJ.

Koch, I., Junker, B.H., and Heiner, M. (2005). Application of Petri net theory for modeling and validation of the sucrose breakdown pathway in the potato tuber. *Bioinformatics*, (21)7:1219-1226.

Koch, I., Schuster, S., and Heiner, M. (2003). Simulation and analysis of metabolic networks by time dependent Petri nets. *Silico Biology*, 3-31.

Kokoska, S. and Zwillonger, D. (2000). *Standard Probability and Statistical Tables & Formula*. CRC Press, Boca Raton, FL.

Koza, J. R. (1992). *Genetic Programming: On the Programming of Computers by Means of Natural Selection*. MIT Press, Cambridge, MA.

Koza, J.R., Keane, M.A., et al. (2005). *Genetic Programming. IV: Routine Human-competitive Machine Intelligence*. Springer, Science+Business Media, Inc.

Laha, R.G. and Rohatgi, V.K. (1979). Probability Theory, Wiley.

Lai, E. and Qiu, L. (2003). The North's intellectual property rights standard for the South? *Journal of International Economics* 59:183-209.

Lan, K.K.G. and DeMets, D. L. (1983). Discrete sequential boundaries for clinical trials. *Biometrika*, 70:659–663.

Landers, P. (2003). Cost of developing a new drug increases to about $1.7 billion. *Wall Street Journal*, December 8, 2003.

Langdon, W.B. and Poli., R. (2002). *Foundations of Genetic Programming*. Springer-Verlag, Berlin, Heidelberg.

Lee, M.L.T, Chang, M., and Whitmore, G.A. (2008). A threshold regression mixture model for assessing treatment efficacy in a multiple myeloma clinical trial. *J Biopharm Stat.* 2008;18(6):1136-49.

Lehmacher, W. and Wassmer G. (1999). Adaptive sample-size calculations in group sequential trials. *Biometrics*, 55:1286-1290.

Leng, M. and Parlar, M. (2006). Game-theoretic analysis of an ancient Chinese horse race problem. *Computers & Operations Research* 33:2033-2055.

Lenk, P. J. and Rao, A.G. (1990). New models from old: Forecasting product adoption by hierarchical Bayes procedures. *Marketing Science*, 9(1):42-57.

Lévy, P. (1925). *Calculdes Probabilites*, Gauthier Villars.

Lewis, J. (2002). *Fundamentals of Project Management* (2nd ed). American Management Association.

Li, H. and Li, C. (2004). Word translation disambiguation using bilingual bootstrapping. *Computational Linguistics*, v. 30 n. 1, p. 1-22.

Lipinski, C.A., et al. (1997). Experimental and computational approaches to estimate solubility and permeability in drug discovery and development settings. *Advanced Drug Delivery Reviews*, 23:3-25.

Lipkus, A. (1999). A proof of the triangle inequality for the Tanimoto distance. *J. Math. Chem.*, 26:263-265.

Liu, J.S. (2003). *Monte Carlo Strategies in Scientific Computing.* Springer, New York.

Lollini, P.L., et al. (2006). Discovery of cancer vaccination protocols with a genetic algorithm driving an agent-based simulator. *BMC Bioinformatics* 7:352.

Macheras, P. and Iliadis, A. (2006). *Modeling in Biopharmaceutics, Pharmacokinetics and Pharmacodynamics: Homogeneous and Heterogeneous Approaches* (1st ed). Springer, New York.

Mahajan, V., Muller, E., and Bass, F.M. (1990). New-Product Diffusion Models in Marketing: A

Mahmood, I. (2000). Critique of prospective allometric scaling: Does the emperor have clothes? *J. Clin. Pharmacol.* 40:671-674.

Manchanda, P., Rossi, P.E., and Chintagunta, P.K. (2003). Response modeling with non-random marketing mix variables. Forthcoming, *Journal of Marketing Research*.

Marin A. (2009). *On the relations among product-form stochastic models*. Ph.D. Thesis. Dipartimento di Informatica. Universit'a Ca' Foscari di Venezia. Via Torino, Italia.

Marwan, W., Sujathab, A., and Starostzik, C. (2005). Reconstructing the regulatory network controlling commitment and sporulation in Physarum polycephalum based on hierarchical Petri net modeling and simulation. *Journal of Theoretical Biology*, 236:349-365.

Materi, W. and Wishart, D.S. (2007). Computational systems biology in drug discovery and development: methods and applications. *Drug Discovery Today*, Volume 12, Numbers 7/8, April 2007.

Mathieu, M. (2003). *New Drug Development: A Regulatory Overview*, PAREXEL International.

Matsuno, H., et al. (2003) Biopathways representation and simulation on hybrid functional Petri net. *Silico Biol.* 3:389-404.

McCain, R. (2009). *Strategy and Conflict: An Introductory Sketch of Game Theory.* http://william-king.www.drexel.edu/top/eco/game/game.html. (March 20, 2009)

McCulloch, J.H. (1996). Financial Applications of Stable Distributions, in G.S. Maddala, C.R. Rao (Eds), *Handbook of Statistics*, Vol. 14, Elsevier, pp. 393-425.

McEntegart, D. (2003). Forced randomization when using interactive voice response systems. *Applied Clinical Trials*, October 2003, 50-58.

McLeish, D.L. (2005). *Monte Carlo Simulation and Finance.* Wiley & Sons, NJ.

Mendes, P. and Kell, D. (1998). Nonlinear optimization of biochemical pathways: applications to metabolic engineering and parameter estimation. *Bioinformatics.* 14(10):869-883.

Meng, E.C., Shoichet, B.K., and Kuntz, I.D. (2004). Automated docking with grid-based energy evaluation. *Journal of Computational Chemistry*, 13(4):505-524.

Metha, C. R., Patel, N. R., and Senchaudhuri, P. (1988). Importance sampling for estimating exact probabilities in permutational inference. *J. Am. Statist. Assoc.*, 83(404):999-1005.

Meyn, S. P. (2007). *Control Techniques for Complex Networks.* Cambridge University Press.

Michael, J.R., Schucany, W.R., and Haas, R.W. (1976). Generating random variates using transformations with multiple roots. *American Statistician,* 30-2, 88-90.

Microsoft (2005). *Simplifying Clinical Trial Management Using the Microsoft Office System.* www.microsoft.com/office/showcase/ctm/default.mspx.

Milosevic, D. Z. (2003). *Project Management ToolBox: Tools and Techniques for the Practicing Project Manager.* Wiley.

Minority Staff Special Investigations Division Committee on Government Reform U.S. House of Representatives. (2001). Prescription Drug Prices in Canada, Europe, and Japan - Prepared by Minority Staff Special Investigations Division Committee on Government Reform U.S. House of Representatives. April 11, 2001. http://oversight.house.gov/documents/20040629103247-74022.pdf.

Mittenthal, J.E., Yuan, A., et al. (1998). Designing metabolism: alternative connectivities for the pentose phosphate pathway. *Bulletin of Mathematical Biology.* Vol. 60. p. 815-856.

Miyamoto, S. and Kollman, P.A. (1993). Absolute and relative binding free energy calculations of the interaction of biotin and its analogs with streptavidin using molecular dynamics/free energy perturbation approaches. *Proteins,* 16, 226-45.

Moore, A.W. (2002). *Markov Systems, Markov Decision Processes, and Dynamic Programming.* www.cs.cmu.edu/~awm.

Mordenti, J. and Chappell, W. (1989). The use of interspecies scaling in toxicology. In Yacobi, A., Skelly J.P., Batra, V.K. (Eds). *Toxicokinetic and Drug Development.* Pergamon, New York.

Morris, G.M., et al. (1998). Automated docking using a Lamarckian genetic algorithm and an empirical binding free energy function. *Journal of Computational Chemistry,* 19(14):1639-1662.

Morrison, A. L. (1999). *The Antidepressant Sourcebook: A User's Guide for Patients and Families.* Main Street Books, Mansfield, OH.

Müller, H.H. and Shäfer, H. (2001). Adaptive group sequential designs for clinical trials: Combining the advantages of adaptive and classical group sequential approaches. *Biometrics,* 57:886-891.

Müller, H.H. and Shäfer, H. (2004). A general statistical principle of changing a design any time during the course of a trial. *Statist. Med.,* 23:2497-2508.

Muller, M.E. (1956). Some continuous Monte Carlo methods for the Dirichlet problem. *Ann. Math. Stat.,* 27:569-589.

Muresan, S. and Sadowski, J. (2005). "In-house likeness": comparison of large compound collections using artificial neural networks. *Journal of Chemical, linfonnation* and Modeling, 45:888-93.

Muryshev, A. E., et al. (2003). Comparing protein-ligand docking programs is difficult. *Comput. Aided Mol. Des.,* 17:597.

Narayanan, S., Desiraju, R., and Chintagunta, P. (2002). ROI implications for pharmaceutical promotional expenditures: The role of marketing mix interactions. Forthcoming, *Journal of Marketing.*

Nash, J. (1951). Non-cooperative games. *Annals of Mathematics,* 5:286-295.

Neelamegham, R. and Chintagunta, P. (1999). A Bayesian model to forecast new product performance in domestic and international markets. *Marketing Science*, 18(2):115-136.

Nevo, A. (2003). Measuring market power in the ready-to-eat cereal industry. *Econometrica*, 69(2):307-342.

Ng, R. (2005). *Drugs, from Discovery to Marketing.* John Wiley.

Norwich, K.H. (1997). Noncompartmental models of whole-body clearance of tracers: A review. *Annals of Biomedical Engineering*, vol. 25, no. 3, pp. 421-439.

Noyes, A.A. and Whitney, W.R. (1897). *Journal of the American Chemical Society*, 19:930-934.

O'Brien, P.C. and Fleming, T.R. (1979). A multiple testing procedure for clinical trials. *Biometrika* 35:549–556.

Oliveira, J.S., Bailey, C. G., et al. (2003). A computational model for the identification of biochemical pathways in the Krebs cycle. *Journal of Computational Biology*, (10)1:5782.

Paich, M., Peck, C., and Valant, J. (2009). *Pharmaceutical Product Branding Strategies - Simulating Patient Flow and Portfolio Dynamics* (2nd ed). Informa Healthcare, New York.

Pammolli, F. and Riccaboni, M. (2007). *Innovation and Industrial Leadership, Lessons from Pharmaceuticals.* Center for Transatlantic Relations, The Johns Hopkins University.

Paolini, G.V., et al. (2006). Global mapping of pharmacological space, *Nature Biotechnology*, 24: 805-15.

Patel, N.R. (2009). *The New Role of Drug Supply Planning in Adaptive Trials.* Clinical Supply Forecasting Summit, Philadelphia, April 2009.

Pearlman, J.B. (2007). *The Commercialization of Medicine.* http://www.google.com.

Peer, M.A., et al. (2004). Cellular automata and its advances to drug therapy for HIV infection. *Indian J. Exp. Biol.* 42:131-137.

Pitman, E. J. G. (1937). Significance tests which may be applied to samples from any population. *Royal Statistical Society Supplement*, 4:119-130 and 225-32 (parts I and II).

Pitman, E. J. G. (1938). Significance tests which may be applied to samples from any population. Part III. The analysis of variance test. *Biometrika*, 29:322-335.

Pocock, S.J. (1977). Group sequential methods in the design and analysis of clinical trials. *Biometrika.* 64:191-199.

Poli, R., Langdon, W.R., and McPhee, N.F. (2008). A field guide to genetic programming, Creative Commons Attribution. UK: England & Wales License.

Politopoulos, I. (2007). *Review and Analysis of Agent-based Models in Biology.* University of Liverpool, Liverpool, United Kingdom.

Powell, W.B. (2007). *Approximate Dynamic Programming: Solving the Curses of Dimensionality.* Wiley-Interscience, New York.

Press, W.H., et al. (2007). *Numerical Recipes* (3rd ed). Cambridge University Press, New York.

Price, G. R. (1970). Selection and covariance. *Nature*, 227:520-521.

Project Management Institute (2003). *A Guide to the Project Management Body of Knowledge* (3rd ed). Project Management Institute.

Proschan, M.A. and Hunsberger, S.A. (1995). Designed extension of studies based on conditional power. *Biometrics*, 51:1315-1324.

Proschan, M.A., Lan, K.K.G., and Wittes, J.T. (2006). *Statistical Monitoring of Clinical Trials, a Uniform Approach*. Springer, New York.

Puterman, M. L. (1994). *Markov Decision Processes*. John Wiley.

Putsis, W. P. and Srinivasan, V. (2000). Estimation Techniques for Macro Diffusion Models. In Mahajan, V., Muller, E., and Wind, Y. (Eds), *New-Product Diffusion Models* (pp. 263-291). Kluwer Academic Publishers, Boston, MA.

Rachev, S. and Mittnik, S. (2000). *Stable Paretian Models in Finance*. Wiley.

Rasiel, E.M. (1999). *The McKinsey Way: Using the Techniques of the World's Top Strategic Consultants to Help You and Your Business*. McGraw-Hill, New York.

Readdy, M.B., et al. (2005). *Physiologically Based Pharmacokinetic Modeling*. John Wiley & Sons, New Jersey.

Reddy, V. N. (1994). *Modeling biological pathways: A discrete event systems approach*. University of Maryland, College Park, MD, Master's Thesis, May 1994.

Reddy, V. N., Mavrovouniotis, M. L., and Liebman, M. N. (1993). Petri net representations in metabolic pathways. In Proceedings of the 2nd International Conference on Intelligent Systems in *Molecular Biology* (ISMB 93), pp. 328-336.

Review and Directions for Research. *Journal of Marketing*, 54(1):1-26.

Rishton, G.M. (1997). Reactive compounds and in vitro false positives in HTS. *Drug Discovery Today*, 2:382-84.

Ritschel, W.A. and Banerjee, P.S. (1986). Physiological pharmacokinetic models: Principles, applications, limitations and outlook. *Meth. Find. Exp. Clin. Pharmacol.*, 8:603-614.

Rizzo, J. A. (1999). Advertising and competition in the ethical pharmaceutical industry: The case of antihypertensive drugs. *Journal of Law and Economics*, XLII(1):89-116.

Robbins, H. and Monro, S. (1951). A stochastic approximation method. *Annals of Mathematical Statistics*, 22:400-407.

Roche, O. and Guba, W. (2005). Computational chemistry as an integral component of lead generation. *Journal of Medicinal Chemistry*, S. 677-83.

Rognan, D., et al. (1999). Predicting binding affinities of prote in ligands from three-dimensional coordinates: application to peptide binding to class I major histocompatibility proteins. *Journal of Medicinal Chemistry*, 42:4650-58.

Romero, J. and Machdo, P., eds. (2008). *The Art of Artificial Evolution*. Springer-Verlag, Berlin Heidelberg.

Rosenthal, M. B., Berndt, E.R., Donohue, J.M., Epstein, A.E., and Frank, R.G. (2002). *Demand Effects of Recent Changes in Prescription Drug Promotion*. Working paper.

Ross, S. M. (1983). *Introduction to Stochastic Dynamic Programming*. Academic Press, UK.

Rossi, P. and Allenby, G. (2003). Bayesian statistics and marketing. *Marketing Science*, 22(3):304-328.

Rowe, R. (2001). *Machine Musicianship*. MIT Press, Cambridge, MA.

Rowland, M. and Tozer, T.N. (1995). *Clinical Pharmacokinetics, Concepts and*

Applications (3rd ed). Lippincott Williams & Williams, Philadephia.

Sadowski, J. and Kubinyi, H. (1998). A scoring scheme for discriminating between drugs and non-drugs, *J. Med. Chem.*, 41:3325-3329.

Sakamoto, K., et al. (2007). A Structural Similarity Evaluation by SimScore in a Teratogenicity Information Sharing System. *J. Comput. Chem.* Jpn., Vol. 6, No. 2, pp. 117-122.

Sampson, A. and Sill, M.W. (2005). Drop-the-losers design: Normal case. *Biometrical Journal*, 47:257-268.

Schneider, G. and Baringhaus, K.H. (2008). *Molecular Design: Concepts and Applications*. Wiley-VCH Verlag, Frankfurt.

Schondelmeyer, S.W. and Wrobel, M.V. (2004). *Medicaid and Medicare Drug Pricing: Strategy to Determine Market Prices*. PRIME Institute, University of Minnesota and Abt Associates Inc., Cambridge, MA.

Schweizer, L. (2005). Concept and evolution of business models. *Journal of General Management*, 31(2):37-56.

Scripture, C.D. and Figg, W.D. (2006). Drug interactions in cancer therapy: Pharmacodynamic drug interactions. *Nat. Rev. Cancer.* 2006;6(7):546-558.

Scsibrany, H., et al. (2003). Clustering and similarity of chemical structures represented by binary substructure descriptors. *Chemom. Intell. Lab. Syst.*, 67:95-108.

Selection Model. *Econometrica*, 71 (4), 1215-1238.

Shao, J. and Tu, D. (1995). *The Jackknife and Bootstrap*. Springer-Verlag, New York.

Shapiro, R. and Vallee, B.L. (1991). Interaction of human placental ribonuclease with placental ribonuclease inhibitor. *Biochemistry.* 26;30(8):2246-55.

Shargel, L., Wu-Pong, S., and Yu, A.B.C. (2005). *Applied Biopharmaceutics & Pharmacokinetics* (5th ed). The McGraw-Hill Companies, New York.

Shubik M. (1982). *Game Theory in the Social Sciences*. The MIT Press, Cambridge, MA.

Simao, E., Remy, E. et al. (2005). Qualitative modeling of regulated metabolic pathways: Application to the tryptophan biosynthesis in E. coli. *Bioinformatics* 21(Suppl 2):ii191-ii196.

Simon, F. and Kotler, P. (2003). *Building Global Biobrands: Taking Biotechnology to Market*. Simon & Schuster, New York.

Singh, K. (1981). On the asymptotic accuracy of Efron's bootstrap. *Ann. Statist.*, 9, 1187-1195.

Slatkin, M. (1970). Selection and polygenic characters. *Proceedings of the National Academy of Sciences* U.S.A., 66:87-93.

Spiegelhalter, D.J., Thomas, A., Best, N.G., and Gilks, W.R. (1994). BUGS: Bayesian Inference Using

Srivastava, R., Peterson, M.S., and Bentley, W.E. (2001). Stochastic kinetic analysis of the Escherichia coli stress circuit using sigma(32)-targeted antisense. Biotechnol. Bioeng., 5;75(1):120-9.

Stark, N.J. (2009). *Top Twelve Mistakes Monitors Manage.* www.clinicaldevice.com.

Steggles, L.J., Banks, R. and Wipat, A. (2006). Modeling and analyzing genetic networks: From Boolean networks to Petri nets. In *Proceedings of Computa-*

tional Methods in Systems Biology (CMSB 06), volume 4210 of LNCSILNBI, pp. 127-141, Springer.

Straffin, P.D. (1993). *Game Theory and Strategy*. The Mathematical Association of America, Washington, DC.

Sutton, R. S. and Barto A. G. (1998). *Reinforcement Learning: An Introduction*. The MIT Press, Cambridge, MA.

Szirtes, T. (2007). *Applied Dimensional Analysis and Modeling* (2nd ed). Elsevier Inc., Oxford, UK.

Talukdar, D., Sudhir, K. and Ainslie, A. (2002). Investigating new product diffusion across products and countries. *Marketing Science*, 21(1):97-114.

Taylor, P. D. (1988). Inclusive fitness models with two sexes. *Theoretical Population Biology*, 34:145-168.

Tegart, G. (2003). *Nanotechnology: The Technology for the 21st Century*. The APEC Center for Technology Foresight. Bangkok, Thailand. Presented at the Second International Conference on Technology Foresight, Tokyo, Feb. 27-28, 2003.

The Royal Society (2004). *Nanoscience and Nanotechnologies: Opportunities and Uncertainties*. www.nanotec.org.uk/finalReport.htm.

Thiers, F.A. (2008). Trends in the globalization of clinical trials. *Natural*, 7:12.

Thoelke, K.R. (2008). *Implication of the Globalization of Clinical Trials and Drug Development*. BayBio 2008. San Francisico, April 17, 2008.

Thompson Medstat Report Using Data and Metrics for Clinical Trials (2004). www.decisionviewsoftware.com.

Tijms, H.C. (2003). *A First Course in Stochastic Models*. John Wiley.

Tufts Center for the Study of Drug Development. (2008). http://www.csdd.tufts.edu.

Uyenoyama, M. K. (1988). On the evolution of genetic incompatibility systems: Incompatibility as a mechanism for the regulation of outcrossing distance. In R. E. Michod and B. R. Levin (Eds). *The Evolution of Sex*. Sinauer Associates, Sunderland, MA, pp. 212-232.

Van den Bulte, C. and Lilien, G.L. (1997). Bias and systematic change in the parameter estimates of macro-level diffusion models. *Marketing Science*, 16(4):338-353.

Van den Bulte, C. (2000). New product diffusion acceleration: Measurement and analysis. *Marketing Science*, 19(4):366-380.

Van Nunen, J.A. (1976). A set of successive approximation methods for discounted Markovian decision problems. Z. *Operations Research*, 20:203-208.

Verdonk, M.L., Cole, J.E., Hartshorn, M., et al. (2003). Improved protein-ligand docking using GOLD *Proteins*, 52:609-23.

Virine, L. and Trumper, M. (2007). *Project Decisions: The Art and Science*. Management Concepts.

von Neumann, J. (1966). *The Theory of Self-Reproducing Automata*. Burks, A. (Ed), University of Illinois Press.

Voss, K., Heiner, M., and Koch, I. (2003). Steady state analysis of metabolic pathways using Petri nets. *Silico Biology*, 3(31):367-87.

Wade, M. J. (1985). Soft selection, hard selection, kin selection, and group selection. *American Naturalist*, 125:61-73.

Walker, D. C., Hill, G., and Wood, et al. (2004). Agent-based computational modelling of wounded epithelial cell monolayers. *IEEE Transactions in Nanobioscience*, 3:153-163.

Walley, T., Haycox, A., and Boland, A. (2004). *Pharmacoeconomics*. Elsevier Science Limited, London, UK.

Wang, D. and Bakhai, A. (2006). *Clinical Trials, A Practical Guidance to Design, Analysis, and Reporting*. Remedica, London, UK.

Wang, S.K. and Tsiatis, A.A. (1987). Approximately optimal one-parameter boundaries for a sequential trial. *Biometrics*, 43:193-200.

Watkins C. and Dayan, P. (1992). *Technical Note, Q,-Learning. Machine Learning*, 8:279-292.

Watkins, C.J.C.H. (1989). *Learning from delayed rewards*. PhD Thesis, University of Cambridge, England.

Watson, J. (2008). *Strategy*. W.W. Norton & Company, p. 159-160.

Weron, R. (2004). Computationally Intensive Value at Risk Calculations, in G. Gentle, et al. (Eds), *Handbook of Computational Statistics*. Springer, p. 914.

When the Regressors Include Lagged Dependent Variables. *Econometrica*, 46(6):1293-1302.

Wishart, D.S. et al. (2005). Dynamic cellular automata: An alternative approach to cellular simulation. *Silico Biol.*, 5:139-161.

Wittink, D. R. (2002). Analysis of ROI for Pharmaceutical Promotions (ARPP). Presentation to the Wolfram, S. (2002). *A New Kind of Science*. Wolfram Media.

Woodcock, J., Deputy Commissioner/Chief Medical Officer, FDA (2008). FDA Update. www.ainbe.org.

Woolf, M.B. (2007). *Faster Construction Projects with CPM Scheduling*. McGraw-Hill.

Wosinska, M. (2002). *Just What the Patient Ordered? Direct-To-Consumer Advertising and the Demand for Pharmaceutical Products*. Harvard Business School.

Zygourakis, K. and Markenscoff, P.A. (1996). Computer-aided design of bioerodible devices with optimal release characteristics: a cellular automata approach. *Biomaterials*, 17: 125-135.

Index